Trends in Inflammatory Bowel Disease Therapy 1999

Trends in Inflammatory Bowel Disease Therapy 1999

Edited by

C.N. Williams
Division of Gastroenterology
Department of Medicine
Dalhousie University
Halifax
Nova Scotia, Canada

R.F. Bursey
Memorial University of Newfoundland
Faculty of Medicine
The Health Sciences Centre
St John's
Newfoundland, Canada

R.S. McLeod
University of Toronto
Mount Sinai Hospital
Toronto
Ontario, Canada

D.G. Gall
Faculty of Medicine
The University of Calgary
Alberta, Canada

L.R. Sutherland
Faculty of Medicine
The University of Calgary
Alberta, Canada

F. Martin
University of Montreal
Canada

J.L. Wallace
Faculty of Medicine
The University of Calgary
Alberta, Canada

*The proceedings of a symposium organized by AXCAN PHARMA,
held in Vancouver, BC, August 27–29, 1999*

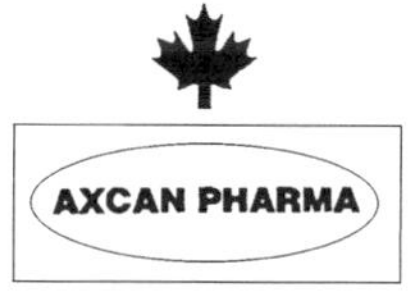

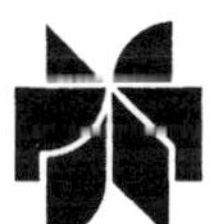

KLUWER ACADEMIC PUBLISHERS
DORDRECHT / BOSTON / LONDON

A C.I.P. Catalogue record for this book is available from the Library of Congress

ISBN 0-7923-8762-7

Published by Kluwer Academic Publishers,
P.O. Box 17, 3330 AA Dordrecht, The Netherlands

Sold and distributed in North, Central and South America
by Kluwer Academic Publishers,
101 Philip Drive, Norwell, MA 02061, U.S.A.

In all other countries, sold and distributed
by Kluwer Academic Publishers,
P.O. Box 322, 3300 AH Doredrecht, The Netherlands.

Printed on acid-free paper

Printed and bound in Great Britain by Antony Rowe Limited.

Contents

List of Principal Authors

viii

Preface
CN Williams

xv

Section I: GENETICS

1 Genetics of inflammatory bowel disease: where are we?
MS Silverberg, A-K Somani and KA Siminovitch

3

2 Genetics of inflammatory bowel disease: why is it important?
DP Jewell

13

3 Genetics of IBD: impact on immune function
C Fiocchi

23

Section II: PATHOGENESIS

4 Bacterial factors in inflammatory bowel disease pathogenesis
WF Doe

39

5 Inflammatory bowel disease: autoimmunity or chronic
inflammation?
L Mayer

46

6 Neutrophil–epithelial interactions, and efforts to down-regulate
them, in inflammatory bowel disease
AT Gewirtz and JL Madara

54

7 Understanding inflammatory bowel disease at the millennium:
tentative answers and future questions
DK Podolsky

61

CONTENTS

Section III: CLINICAL CHALLENGES IN INFLAMMATORY BOWEL DISEASE

8 Diagnosis of inflammatory bowel disease: an update
M Robinson   73

9 Recent developments in the diagnosis and management of paediatric inflammatory bowel disease
EG Seidman, M Dubinsky, H Patriquin, G Marx and Y Théorêt   87

10 Inflammatory bowel disease in the elderly
GR Greenberg and I Tai   96

Section IV: CURRENT THERAPY IN INFLAMMATORY BOWEL DISEASE

11 Induction of remission in ulcerative colitis
SB Hanauer   107

12 Remission maintenance in ulcerative colitis
J Schölmerich   117

13 Induction therapy for Crohn's disease
AH Steinhart   128

14 Maintenance of remission in Crohn's disease
P Rutgeerts   137

Section V: BONE DISEASE IN INFLAMMATORY BOWEL DISEASE

15 Risk factors and prevalence of bone disease in inflammatory bowel disease
CN Bernstein   147

16 Management of low bone mass in patients with inflammatory bowel disease
A Tenenhouse   163

17 Steroid-induced osteonecrosis in inflammatory bowel disease: Canadian legal status
RM Carter and MGA Grace   173

CONTENTS

Section VI: ALTERNATIVE THERAPY

18 Psychotherapy for inflammatory bowel disease:
new prospects
RG Maunder   185

19 The use of complementary and alternative medicine by
patients with inflammatory bowel disease
RJ Hilsden and MJ Verhoef   194

20 Gut inflammation: is there a role for herbal medicines?
MJS Miller   201

21 The role of nutrition in the treatment of inflammatory
bowel disease
MA Gassull   207

Section VII: NEW THERAPEUTIC APPROACHES

22 Antibodies to proinflammatory cytokines
LC Karp and SR Targan   219

23 Immunomodulation of Crohn's disease
C van Montfrans, T ten Hove and SJH van Deventer   227

24 Application of recombinant DNA technology to the
identification of novel therapeutic targets in inflammatory
bowel disease
*GE Wild, J Hasan, MJ Ropeleski, KA Waschke, C Cossette,
L Dufresne, BQH Le and ABR Thomson*   234

25 The use of probiotics in inflammatory bowel disease
M Campieri, P Gionchetti, F Rizzello and A Venturi   252

Index   259

List of Principal Authors

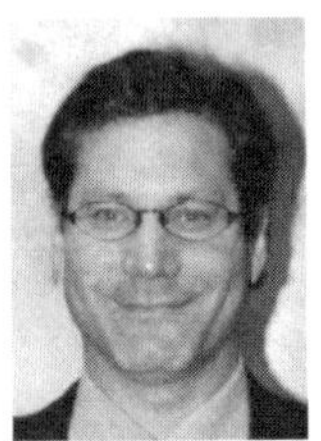

C. N. BERNSTEIN
University of Manitoba
Section of Gastroenterology
GB-443 Health Sciences Centre
820 Sherbrook Street
Winnipeg MB R3A-1R9
Canada

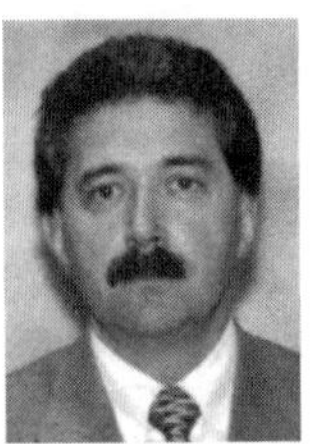

R. F. BURSEY
Department of Medicine "Gastroenterology"
Memorial University of Newfoundland
Faculty of Medicine
The Health Sciences Centre
St. John's, NFLD
A1B 3B6
Canada

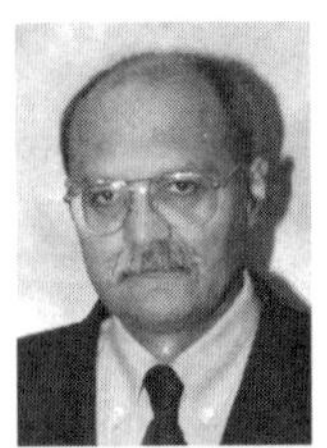

M. CAMPIERI
Policlinico S. Orsola
Department of Internal Medicine & Gastroenterology
University of Bologna
Policlinico Sant'Orsola-Malpighi
via Massarenti, 9
40138 Bologna
Italy

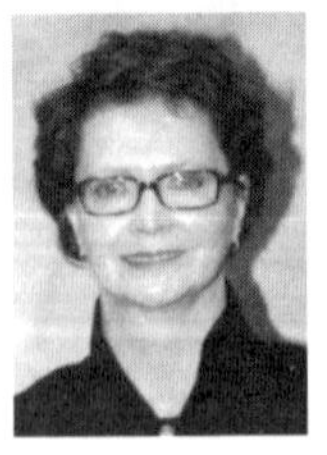

R. M. CARTER
Bennett Jones
Barristers and Solicitors
1000, 10035—105 Street
Edmonton
AB T5J 3T2
Canada

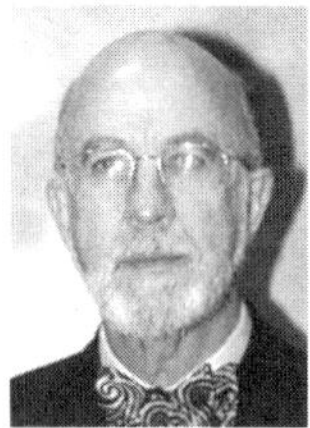

W. F. DOE
University of Birmingham
Medicine, Dentistry & Health Sciences
The Medical School
Edgbaston
Birmingham
B15 2TT
UK

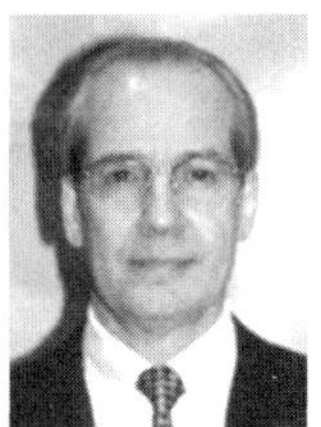

C. FIOCCHI
Division of Gastroenterology
University Hospitals of Cleveland and Case Western Reserve
School of Medicine (BRB)
10900 Euclid Avenue
Cleveland, OH 44106-4952
USA

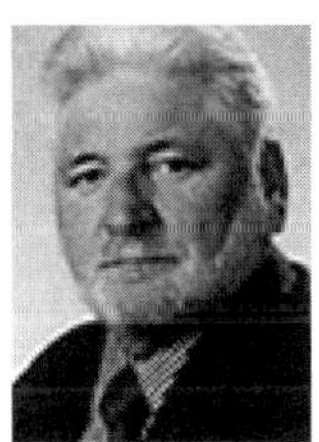

D. G. GALL
Faculty of Medicine
The University of Calgary
3330 Hospital Dr. NW
Calgary, AB
T2N 4N1
Canada

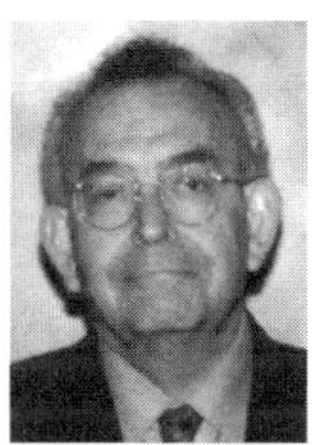

M. A. GASSULL
Department of Gastroenterology
Hospital Universitari Germans Trias i Pujol
Carretera del Canyet s/n
08916 Badalona
Catalonia
Spain

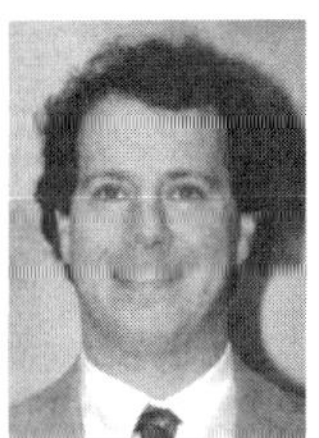

A. T. GEWIRTZ
Epithelial Pathobiology Unit
Department of Pathology and Laboratory Medicine
Emory University School of Medicine
1364 Clifton Road, NE
Atlanta, GA 30322
USA

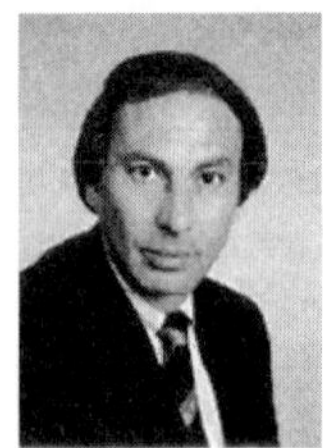

G. R. GREENBERG
Mount Sinai Hospital
Room 445
600 University Avenue
Toronto
ON, M5G 1X5
Canada

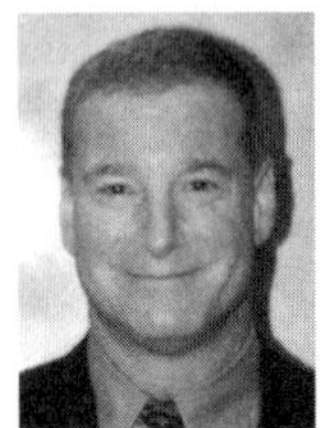

S. B. HANAUER
University of Chicago
Medical Centre
Pritzker School of Medicine
5841 Maryland Avenue
Chicago
IL 60637
USA

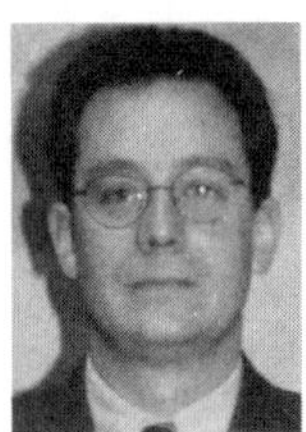

R. J. HILSDEN
Department of Community Health Sciences
Room 1751
3330 Hospital Drive NW
Calgary
AB T2N 4N1
Canada

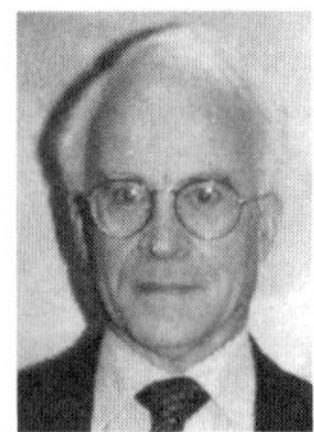

D. P. JEWELL
Gastroenterology Unit
The Radcliffe Infirmary
Woodstock Road
Oxford
OX2 6HE
UK

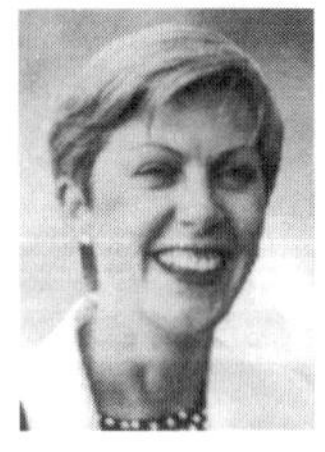

R. S. McLEOD
University of Toronto
Mount Sinai Hospital
600 University Avenue, Room #449
Toronto, ON
M5G 1X5
Canada

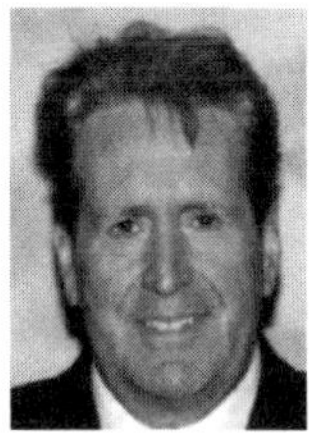

F. MARTIN
Honorary Professor of Medicine
University of Montreal
Vice-President, Scientific Affairs
Axcan Pharma Inc.
Canada

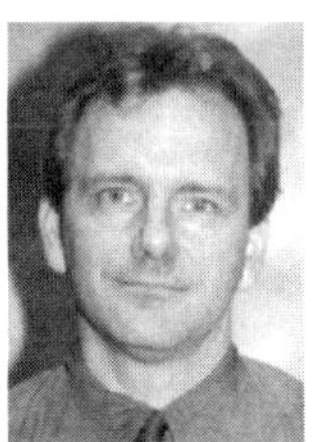

R. G. MAUNDER
Department of Psychiatry
Mount Sinai Hospital
600 University Avenue
Room #1401
Toronto
On M5G 1X5
Canada

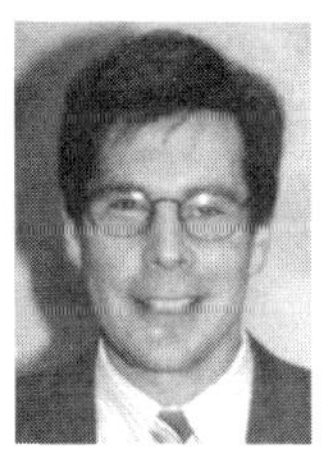

L. MAYER
The Mount Sinai Medical Center
Annenberg 23-16 — Box 1089
1425 Madison Avenue
New York
NY 10029
USA

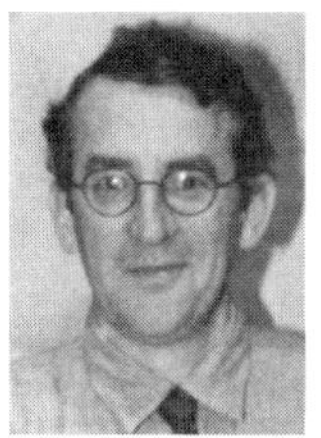

M. J. S. MILLER
Albany Medical College
Department of Pediatrics
47 New Scotland Avenue
Albany
NY 12208
USA

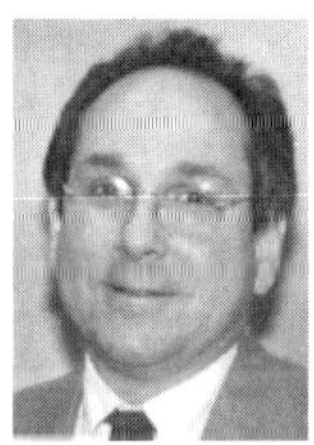

D. K. PODOLSKY
Gastrointestinal Unit & Center for the Study of IBD
Massachusetts General Hospital
Harvard Medical School
Boston, MA 02114
USA

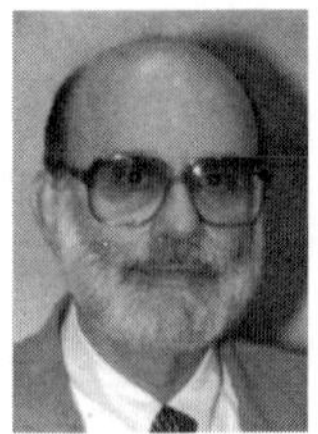

M. ROBINSON
The Oklahoma Foundation for Digestive Research
711 Stanton L. Young Blvd, Suite 619
Oklahoma City, OK 73014
USA

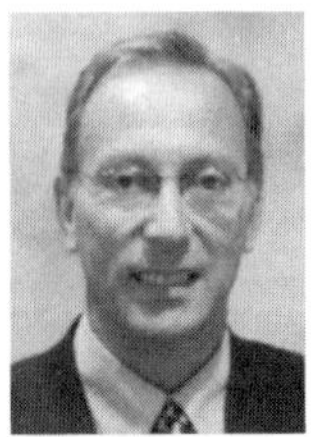

P. RUTGEERTS
Department of Medicine
University Hospital of Leuven
Herestraat 49
B3000 Leuven
Belgium

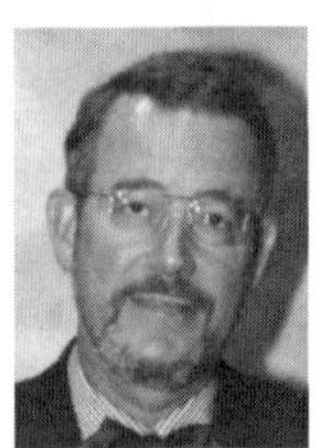

J. SCHÖLMERICH
Klinik und Poliklinik für Innere Medizin I
Universität Regensburg
D-93042 Regensburg
Germany

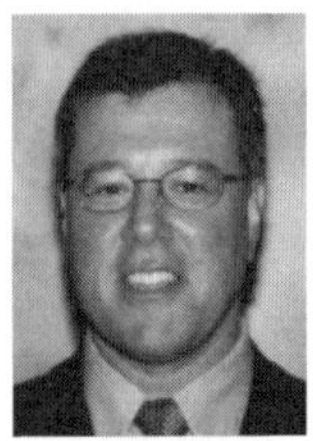

E. G. SEIDMAN
Division of Gastroenterology & Nutrition
Sainte-Justine Hospital
3175 Côte Ste-Catherine Rd
Montreal
QC H3T 1C5
Canada

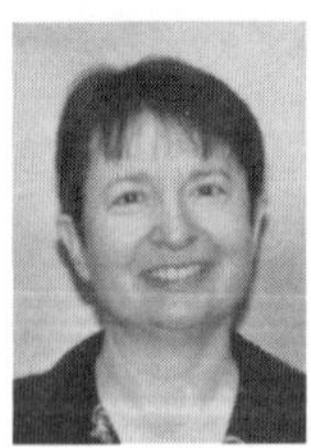

K. SIMINOVITCH
Mount Sinai Hospital
656A-600 University Avenue
Toronto
ON M5G 1X5
Canada

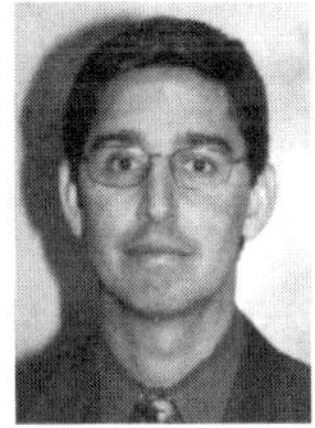

A. H. STEINHART
Inflammatory Bowel Disease Centre
Mount Sinai Hospital
Suite 445, 600 University Avenue,
Toronto, ON M5G 1X5
Canada

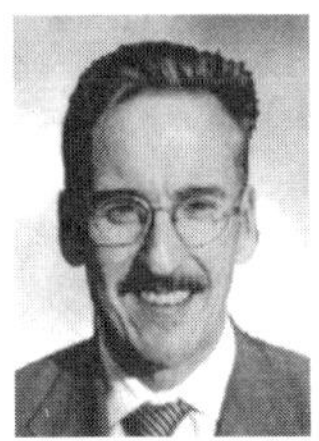

L. R. SUTHERLAND
Department of Community Health Sciences
University of Calgary
3330 Hospital Drive NW, Room 1751
Calgary, AB
T2N 4N1
Canada

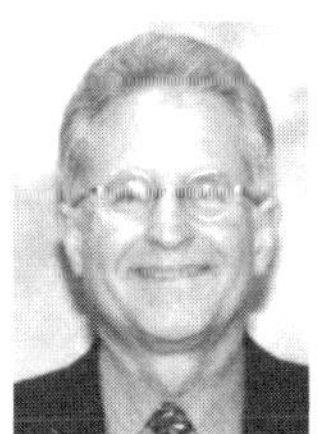

S. R. TARGAN
Cedars-Sinai Division of Gastroenterology and Inflammatory
Bowel Disease Center
Suite D4063
8700 Beverly Blvd
Los Angeles
CA 90048 1804
USA

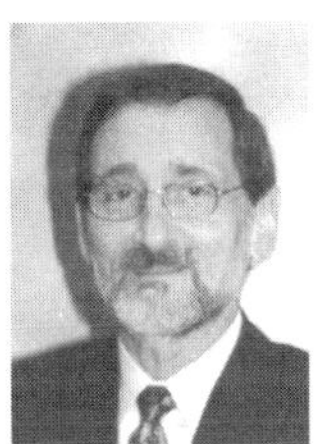

A. TENENHOUSE
Bone Disease Department
Montreal General Hospital
Room L8-121
1650 Cedar Avenue
Montreal, QC H3G 1A4
Canada

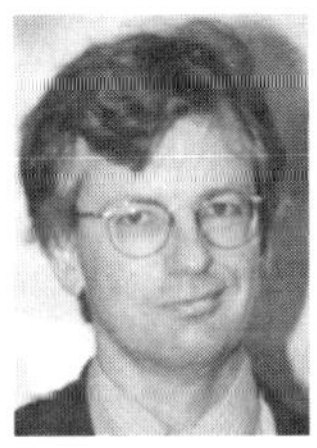

S. Z. H. VAN DEVENTER
Laboratory of Experimental Internal Medicine
Academic Medical Center
G2-105
Meibergdreef 9
1105 AZ Amsterdam
The Netherlands

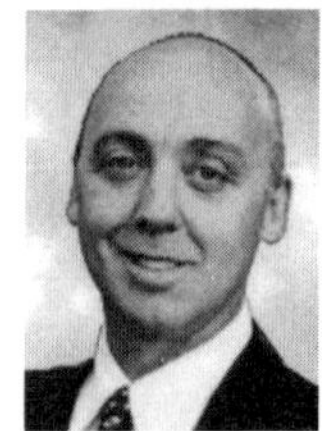

J. L. WALLACE
Department of Physiology and Medicine
University of Calgary
Health Sciences Centre
3330 Hospital Drive NW
Calgary, AB
T2N 4N1
Canada

Preface

This Trends in Inflammatory Bowel Disease Therapy Symposium was held in Vancouver, British Columbia, Canada, 27–29 August 1999. This is the seventh international symposium, sponsored by Axcan Pharma Canada Inc., since the first symposium in 1986. The Canadian Association of Gastroenterology has co-sponsored these symposia since 1990. Each symposium has been published, and reflects and updates the extensive research and education, and the understanding of the mechanisms and treatment of inflammatory bowel disease. From the beginning, Canadian and international experts have been involved, maintaining a consistently high quality, both in their presentations, during discussions, and the subsequent publication of their work. There have been major advances since the symposium held two years ago, and these are presented in this book. In keeping with modern educational practice, objectives are provided, and all presentations were subject to written independent evaluation. All participants are asked to declare any conflicts of interest. MOCOMP and educational credits are available.

The general objective is to provide an update in the aetiology, pathogenesis and treatment of inflammatory bowel disease. The specific objectives are as follows: (1) to inform the participants of the current information concerning the genetic basis for inflammatory bowel disease and its impact on immune function; (2) to explore the pathogenesis of inflammatory bowel disease under the headings of *bacterial factors, autoimmunity, neutrophil–epithelial interactions*, with an *overview of present and future trends*; (3) to discuss up-to-date information on clinical challenges in inflammatory bowel disease and adults with diagnostic issues, as well as specific issues that impact on children and the elderly; (4) to discuss cases showing features of proctitis, terminal ileal disease, colonic dysplasia, and to generate interactive discussion with a panel and audience using touch-pad question/answers and by verbal communication; (5) to learn the latest information on the induction and maintenance of remission in ulcerative colitis and in Crohn's disease; (6) to explore the increasingly important topic of bone disease in inflammatory bowel disease, including risk factors, prevalence, treatment, prevention and steroid risk and the law; (7) to understand the current view on alternative therapy under the topics of *psychotherapy, web therapies* and *complementary therapies*, and the place of nutrition in inflammatory bowel disease; and finally, (8) to understand the latest information applying recombinant DNA technology to identify novel therapeutic targets and the exciting new treatment modalities, with new biological agents (anti-inflammatory cytokines, interleukin-10), and the significant advance in treatment using chimaeric antibody to tumour necrosis factor alpha in patients with intractable Crohn's disease. New information concerning probiotics in ulcerative colitis is presented.

Finally, there were three posters chosen as the best clinical and basic research posters from those submitted, which are also included.

I wish to acknowledge the excellent contributions and presentations of the speakers, and their diligence in providing manuscripts in a timely fashion for this report of the conference. The Scientific Organizing Committee, consisting of Lloyd Sutherland, Francois Martin, Robin McLeod, John Wallace, Ford Bursey and Miguel Gassull have given sterling service in the organization of this meeting and the publication of these proceedings. Grant Gall provided knowledge and input in coordinating this symposium as part of the Digestive Disease Week of the Canadian Association of Gastroenterology.

I would like to acknowledge and express the Scientific Organizing Committee's and my own appreciation to Leon and Diane Gosselin and the employees of Axcan Pharma Canada Inc., not only for making this meeting financially possible, in providing the wherewithal to attract this excellent panel of international and local speakers, but also for their major role in the support of education and research activities in the field of inflammatory bowel disease in Canada.

C. Noel Williams, FRCPC
Chairman, Scientific Organizing Committee
Trends in Inflammatory Bowel Disease Therapy 1999

Section I
Genetics

Moderators: **S. Peña,** Amsterdam
                   C. N. Williams, Halifax

1
Genetics of inflammatory bowel disease: where are we?

M. S. SILVERBERG, A.-K. SOMANI AND K. A. SIMINOVITCH

ABSTRACT

Recent advances in recombinant DNA technology have rendered feasible the application of a positional cloning strategy to the identification of inflammatory bowel disease (IBD) susceptibility genes. In this context many groups have now performed genome-wide scans on multi-case IBD families so as to identify chromosomal loci showing linkage with IBD. The results of such studies have revealed a number of suggestive susceptibility loci, some of which have been independently replicated, but none of which has been found uniformly in all studies. At present the reasons for such disparities remain unclear, but the available linkage data suggest that IBD gene discovery can be achieved by positional cloning. It seems likely, however, that this work will be greatly expedited through the use of several technologies which complement the positional cloning approach, including, for example, expression array and candidate gene analysis. Availability of these strategies together with the progress already made in relation to the genetics of IBD should render feasible relatively rapid isolation of IBD susceptibility genes and the translation of such information to clinical benefit.

INTRODUCTION

Among the many clinical benefits to be realized from recombinant DNA technology, the identification of the genes responsible for disease represents one of the achievements with the most potential to impact upon clinical care. Identification of genes responsible for 'single' gene diseases with a Mendelian pattern of inheritance has proceeded at a remarkable pace and these successes, together with a myriad of advances in robotics, bioinformatics and other technologies that facilitate 'high throughput' genetic analyses, have paved the way for the identification of genes underlying more complex genetic disorders[1]. In this context, intensive research effort is now being directed towards the isolation of susceptibility genes for complex diseases such as asthma, type II diabetes mellitus, multiple sclerosis and, as detailed below, inflammatory bowel disease.

GENETIC CONTRIBUTION TO IBD

As compared to single-gene disorders with simple Mendelian inheritance, IBD and the majority of other human diseases represent complex genetic disorders[2]. Such diseases reflect an interplay between multiple genetic and environmental factors; thus, definition of aetiology has, for the most part, remained elusive (Figure 1). Further complicating attempts to understand disease pathogenesis is the fact that conditions such as IBD may not only be polygenic (i.e. caused by multiple genetic 'hits'), but may also be genetically heterogeneous (i.e. caused by different genes in different individuals) and involve genetic lesions that are often not fully penetrant (implying that apparently healthy individuals may carry the disease susceptibility alleles).

Despite the multifactorial aetiology of IBD, epidemiological data provide support for a major aetiological role for heritable factors[2]. For example, monozygotic twin concordance rates for IBD are 40–50% as compared to a dizygotic twin concordance rate of about 8%[3]. In addition, the prevalence of IBD is increased in first-degree relatives of affected individuals (10–20%) but not in spouses of these individuals[4,5]. The prevalence is also increased in particular racial and ethnic groups such as in Ashkenazi Jews[2] (2–8 times greater risk as compared to non-Jewish Caucasians), which represents a more genetically homogeneous group. The λ_s (relative risk of disease in a sibling of an

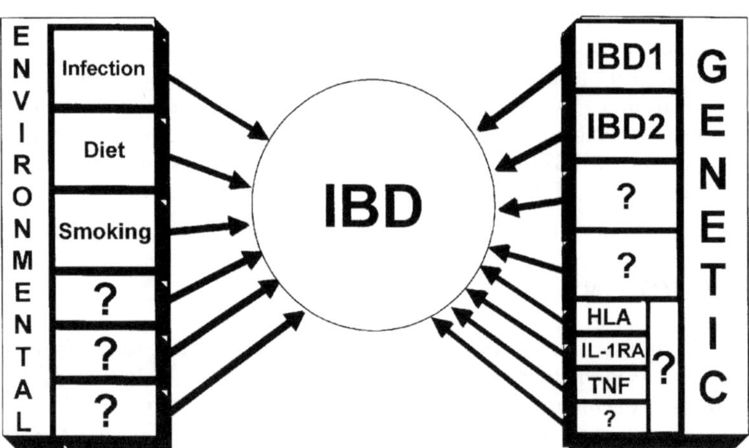

Figure 1 Multiple variables contribute to the complex aetiology of inflammatory bowel disease. These variables are likely to include environmental 'triggers' such as infectious organisms, dietary components or exposure to toxins. Expression of IBD is also likely to involve multiple genetic 'hits', for example, from potential susceptibility loci such as IBD1 and IBD2 or from modifier genes such as the HLA genes

affected individual versus the population prevalence) is estimated to be 20–30 for Crohn's disease (CD) and 8–16 for ulcerative colitis (UC), an observation which implies a stronger role for genetic predisposition in the expression of CD as compared to UC[6]. Despite this finding, and the clinical differences between CD and UC, these conditions probably share at least some genetic alterations as the risk of CD is increased in relatives of UC patients and vice-versa[5]. These epidemiological data provide the incentive for current efforts to isolate IBD susceptibility genes. As outlined below, identification of IBD genes is being attempted utilizing two different strategies: the positional cloning and candidate gene approaches.

POSITIONAL CLONING

Positional cloning represents a disease gene-hunting strategy which allows disease susceptibility genes to be identified in the absence of knowledge of disease pathogenesis or mode of inheritance. The methodology involves analysis of multicase families for the segregation of chromosome-specific markers so as to identify the chromosomal regions which contain genes of interest[7]. To this end, DNA is prepared from multi-case families (such as sib-pair families in which at least two siblings are affected) and then subjected to genotype analysis using sets of microsatellite markers (highly polymorphic markers usually found in non-coding DNA) which represent chromosomal sites spaced at relatively even intervals throughout the entire genome. Linkage analysis is then carried out using statistical software that allows for an analysis of the extent to which particular marker alleles segregate with disease[7]. For example, in affected sibling studies the possibility that affected siblings share alleles more often than expected by chance is evaluated (Figure 2).

Some controversy exists, however, as to what constitutes meaningful linkage data in relation to genome-wide scans carried out in the context of a complex disease. The most widely followed guidelines are those proposed by Lander and Kruglyak[8], in which a LOD (logarithm of the odds) of > 2.2 or $p<7 \times 10^{-4}$ is considered to be *suggestive* of linkage and a LOD > 3.6 or $p<2 \times 10^{-5}$ is considered to represent *significant* linkage. To *confirm* previously reported linkage results, *replication* data are required in which the *p*-value for linkage obtained by analysis of an independent population for the region of interest is < 0.01. Using this strategy a particular locus can be determined to be 'linked' to disease based on the finding that a marker allele at that locus segregates with disease affectation status. Once such a chromosomal locus or region has been identified, physical mapping studies are carried out so as to elucidate candidate genes in the region of interest. The status (i.e. sequence/expression) of each of these genes is then compared between patients and healthy controls so as to identify a defective or variant allele found more frequently or even exclusively in affected individuals (Figure 2).

A number of studies reporting data from genome-wide scans or, alternatively, attempts to replicate such data, have now been published. The first such report was from Hugot *et al*[9] who published data suggesting linkage between CD (European population) and a marker *D16S409* which maps to the

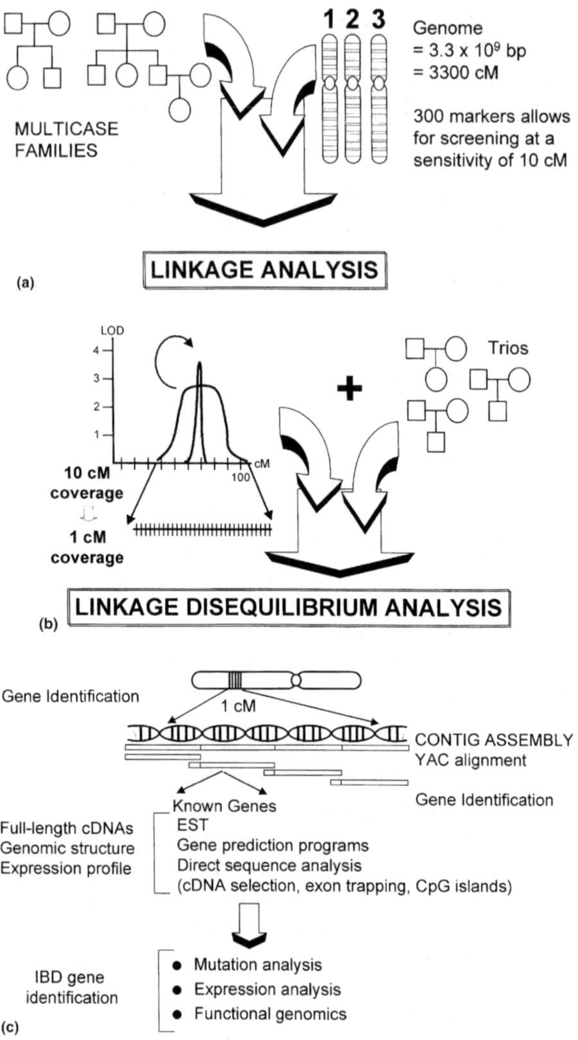

Figure 2 (**a**) Multi-case family collections are required to achieve the disease gene localization integral to positional cloning. Genotyping is performed on each individual using approximately 300 microsatellite markers that span the entire genome at 10 centiMorgan (cM) or 10 million base pair (bp) intervals. Marker–disease cosegregation can then be assessed so as to elucidate loci linked with disease expression. (**b**) Linkage analysis allows disease genes to be mapped to broad (> 5 cM) chromosomal regions that must then be refined to allow disease gene identification. Such refinement is achieved by genotyping with a more dense marker set that provides at least 1 cM coverage of the region of interest. Improved localization of the gene of interest may also be obtained using additional statistical approaches such as the transmission disequilibrium test (TDT), a test in which trios (one affected child and both parents) are evaluated for evidence of marker linkage disequilibrium (i.e. transmission of a particular marker allele to affected offspring more frequently than expected by chance). (**c**) Once a chromosomal region has been sufficiently refined to make gene identification feasible (<1 cM), various techniques are employed to identify genes in this region. The sequences and expression of these genes are then studied in patients and controls so as to identify the disease-causing gene

pericentromeric region of chromosome 16 (LOD 2.04). This locus was designated as *IBD1* and this observation was subsequently replicated in studies of CD families from the USA, Europe and Australia[10–13], the last of which elucidated a LOD of 6.3 in relation to the CD–*IBD1* linkage[13]. Data from one study[14] have also suggested UC to be linked to the *IBD1* locus, but this finding has not been confirmed by others. Moreover, data from two large IBD linkage studies carried out in the UK[15] and Canada[16] revealed no evidence for linkage between IBD and representative loci on chromosome 16. The second report describing results of a genome-wide scan on IBD families was from Satsangi *et al.*[15] and included data ascertained from a UK population demonstrating linkage between IBD (CD and UC) and regions on chromosomes 12q (*D12S83*, LOD 5.47, $p=2.66 \times 10^{-7}$), 7q (*D7S669*, LOD 3.08, $p=8.2 \times 10^{-5}$) and 3p (*D3S1573*, LOD 2.69, $p = 2.1 \times 10^{-4}$). The chromosome 12 localization, designated *IBD2*, has since been replicated by Duerr *et al.*[17] (American IBD population) and by Hampe *et al.*[18] (European CD population), but other linkage data obtained from analysis of American[11] and Canadian[16] populations do not support this finding. Results of two other genome-wide scans involving analysis of American[19] and European[18] populations have also been published, and these linkage data have revealed potential IBD susceptibility loci on chromosomes 1p, 1q, 3q, 6p and 10. The locus on chromosome 6p is of particular interest in view of the localization of the MHC gene cluster and the *TNF*-α gene in this vicinity. Two other recent reports have also revealed this region on 6p to be linked to IBD[20,21].

At present, the reasons for failures to replicate IBD linkage data are unclear. However, the situation is likely to reflect, at least in part, the clinical and genetic heterogeneity of IBD. Thus, for example, patients displaying specific presentations such as fistulizing disease, extraintestinal features or unusually severe, unremitting disease necessitating surgery may represent not only clinical, but also genetic, subsets whose IBD susceptibility gene profiles differ from those of other patients. It is also very likely that the disease reflects many different combinations of susceptibility genes and that these combinations vary among different ethnic, racial and geographic groups. Errors in classification or diagnosis may also affect results significantly as some patients, particularly those initially diagnosed with UC, may in reality have either Crohn's colitis or even a self-limited infectious colitis. Similarly, differences in the diagnostic criteria used by various groups may also account for discrepancies in linkage findings. Finally, there remains some disagreement as to what constitutes significant linkage in relation to complex genetic disease, and the possibility exists that the threshold used to declare linkage has been too low in some of the IBD studies. Despite these problems, however, for at least two of the putative IBD loci (chromosomes 12 and 16), the replication data have been sufficiently consistent to provide an incentive for many of the groups studying IBD genetics to pool their linkage data under a collaboration known as the IBD International Genetic Consortium (http://Rpride.anu.edu.au/~ibd/index.html) and to determine whether collective data will confirm and/or refine these localizations.

CANDIDATE GENE STUDIES

As the data from the human genome project continue to amass, it is becoming increasingly attractive to apply a candidate gene approach to IBD gene identification[22]. This strategy involves the analysis of known genes which are selected for testing based on the function of their protein products and the prediction that such products play a role in IBD susceptibility. Once an appropriate candidate is selected, a case–control association analysis is performed wherein the frequency of a particular allele(s) of the gene of interest is compared between patients and matched controls (Figure 3).

A good example of the candidate gene approach is provided by the evaluation of HLA class II genes among IBD patients. The HLA class II genes have been studied extensively in IBD and negative and positive associations have been reported for many antigen groups and alleles[23–37]. These findings have, however, been highly variable depending on the technique used (serological vs molecular testing) and populations studied. Some of the more consistent results include the demonstration that HLA DR2 (specifically the DRB1*1502 allele) and DRB1*0103 are positively associated while DR4 is negatively associated with UC[23–30]. The DR2 association with UC appears to be particularly strong among both Japanese[23,28] and Jewish[24] patients. There is also a suggestion that UC-affected individuals carrying the DRB1*0103 allele are likely to manifest more extensive disease[29]. Results in CD have been considerably more variable. CD has been reported to be positively associated with DR7, DRB1*0103, DRB3*0301 and DQ4 and negatively associated with DR2 and DR3[31–34,36]. Despite the variable results and relatively minor role the HLA genes appear to play in conferring susceptibility to IBD, it seems likely that these genes impact upon expression of IBD, perhaps by modifying disease severity (as suggested

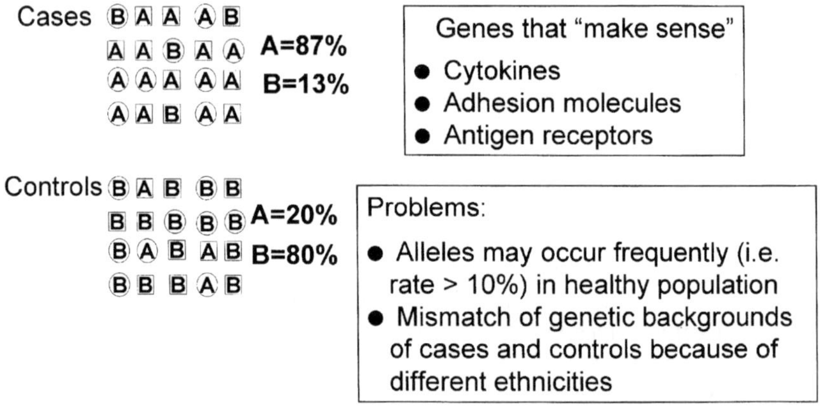

Figure 3 Candidate genes which 'make sense' in terms of their relevance to disease pathophysiology are identified and an association study is performed to determine whether a particular allele is more likely to be found in affected individuals versus a matched control population. Positive results can be verified by analysis of allele transmission from heterozygous parents to affected and unaffected children

by the association of the DRB1*0103 allele with extensive disease in UC). This conclusion is also supported by recent linkage data revealing IBD to be linked to the chromosomal region on 6p which contains the MHC gene cluster[20,21]. These data suggest that an important susceptibility gene may map within this region in linkage disequilibrium with the HLA genes[38].

In addition to the HLA genes, other genes, most notably the cytokine genes, have also been investigated as candidate IBD genes, but the data from such studies have, for the most part, shown little reproducibility or statistical significance. One gene that has been particularly targeted for study is the gene encoding tumour necrosis factor (TNF). For example, one particular TNF haplotype (TNF a2b1c2d4e1) has been shown to be present in 24% of American CD patients as compared to 4.1% of UC patients (p=0.001) and 6.7% of control subjects ($p = 0.01$)[39]. In addition, an association between two polymorphisms in the 5'-flanking region of the *TNF-*α gene (–1031, –863) and CD has been detected in a study of Japanese patients, the conclusion being that these polymorphisms may be associated with higher levels of TNF-α production[40]. A polymorphism in the gene encoding ICAM-1 has also been found to be associated with ANCA-negative UC and with ANCA-positive CD, and on this basis has been postulated to underlie some of the heterogeneity found among CD and UC patients[41]. The IL-1 receptor antagonist gene has also been studied as an IBD candidate gene[42–44], with some reports suggesting that an allele of this gene occurs more frequently in UC patients, particularly those with extensive colitis[42] and in those who are Jewish[43]; these results, however, have not been confirmed by others[44]. Another more recently described IBD–gene association involves rare alleles of the MUC3 gene, a gene controlling intestinal mucin production, and indicates that these alleles are more prevalent in UC patients of both Japanese and Caucasian background (OR 2.64, 95% CI 1.60–4.33, P=0.0001)[45]. These data are particularly intriguing as MUC3 maps to a region on chromosome 7q that has been shown to be linked to IBD[15].

As is evident from the above, data from candidate gene studies have not yet had a large impact on the understanding of the genetic contribution to IBD. However, as progress is made towards identifying susceptibility genes on chromosomal regions and specific environmental triggers, these genes may need to be re-examined for their potential roles in disease predisposition and/or modification. This understanding may provide the ability to introduce early therapeutic intervention in individuals prone to more aggressive disease or particular IBD-associated complications such as colorectal cancer or osteoporosis.

FUTURE DIRECTIONS

The identification of susceptibility genes for IBD is closer to becoming a reality. In addition to the positional cloning techniques and candidate gene testing currently in use for IBD gene identification, new molecular technologies, such as microexpression arrays, will probably markedly expedite this effort. Isolation of susceptibility genes will not only lead to a better understanding of disease pathogenesis, but will also provide the framework for identifying environmental triggers and gene–environment interactions that lead to disease. Information garnered as a result of such a discovery will also yield improvements in diagnostic testing and, ultimately, allow the application of such information to the design of more effective and less toxic therapeutic strategies and possibly disease prevention.

Acknowledgements

This work was supported by a grant from the Crohn's and Colitis Foundation of Canada. Mark Silverberg is a recipient of a Canadian Association of Gastroenterology/Medical Research Council of Canada/Axcan Pharma Fellowship Award, Ally-Khan Somani is a recipient of an NCIC Steve Fonyo Studentship Award, and Katherine Siminovitch is an Arthritis Society of Canada Research Scientist.

References

1. Lander ES, Schork NJ. Genetic dissection of complex traits. Science 1994;265:2037–48.
2. Yang H, Rotter JI. Genetics of inflammatory bowel disease. In: Targan SR, Shanahan F, editors. Inflammatory Bowel Disease: from bench to beside. Baltimore, MD: Williams & Wilkins, 1994:5–30.
3. Tysk C, Lindberg E, Jarnerot G, Floderus-Myrhed B. Ulcerative colitis and Crohn's disease in an unselected population of monozygotic and dizygotic twins. A study of heritability and the influence of smoking. Gut 1988;29:990–6.
4. Orholm M, Munkholm P, Langholz E, Nielson OH, Sorensen IA, Binder V. Familial occurrence of inflammatory bowel disease. N Engl J Med 1991;324:84–8.
5. Mayberry JF, Rhodes J, Newcombe RG. Familial prevalence of inflammatory bowel disease in relatives of patients with Crohn's disease. Br Med J 1980;280:84.
6. Satsangi J, Jewell DP, Bell JI. The genetics of inflammatory bowel disease. Gut 1997;40:572–4.
7. Kruglyak L, Lander ES. Complete multipoint sib-pair analysis of qualitative and quantitative traits. Am J Hum Genet 1995;57:439–54.
8. Lander ES, Kruglyak L. Genetic dissection of complex traits: guidelines for interpreting and reporting linkage results. Nat Genet 1995;11:241–7.
9. Hugot JP, Laurent-Puig P, Gower-Rousseau C et al. Mapping of a susceptibility locus for Crohn's disease on chromosome 16. Nature 1996;379:821–3.
10. Ohmen JD, Yang H, Yamamoto KK et al. Susceptibility locus for inflammatory bowel disease on chromosome 16 has a role in Crohn's disease, but not in ulcerative colitis. Hum Mol Genet 1996;5:1679–83.
11. Brant SR, Fu Y, Fields CT et al. American families with Crohn's disease have strong evidence for linkage to chromosome 16 but not chromosome 12. Gastroenterology 1998;115:1056–61.
12. Curran ME, Lau KF, Hampe J et al. Genetic analysis of inflammatory bowel disease in a large European cohort supports linkage to chromosomes 12 and 16. Gastroenterology 1998;115:1066–71.
13. Cavanaugh JA, Callen DF, Wilson SR et al. Analysis of Australian Crohn's disease pedigrees refines the localization for susceptibility to inflammatory bowel disease on chromosome 16. Ann Hum Genet 1998;62:291–8.
14. Mirza MM, Lee J, Teare D et al. Evidence of linkage of the inflammatory bowel disease susceptibility locus on chromosome 16 (IBD1) to ulcerative colitis. J Med Genet 1998;35:218–21.
15. Satsangi J, Parkes M, Louis E et al. Two stage genome-wide search in inflammatory bowel disease provides evidence for susceptibility loci on chromosome 3, 7 and 12. Nat Genet 1996;14:199–202.
16. Rioux JD, Daly MJ, Green T et al. Absence of linkage between inflammatory bowel disease and selected loci on chromosomes 3, 7, 12, and 16. Gastroenterology 1998;115:1062–5.
17. Duerr RH, Barmada MM, Zhang L et al. Linkage and association between inflammatory bowel disease and a locus on chromosome 12. Am J Hum Genet 1998;63:95–100.
18. Hampe J, Schreiber S, Shaw SH et al. A genomewide analysis provides evidence for novel

linkages in inflammatory bowel disease in a large European cohort. Am J Hum Genet 1999;64:808–16.

19. Cho JH, Nicolae DL, Gold LH *et al*. Identification of novel susceptibility loci for inflammatory bowel disease on chromosomes 1p, 3q, and 4q: evidence for epistasis between 1p and IBD1. Proc Natl Acad Sci USA 1998;95:7502–7.

20. Silverberg MS, Steinhart AH, McLeod RS *et al*. Evidence for linkage between Crohn's disease and a locus near the major histocompatibility complex on chromosome 6 in a Canadian inflammatory bowel disease population. Gastroenterology 1999;116:A820 (abstract).

21. Hampe J, Schreiber S, Lantermann A *et al*. The chromosome 6 susceptibility gene for inflammatory bowel disease localizes outside the TNF-α gene. Gastroenterology 1999;116:A730 (abstract).

22. Todd JA. Interpretation of results from genetic studies of multifactorial diseases. Lancet 1999;354(Suppl. I):15–16.

23. Sugimura K, Asakura H, Mizuki N *et al*. Analysis of genes within the HLA region affecting susceptibility to ulcerative colitis. Hum Immunol 1993;36:112–18.

24. Toyoda H, Wang SJ, Yang HY *et al*. Distinct associations of HLA class II genes with inflammatory bowel disease. Gastroenterology 1993;104:741–8.

25. Yang H, Rotter JI, Toyoda H *et al*. Ulcerative colitis: a genetically heterogeneous disorder defined by genetic (HLA class II) and subclinical (antineutrophil cytoplasmic antibodies) markers. J Clin Invest 1993;92:1080–4.

26. Satsangi J, Welsh KI, Bunce M *et al*. Contribution of genes of the major histocompatibility complex to susceptibility and disease phenotype in inflammatory bowel disease. Lancet 1996;347:1212–17.

27. De La Concha EG, Fernandez-Arquero M, Santa-Cruz S *et al*. Positive and negative associations of distinct HLA-DR2 subtypes with ulcerative colitis (UC). Clin Exp Immunol 1997;108:392–5.

28. Futami S, Aoyama N, Honsako Y *et al*. HLA-DRB1*1502 allele, subtype of DR15, is associated with susceptibility to ulcerative colitis and its progression. Dig Dis Sci 1995;40:814–18.

29. Roussomoustakaki M, Satsangi J, Welsh K *et al*. Genetic markers may predict disease behavior in patients with ulcerative colitis. Gastroenterology 1997;112:1845–53.

30. Silverberg MS, Murphy J, Steinhart AH *et al*. Contribution of HLA Class II genes to susceptibility to ulcerative colitis in a Canadian inflammatory bowel disease population. Gastroenterology 1998;114:A2946.

31. Danze PM, Columbel JF, Jacquot S *et al*. Association of HLA class II genes with susceptibility to Crohn's disease. Gut 1996;39:69–72.

32. Forcione DG, Sands B, Isselbacher KJ, Rustgi A, Podolsky DK, Pillai S. An increased risk of Crohn's disease in individuals who inherit the HLA class II DRB3*0301 allele. Proc Natl Acad Sci USA 1996;93:5094–8.

33. Nakajima A, Matsuhashi N, Kodama T, Yazaki Y, Takazoe M, Kimura A. HLA-linked susceptibility and resistance genes in Crohn's disease. Gastroenterology 1995;109:1462–7.

34. Reinshagen M, Loeliger C, Kuehnl P *et al*. HLA class II gene frequencies in Crohn's disease: a population based analysis in Germany. Gut 1996;38:538–42.

35. Naom I, Lee J, Ford D *et al*. Analysis of the contribution of HLA genes to genetic predisposition in inflammatory bowel disease. Am J Hum Genet 1996;59:226–33.

36. Silverberg M, Murphy J, Mirea L *et al*. The HLA DRB1*0103 allele is associated with Crohn's disease in a Toronto inflammatory bowel disease population. Gastroenterology 1999;116:A820 (abstract).

37. Stokkers PCF, Reitsma PH, Tytgat GNJ, van Deventer SJH. HLA-DR and -DQ phenotypes in inflammatory bowel disease: a meta-analysis. Gut 1999;45:395–401.

38. Tomlinson IPM, Bodmer WF. The HLA system and the analysis of multifactorial genetic disease. Trends Genet 1995;11:493–8.

39. Plevy SE, Targan SR, Yang H, Fernandez D, Rotter JI, Toyoda H. Tumor necrosis factor microsatellites define a Crohn's disease-associated haplotype on chromosome 6. Gastroenterology 1996;110:1053–60.

40. Negoro K, Kinouchi Y, Hiwatashi N *et al*. Crohn's disease is associated with novel polymorphisms in the 5' flanking region in the tumor necrosis factor gene. Gastroenterology 1999;117:1062–8.

41. Yang H, Vora DK, Targan SR, Toyoda H, Beaudet AL, Rotter JI. Intercellular adhesion molecule 1 gene associations with immunologic subsets of inflammatory bowel disease. Gastroenterology 1995;109:440–8.
42. Mansfield JC, Holden H, Tarlow JL *et al*. Novel genetic association between ulcerative colitis and the anti-inflammatory cyokine interleukin-1 receptor antagonist. Gastroenterology 1994;106:637–42.
43. Tountas NA, Casini-Raggi V, Yang H *et al*. Functional and ethnic association of allele 2 of the interleukin-1 receptor antagonist gene in ulcerative colitis. Gastroenterology 1999;117:806–13.
44. Louis E, Satsangi J, Roussomoustakaki M *et al*. Cytokine gene polymorphisms in inflammatory bowel disease. Gut 1996;39:705–10.
45. Kyo K, Parkes M, Takei Y *et al*. Association of ulcerative colitis with rare VNTR alleles of the human intestinal mucin gene, MUC3. Hum Mol Genet 1999;8:307–11.

2
Genetics of inflammatory bowel disease: why is it important?

D. P. JEWELL

ABSTRACT

A genetic susceptibility to inflammatory bowel disease (IBD) is suggested by the familial incidence of 15–20%, disease concordance within monozygotic twins (especially for Crohn's disease), and a remarkable concordance of disease characteristics within individual families. However, the pattern of inheritance is complex and data from genome-wide searches using microsatellite markers suggest that there are multiple susceptibility genes involved. Patients with ulcerative colitis or Crohn's disease may share many of these but the precise clinical phenotype may be determined by the number and nature of these genes possessed by any one individual, as well as by the inheritance of disease-specific genes. Current evidence suggests that susceptibility genes for IBD overall are located on chromosomes 3, 7 and 12 but that there specific susceptibility genes for Crohn's disease on chromosome 16 (and also probably on chromosomes 1 and 4) and for ulcerative colitis on chromosomes 2 and 6. The regions of linkage are large but are being progressively narrowed using large family collections (affected sibling pairs or multiply-affected families) and family-based association studies. The results of these studies have become important to many groups, including patients, clinical investigators, the practising physician, and the pharmaceutical industry.

Patients have become aware of the genetic susceptibility and are keen to know the risk of their siblings or children developing IBD. These risks have now been calculated and for IBD overall the relative risk for siblings is about 25 and slightly less for offspring. However, the absolute risk is still small given the low incidence of IBD.

Clinical investigators: the human genome is thought to contain 80 000–100 000 genes – a formidable number – and this provides a daunting task to sort out polygenic diseases. The ability to use microsatellite markers (dinucleotide repeats which are scattered throughout the genome) as polymorphic alleles (the length of the repeat being the polymorphism) has allowed linkage studies to be performed using techniques such as allele sharing in affected sibling pairs. In contrast to many other polygenic diseases, linkage studies in IBD have been replicated to a remarkable degree and the linkage with regions on chromosomes 12 and 16 are now regarded as established. As these regions of linkage are being narrowed (for chromosome 12 it is now down to 0.5 cM), physical mapping strategies can begin in order to identify precise genes. Many of these regions of linkage are known to contain genes of considerable relevance to a chronic inflammatory disease (e.g. genes for growth factors, cytokines, chemokines and their receptors). Identification of polymorphisms within these genes and their relation to disease may provide new information on disease pathogenesis, as well as providing a means of narrowing regions of linkage by using them as positional candidates.

Clinicians will need to be aware of the risk to family members but will also need to be aware that genetic information may predict disease behaviour (e.g. extent of disease predicted by HLA DR3, DQ2, severity predicted by HLA DR103), the chance of developing extraintestinal manifestations and the possible response to treatment (e.g. response to anti-TNF antibody).

The pharmaceutical industry: genetic susceptibility to IBD might be mediated at various levels which include intestinal epithelial cell biology, mucus synthesis, and mucosal immunoregulation. Identification of susceptibility genes and knowledge of their function offers potential hope for pharmaceutical intervention.

INTRODUCTION

The occasional occurrence of either Crohn's disease or ulcerative colitis in a relative of a patient with disease has long been recognized, and familial prevalence has even reached 30% or so in some early series[1]. However, the failure to detect any obvious pattern of inheritance, and the very discrepant early studies on HLA associations, provided no encouragement for further study. Two events then occurred which stimulated further interest and allowed great progress to be made during the 1990s. This progress has raised real hopes that susceptibility genes may be identified early in the next millennium. The first concept was that ulcerative colitis and Crohn's disease may be clinically heterogeneous, i.e. they may reflect a variety of disease, and that the exact phenotype might be influenced by specific genes which may not necessarily influence overall susceptibility to developing chronic inflammatory disease. This realization has led to the study of large numbers of patients to allow adequate analysis of genotype–phenotype relationships. The second event that allowed progress to develop so quickly was the seminal paper of Weissenbach et al.[1] that demonstrated how diseases of unknown heritability could be studied by linkage analysis using polymorphic dinucleotide repeats which are found throughout the genome. As discussed in Chapter 1, both ulcerative colitis and Crohn's disease have been linked to regions on several chromosomes. There has been considerable, though not complete, agreement about linkage to chromosome 12. Furthermore, the region of linkage has been progressively narrowed to the point where gene identification studies can begin. Confirmation of the original linkage found on chromosome 7 has recently been found, but this is awaited for other reported loci on chromosomes 1,3,4,10 and 22. In

Table 1 The relative risk of developing IBD in the first-degree relatives of an affected individual

	Siblings	*Parents*	*Offspring*
Oxford[2]	24.7	12.5	4.4
Leicester[3]	34.7	17.1	29.1
Leuven[4]	20.0	8.9	15.0

addition, there has also been remarkable agreement about the possibility of a susceptibility gene(s) on chromosome 16 for Crohn's disease, whereas the HLA region on the short arm of chromosome 6 may be more relevant for ulcerative colitis than Crohn's disease. Thus, it appears that these diseases are polygenic and that they share some susceptibility genes but differ for others. If this model is correct it provides a plausible explanation for the similarity, and also the frequent dissimilarity, of the clinical features.

These observations have generated intense interest and have major implications for probands and their families, clinicians looking after patients with IBD, geneticists and, not least, the pharmaceutical industry.

IMPORTANCE FOR PATIENTS

A common question in the clinic from a newly diagnosed young patient is: 'What is the chance of my children developing the disease?' Recent studies of familial disease have partly answered this[2-4]. Table 1 lists the relative risks of either ulcerative colitis or Crohn's disease for the first-degree relatives of a proband. There is clearly an increased risk, which appears greatest within siblings, but the low incidence of the diseases makes the absolute risk still quite small. Thus, if the combined incidence of both diseases in the Western world is about 20 new cases per 100 000 of the population per year, a 10-fold increased risk provides an incidence of 200 per 100 000 per year, i.e. 0.2% per year. However, since the onset of disease is not linear over time, this can in no way be regarded as the basis for cumulative risk.

A familial study from Baltimore suggests that there is a greater risk of a child developing more extensive disease if the father has the disease rather than the mother[5]. However, this has not been a consistent finding in other populations and it is not clear, at the present time, whether the Baltimore data are specific for that particular population (with a high proportion of Ashkenazi Jews) or whether it is a 'false-positive' which occurred by chance. Nevertheless, virtually all the family studies have shown a high degree of concordance for disease type (ulcerative colitis or Crohn's disease) and disease behaviour (e.g. extent, severity, presence of extraintestinal manifestations) within families[4,6-8]. So although mixed families occur in which both diseases are present in different members, it is more likely that disease type runs true within a given family. However, there seems little difference between the characteristics of either disease when they occur in families compared with the characteristics of sporadic disease[9,10]. One particular feature of familial disease has been that offspring develop their disease about 15 years of age younger than the affected parent[5,6]. The explanation for this very consistent observation is not entirely clear, but may be explained by ascertainment bias[11] and possibly by a greater genetic load, i.e. an individual is more likely to inherit more susceptibility genes for IBD if one parent has the disease than if both parents are healthy.

There has been considerable anxiety about the role of measles and Crohn's disease, either because of intrauterine infection or perhaps because of vaccination with the MMR vaccine. Thus, another question that frequently arises is whether the risk is even higher if other members of the family are already known to have ulcerative colitis or Crohn's disease. This cannot be accurately answered. However, a careful review by the Medical Research Council of the UK, of all the available data on measles and measles vaccine, concluded that there was no convincing evidence to link these with the subsequent development of Crohn's disease. Hence there is no reason not to vaccinate young children, as the risk of neurological damage, or even death, from measles early in life far outweighs an unproven risk of IBD following vaccination.

IMPORTANCE FOR CLINICIANS

The data on familial incidence and the risk to other family members are clearly important for clinicians to know, especially if they are caring for large numbers of these patients. However, it is possible that, within the foreseeable future, molecular genetics may allow the clinician to predict behaviour of disease and even response to treatment.

Recent studies of HLA antigens in large numbers of patients have suggested that they may influence disease phenotype, especially in ulcerative colitis. Several studies from Japan have shown an association between ulcerative colitis and the HLA DRB1*1502 allele of HLA DR2[12–14]. A similar finding has also been reported from a Californian population which was predominantly Jewish[15]. Japanese colitics possessing this allele were more likely to require surgery than colitics who did not have this allele. In Oxford no association with DRB1*1502 was found, but severe disease coming to colectomy was associated with HLA DRB1*0103[16,17]. This rare allele of HLA DR1 is found in only 3% of the general population but is present in about 14% of those requiring colectomy for severe disease, a finding that has been confirmed both in Pittsburgh and in Holland[18,19]. Whether the HLA DRB1*0103 molecule is responsible for this pattern of disease, perhaps by its ability to present specific antigens to the immune system, or whether it is in linkage disequilibrium with another gene which is more relevant is currently unknown. Disease extent may also be influenced by Class II antigens. It is a well-known clinical observation that patients with primary sclerosing cholangitis (PSC) usually have a mild, often asymptomatic, colitis which characteristically affects the whole colon. It is also known that the majority of patients with PSC have the HLA DR3, DQ2 positive haplotype. Thus it was particularly interesting when it was found that, in a large population of patients with ulcerative colitis, extensive disease was associated with this haplotype[16]. Indeed, this haplotype is found in less than

10% of patients with distal disease compared with about 30% of those with extensive (proximal to the splenic flexure) or total colitis. Extensive disease may also be associated with a particular intronic polymorphism (i.e. a non-coding allele) in the IL-1 receptor antagonist gene[20]. However, this last association has been found in only a few centres[21–23] and has not been confirmed in many others[19,24,25]. The discrepancies are not explained but may be due to small sample sizes and, in particular, the criteria on which extent of disease was determined (barium radiology, macroscopic appearances on colonoscopy or histological assessment).

While analysing HLA association data in a cohort of patients who had undergone a restorative proctocolectomy for ulcerative colitis, it was noted that the DRB1*0103 allele was not only associated with severe disease and need of surgery but was particularly prevalent (27.4%) in patients who had had previous extraintestinal manifestations[17]. This has been explored in a much more detailed study, predominantly in those patients with joint complications. Orchard et al.[26], on the basis of a large clinical study, were able to categorize the peripheral joint disease into two main types as determined by distinct clinical characteristics and natural history (patients with simply arthralgia were not included further in the study). Type 1 is a pauciarticular arthropathy affecting mainly large joints in association with active intestinal disease. The joints are hot, swollen and painful and the features are similar to an acute reactive arthropathy. It is non-deforming and seronegative. In contrast, Type 2 arthropathy affects small joints, is much more persistent and is not related to the activity of the intestinal disease. It is also seronegative. These two forms of peripheral arthropathy also have distinct genetic associations[27]. Thus, Type 1 is associated with HLA-B27, B35 and DRB1*0103 whereas Type 2 is associated with HLA-B44. The association of DRB1*0103 with Type 1 arthropathy is particularly strong (40%) compared with a frequency of 10% in a colitic population without joint disease and only 3% in healthy controls. It is possible to calculate predictive values from the data and thus a patient who carries the DRB1*0103 allele has a positive prediction of about 60% for developing Type 1 arthropathy. In contrast, for patients who are not HLA-DRB1*0103, over 90% will not develop this form of joint disease.

There are fewer genetic data for the other extraintestinal manifestations. HLA-B27, found in less than 7% of controls, is associated with ankylosing spondylitis but the frequency (65%) is less than is seen in ankylosing spondylitis not associated with IBD (95%)[27]. Recurrent mouth ulceration is strongly associated with HLA B44[28].

The HLA associations with Crohn's disease have been much more variable than in ulcerative colitis. Despite more consistent associations described from Japan[29], no reproducible findings have been reported from the West even when sufficient patients have been studied to allow subanalysis with respect to phenotype. These negative observations fit the failure to demonstrate linkage to chromosome 6p for Crohn's disease in sib-pair analysis[16]. However, a recent report from Holland suggests that patients with fistulizing Crohn's disease have a decreased frequency of HLA DRB1*0301. The extraintestinal manifestations of Crohn's disease (joint disease, mouth ulcers) have similar HLA associations to those described for ulcerative colitis[27].

IMPORTANCE TO GENETICISTS

Ulcerative colitis and Crohn's disease are examples of complex traits, which means that the phenotype does not exhibit classical Mendelian inheritance, whether dominant or recessive, attributable to a single gene locus. The degree of complexity is shown by: (1) the fact that possession of a predisposing allele may not cause disease in the absence of other (e.g. environmental) factors, (2) there may be genetic heterogeneity insofar as mutation in one of several genes may result in the same phenotype, and (3) simultaneous mutations in several genes may be required before disease develops and phenotype may vary according to how many mutations are present. To begin to analyse complex traits in humans, several methods have been developed: linkage analysis, allele-sharing methods and association methodology (whether as case–control studies or as family-based associations studies forming the basis of the transmission by descent test (TDT))[30]. Allele-sharing methods have become popular because they do not assume a mode of inheritance, i.e. they are nonparametric. The basis of the test is that an allele, or a chromosomal region, is inherited more often in an affected relative than would be expected by simple Mendelian segregation. Affected sibling pairs or relative pairs are usually studied. The use of polymorphic dinucleotide repeats (the length of the repeat being the polymorphism), which are distributed throughout the genome at about 0.4 cM intervals, has allowed genome-wide screens to be performed, as described in Chapter 1. However, several limitations of this methodology have become apparent, since even with hundreds of affected-sibling, or relative, pairs it is difficult to narrow the region of linkage to much less than 1 cM[31]. Thus, in this type of analysis, major susceptibility genes can easily be missed. Furthermore, the data from genome-wide screens can be confounded by both genetic and phenotypic heterogeneity. These reasons are the probable explanation for the considerable variability in the results of genome-wide screens in many other polygenic disorders such as Type I diabetes, multiple sclerosis and bipolar affective disorders. The use of single-nucleotide polymorphisms (SNP), which are found at about 3 kb intervals, should allow better resolution of chromosomal linkage than the more broadly distributed dinucleotide repeats[32].

Inflammatory bowel disease has become important because of the high degree of reproducibility in data reported from different centres, in contrast to the wide variability seen in other polygenic disorders. The linkage between a locus on chromosome 16 and Crohn's disease has been reported in six of 10 studies, and between chromosome 12 and both ulcerative colitis and Crohn's disease in five of nine studies. Furthermore, fine-mapping using a larger set of markers and transmission by descent tests have narrowed the regions of interest on chromosome 12 to less than 0.5 cM[33]. For chromosome 3, the region of interest has been particularly narrowed by the use of a 'positional candidate', namely the CCR5 gene (CCR5 is a chemokine receptor). This gene lies at the peak of the multipoint linkage curve and is known to have a functional polymorphism. A 32 bp deletion abolishes function in individuals homozygous for the deletion, but function is also severely reduced in heterozygotes. The deletion is known to protect lymphocytes from invasion by HIV[34,35], but there is other evidence to implicate the deletion in regulatory function of macrophages

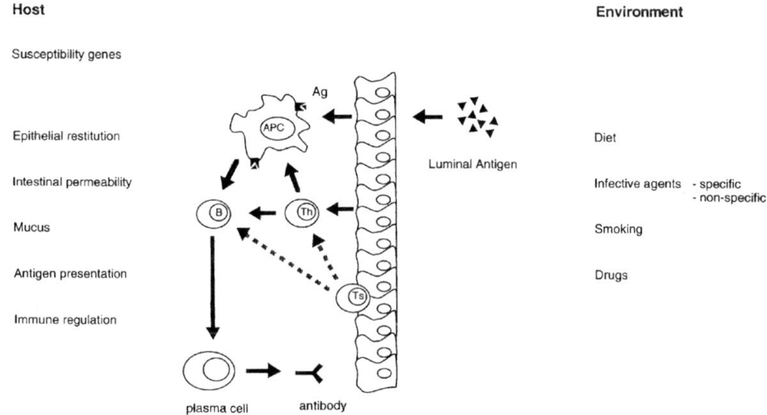

Figure 1   The pathogenesis of IBD. Genetic susceptibility to chronic intestinal inflammation may be mediated via mucosal barrier function or immune events in response to a variety of luminal constituents

and T cells[36]. Recent observations have shown that a significant proportion of IBD patients carry this deletion[37]. The functional significance for IBD is not clear but the observation is strong support for the existence of a susceptibility gene in this region of chromosome 3.

Thus, IBD has almost become a 'model' of complex genetic analysis. The recent setting-up of an international consortium will greatly facilitate combined analysis on large family populations and should allow subanalysis on specific phenotypes.

IMPORTANCE TO THE PHARMACEUTICAL INDUSTRY

Although a number of loci on a variety of chromosomes have been linked to IBD, with loci on chromosomes 12 and 16 having the strongest evidence, precise identification of a susceptibility gene has not yet been achieved. Furthermore, it is by no means certain that, should one or more gene be identified, the function of that gene(s) will be apparent. Nevertheless, there are many potential biological functions of the intestine that might be under genetic control, as shown in Figure 1. Many of the chromosomal regions which may contain susceptibility genes are already known to be rich in genes, which could be highly relevant to intestinal function. Should the polymorphisms in these genes affect function, and be shown to be relevant for disease pathogenesis, then the possibility of pharmaceutical manipulation becomes obvious.

An increasing area of interest is in pharmacogenetics. The possibility that response to a particular therapy could be predicted from knowledge of molecular genetics is becoming apparent. Azathioprine is currently the best example of relevance to IBD since polymorphisms within the gene encoding thiopurine methyl transferase are known to have profound effects on enzyme activity and hence the concentrations of azathioprine metabolites[38]. There are also preliminary data on different tumour necrosis factor (TNF) microsatellite haplotypes influencing response to steroids in ulcerative colitis and to anti-TNF infusions in Crohn's disease[39–41].

CONCLUSIONS

Both ulcerative colitis and Crohn's disease appear to represent an interaction between environmental factors and genetic susceptibility mediated through multiple genes. The pattern of disease that results is also partly determined by the possession of 'phenotype-determining' genes and response to individual therapies may also be determined by genetic polymorphisms. Better knowledge of the actual genes influencing these diseases should allow more accurate prediction of familial risks, of natural history and of disease behaviour. It should also lead to novel therapeutic approaches.

References

1. Weissenbach J, Gyapay G, Dib C et al. A second generation linkage map of the human genome. Nature 1992;359:794–801.
2. Satsangi J, Rosenberg WMC, Jewell DP. The prevalence of inflammatory bowel disease in relatives of patients with Crohn's disease. Euro J Gastroenterol Hepatol 1994;6:413–16.
3. Probert CSJ, Jayanthi V, Pinder D, Wicks AC, Mayberry JF. Epidemiological study of ulcerative proctocolitis in Indian migrants and the indigenous population of Leicestershire. Gut 1992;33:687–93.
4. Peeters M, Nevens H, Baert F et al. Familial aggregation in Crohn's disease: increased age adjusted risk and concordance in clinical characteristics. Gastroenterology 1996;111:597–603.
5. Polito JM, Rees RC, Childs B, Mendeloff AI, Harris ML, Bayless TM. Preliminary evidence for genetic anticipation in Crohn's disease. Lancet 1996;347:798–800.
6. Satsangi J, Grootscholten C, Holt H, Jewell DP. Clinical patterns of familial inflammatory bowel disease. Gut 1996;38:738–41.
7. Bayless TM, Tokayer AZ, Polito JM, Quaskey SA, Mellits ED, Harris ML. Crohn's disease: concordance for site and clinical type in affected family members – potential heriditary influences. Gastroenterology 1996;111:573–9.
8. Lee JCW, Lennard-Jones JE. Inflammatory bowel disease in 67 families each with 3 or more affected first-degree relatives. Gastroenterology 1996;111:587–96.
9. Colombel J-F, Grandbastian B, Gower-Rousseau C et al. Clinical characteristics of Crohn's disease in 72 families. Gastroenterology 1996;111:604–7.
10. Carbonnel F, Macaigne G, Beaugerie L, Gendre JP, Cosnes J. Crohn's disease severity in familial and sporadic cases. Gut 1999;44:91–5.
11. Lee JC, Bridger S, McGregor C, Macpherson AJ, Jones JE. Why children with inflammatory bowel disease are diagnosed at a younger age than their affected parent. Gut 1999;44:808–11.
12. Futami S, Aoyama N, Honsako Y et al. HLA-DRB1*1502 allele, subtype of DR15, is associated with susceptibility to ulcerative colitis and its progression. Dig Dis Sci 1995;40:814–18.
13. Sugimura K, Asakura H, Mizuki N et al. Analysis of genes within the HLA region affecting susceptibility to ulcerative colitis. Hum Immunol 1993;36:112–18.
14. Masuda H, Nakamura Y, Tanaka T, Hayakawa S. Distinct relationship between HLA-DR genes and intractability of ulcerative colitis [see comments]. Am J Gastroenterol 1994;89:1957–62.
15. Toyoda H, Wang S-J, Yang H et al. Distinct association of HLA Class II genes with inflammatory bowel disease. Gastroenterology 1993;104:741–8.
16. Satsangi J, Welsh KI, Bunce M et al. Contribution of genes of the major histocompatibility complex to susceptibility and disease phenotype in inflammatory bowel disease. Lancet 1996;347:1212–17.
17. Roussomoustakaki M, Satsangi J, Landers C et al. Genetics of ulcerative colitis: HLA

DRB1*0103 (DR103) is associated with extra-intestinal manifestations and need for surgery. Gastroenterology 1996;110:A1004.

18. Duerr RH, Chensny LJ. Associations between HLA DR alleles and subsets of ulcerative colitis defined by extent of colitis. Gastroenterology 1997;112:A963.

19. Bouma G, Crusius JB, Garcia-Gonzalez MA *et al.* Genetic markers in clinically well defined patients with ulcerative colitis (UC). Clin Exp Immunol 1999;115:294–300.

20. Mansfield JC, Holden H, Tarlow JK *et al.* Novel genetic association between ulcerative colitis and the anti-inflammatory cytokine interleukin-1 receptor antagonist. Gastroenterology 1994;106:637–42.

21. Tountas NA, Yang H, Coulter DL, Rotter JI, Cominelli F. Increased carriage of allele 2 of IL-1 receptor antagonist in Jewish populations: the strongest known genetic association in ulcerative colitis. Gastroenterology 1996;110:A1029.

22. Tountas NA, Kam L, di Giovine FS, Casini-Raggi V, Cominelli F. Genetic association between allele 2 of IL-1 receptor antagonist (IL-1RA) and ulcerative colitis in a Los Angeles based Hispanic population. Gastroenterology 1995;108:A930.

23. Duerr RH, Tran T. Association between ulcerative colitis and a polymorphism in intron 2 of the interleukin-1 receptor antagonist gene. Gastroenterology 1995;108:A812.

24. Louis E, Satsangi J, Roussomoustakaki M *et al.* Cytokine gene polymorphisms in inflammatory bowel disease. Gut 1996;39:705–10.

25. Andus T, Caesar I, Vogl D, Scholmerich J, Gross V. Association of HLA-DR15, pANCA and IL-1 receptor antagonist allele 2 with ulcerative colitis. Gastroenterology 1995;108:A770.

26. Orchard TR, Wordsworth BP, Jewell DP. Peripheral arthropathies in inflammatory bowel disease: their articular distribution and natural history. Gut 1998;42:387–91.

27. Orchard TR, Thiyagaraja S, Welsh KI, Wordsworth BP, Gaston JSH, Jewell DP. Clinical phenotype is related to HLA genotype in the peripheral arthropathies of inflammatory bowel disease (IBD). Gastroenterology 1999(Submitted).

28. Orchard TR, Vaughan R, Simmons JD, Welsh KI, Jewell DP. MHC Class I like gene-A (MICA) is associated with ulcerative colitis but not Crohn's disease. Gastroenterology 1999;116:A789.

29. Stokkers PC, Reitsma PH, Tytgat GN, van Deventer SJ. HLA-DR and -DQ phenotypes in inflammatory bowel disease: a meta-analysis. Gut 1999;45:395–401.

30. Lander ES, Schork NJ. Genetic dissection of complex traits. Science 1994;265:2037–48.

31. Risch N, Merikangas K. The future of genetic studies of complex human diseases. Science 1996;273:1516–17.

32. Kruglyak L. Prospects for whole-genome linkage disequilibrium mapping of common disease genes. Nat Genet 1999;22:139–44.

33. Parkes M, Vyas P, Satsangi J, Jewell DP. Fine mapping the IBD linkage on chromosome 3. Gastroenterology 1999;116:A792.

34. Samson M, Libert F, Doranz BJ *et al.* Resistance to HIV-1 infection in caucasian individuals bearing mutant alleles of the CCR-5 chemokine receptor gene. Nature 1996;382:722–5.

35. Zimmerman PA, Buckler-White A, Alkhatib G *et al.* Inherited resistance to HIV-1 conferred by an inactivating mutation in CC chemokine receptor 5: studies in populations with contrasting clinical phenotypes, defined racial background, and quantified risk. Mol Med 1997;3:23–36.

36. Zhou Y, Kurihara T, Ryseck RP *et al.* Impaired macrophage function and enhanced T cell-dependent immune response in mice lacking CCR5, the mouse homologue of the major HIV-1 corecptor. J Immunol 1998;160:4018–25.

37. Simmons J, Marshall S, Welsh KI, Jewell DP. C-C Chemokine receptor 5 polymorphism in inflammatory bowel disease. Gastroenterology 1999;116:A821.

38. Spire-Vayron de la Moureyre C, Debuysere H, Mastain B *et al.* Genotypic and phenotypic analysis of the polymorphic thiopurine S-methyltransferase gene (TPMT) in a European population. Br J Pharmacol 1998;125:879–87.

39. Louis E, Dupont P, Depauw A, Croes F, Demolin G, Belaiche J. Rapid anti-inflammatory effect of high dose azathioprine in inflammatory bowel disease: an *in vitro* study. Gastroenterology 1998;114:A1027.

40. Plevy SE, Taylor K, DeWoody KL, Schaible TF, Shealy D, Targan SR. Tumor necrosis factor (TNF) microsatellite haplotypes and perinuclear anti-neutrophil cytoplasmic antibody

(pANCA) identify Crohn's disease (CD) patients with poor clinical responses to anti-TNF monoclonal antibody (cA2). Gastroenterology 1997;112:A1062.

41. Plevy SE, Vasiliauskas EA, Taylor K *et al*. The Crohn's disease associated tumor necrosis factor (TNF) microsatellite A2B1C2D4E1 haplotype and anti-*Saccharomyces cerivisiae* antibody (ASCA) define medically resistant forms of ulcerative colitis. Gastroenterology 1997;112:A1062.

3
Genetics of IBD: impact on immune function

C. FIOCCHI

ABSTRACT

Both forms of inflammatory bowel disease (IBD), Crohn's disease and ulcerative colitis, are complex clinical entities whose aetiopathogenesis involves several components divided into two categories: conditioning factors that are permissive for IBD, and effector mechanisms that mediate tissue damage. Included in the first category are genes, the environment, the enteric flora and possible infectious agents, whereas the second category includes intestinal immune and non-immune systems. Components in both categories must coalesce to induce the clinical manifestations of IBD, but which and how conditioning factors trigger mediator systems is unknown. More specifically, which genes are involved, how they interact with microorganisms or the environment, and how they induce uncontrolled immune activation in the gut is totally unclear.

Studies performed during the past two decades have generated abundant information on the activation and effector function of most types of immune cells in IBD intestine, e.g. T cells, B cells and macrophages, as well as epithelial, endothelial, mesenchymal and nerve cells, and all their products (cytokines, antibodies, cell adhesion molecules, prostanoids, reactive metabolites, etc.). In contrast, investigation of genetics in IBD has just begun, but is proceeding quickly, with an increasingly large number of putative associations and linkages being reported in defined or random patient populations. The consistency and reproducibility of these observations are far from satisfactory, as all but four chromosomes have at least nominal associations with IBD. Many of the associations are probably spurious, casting doubts on their value, and making it difficult to define or even conceive possible consequences on immune reactivity that may lead to gut inflammation. Furthermore, genes may not directly impact on immune function, but on intermediate systems that indirectly affect immune responses.

At the moment the functional relationships between certain 'IBD chromosomes' (2, 3, 6, 7, 12 and 16) and 'immune genes' they may contain are unclear, allowing only theoretical speculations on eventual immune dysfunction. An additional complicating factor is that the human genome varies among all individuals, and until this sequence diversity is fully appreciated and understood, the connection between putative IBD genes and mechanisms of gut inflammation is bound to remain nebulous.

INTRODUCTION: BASIC ISSUES AND DEFINITIONS

The last two decades have witnessed impressive progress in our understanding of the pathogenesis of inflammatory bowel disease (IBD)[1]. This progress is mostly based on expanded knowledge of the basic mechanisms of intestinal inflammation, which largely depends on an inappropriate response of the local immune system. New insights into possible aetiological agents for Crohn's disease (CD) and ulcerative colitis (UC) have been hard to come by, with the normal enteric flora regaining momentum as the main inciter of the altered immune reactivity found in IBD. In addition to immune effector mechanisms and putative aetiological agents, a third component of IBD pathogenesis is receiving more and more attention, e.g. the genetics of patients with IBD and their at-risk relatives[2]. Since the genetic make-up of one individual represents a permanent and indelible imprint of his or her ability to respond to the challenges of the surrounding environment, it is logical to assume that genes might determine the immune-mediated inflammatory response which is ultimately responsible for the initiation of disease and clinical outcome. Based on these premises, the question of what is the impact of IBD genetics on immune function is timely and extremely important. In order to properly answer this critical question, one should be equipped with a baggage of detailed data generated directly from the IBD population. Unfortunately this is not yet the case. Therefore, before discussing what is currently known, and putting forward reasonable but speculative hypotheses of what links might exist between genetics and immune function in IBD, and how they together induce and maintain chronic gut inflammation, some definitions, albeit somewhat arbitrary, are necessary:

1. Genetic disease is defined as a condition in which genes play a role in determining the appearance and outcome of the disease, or at least predisposing to and modifying the disease.
2. Immunological disease is a condition in which an abnormal immune response plays a role in the mechanism of disease and often mediates tissue injury.
3. Environmental disease is a condition in which environmental factors play a role in triggering or modulating the disease.

DISEASE HETEROGENEITY IN IBD: GENETIC, IMMUNOLOGICAL AND CLINICAL

Both CD and UC are entities characterized by an extreme degree of clinical variability, from the age of onset of the initial clinical manifestations to the severity and diversity of the clinical course, response to therapy, need for surgical intervention, and medical as well as surgical complications. It has been proposed that clinical heterogeneity correlates with genetic heterogeneity, and that the heterogeneity of certain immune-mediated diseases reflects genetic differences[3]. This is also probably true for IBD, in which clinical heterogeneity of the intestinal inflammatory response may be a reflection of the patient's genetic heterogeneity, prompting two fundamental questions:

1. Does genetic heterogeneity translate into immune heterogeneity?
2. Does immune heterogeneity translate into clinical heterogeneity?

At the present time there are no objective data that can offer the expected positive reply to both questions. Ongoing studies are trying to address these questions by defining the genetic make-up of the IBD population at large or more homogeneous CD and UC subgroups. The likely outcome of these studies is that the pathogenesis of IBD is based on a heterogeneity triad, composed to a considerable degree of genetic, immunological and clinical variability (Figure 1). How well does this proposed heterogeneity triad fit into current concepts of IBD pathophysiology? It is generally believed that IBD is the result of the close interaction of three basic components: genetic, environmental and immunological[1], which constitute an additional aetiopathogenic triad (Figure 2). Based on this assumption the key components of IBD pathogenesis will yield different outcomes depending on each patient's genetic make-up by determining the type of the immune response and differences in clinical presentation.

LINKING GENES TO A DISEASE PHENOTYPE: INTRINSIC DIFFICULTIES AND THE INFLUENCE OF THE ENVIRONMENT

As proposed by Seldman and co-workers, a sequential series of hypothetical stages links genes to overt clinical manifestations, starting with genetic

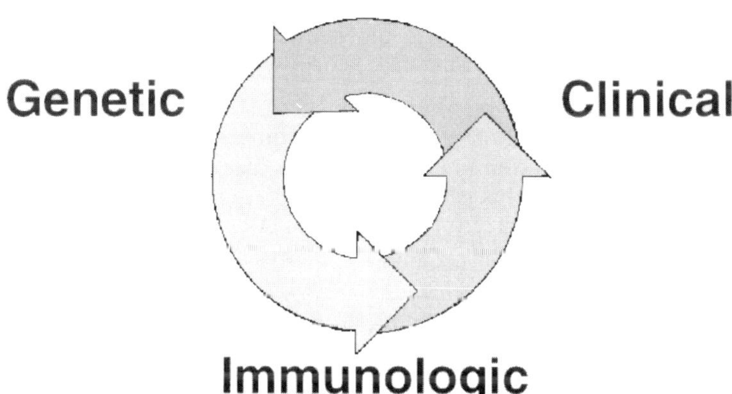

Figure 1 Components of the heterogeneity triad of inflammatory bowel disease

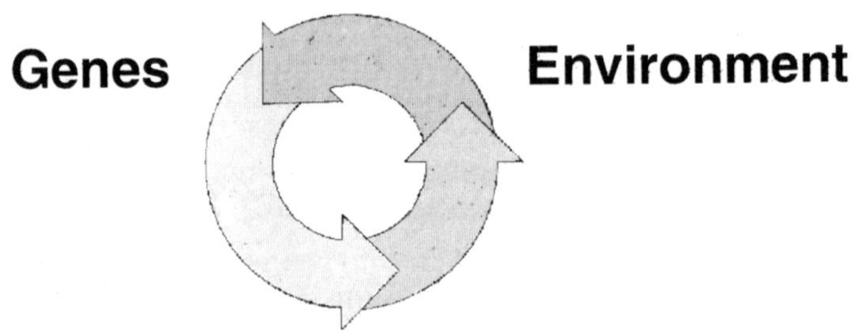

Figure 2   Components of the aetiopathogenic triad of inflammatory bowel disease

susceptibility and going on to exposure to the environment, immunoregulatory imbalance, microscopic disease and finally clinical disease. Scattered along this course of events are priming and triggering events which precede the clinical diagnosis of IBD[4]. Thus, at least in theory, it is possible to follow this successive line and dissect each stage in order to answer the question of how the conditioning power of the genes activates the damaging effector mechanisms of the intestinal immune system. As usual, theory and practice are separated by wide and difficult-to-navigate waters, and to successfully establish a direct connection of a defined gene to a specific disease is still the exception. In principle, one could envision an approach that allows such connection to be firmly established. This could be achieved by the longitudinal follow-up of large, strictly defined IBD populations at a time and place where the disease is appearing in such a population, with the simultaneous evaluation of refined genetic markers, multiple environmental influences, detailed immune function and the correlated phenotypic manifestations that characterize the clinical presentation. To do this is obviously impossible in IBD (or any other common disease); therefore one must revert to more realistic and practical approaches to link genes to a disease:

1.   If the gene(s) is known, find the biochemical correlate.
2.   If the (immune) defect is known, perform segregation analysis.

Either one or both approaches have been successfully utilized to define and connect the genetic to the functional bases of some diseases, but this is almost exclusively relegated to dominant or recessive diseases mediated by simple Mendelian inheritance. This is clearly not the case in IBD, since neither the gene(s) nor the immune defect(s) are known in either CD or UC. Additional, more liberal criteria can then be adopted to link genes to deranged immune function in IBD:

1.   The majority of the patients have the gene or a gene variant.
2.   The function of the gene(s) makes sense in the context of disease pathophysiology.
3.   In either case, gene deletion and overexpression studies *in vitro* or *in vivo* should follow to prove or disprove the relevance of the gene.

Table 1 Problems associated with identification of gene variations in complex polygenic disorders

Correct patient diagnosis and classification often difficult
Replication of results requires multiple repeat analyses
High incidence of disease-prone genes
Small contribution of individual genes
Excessively large suspect genomic regions
Linkage between candidate genes may affect resolution
Discordance between animal models and human disease

Adapted from ref. 6.

Unfortunately, even these criteria are not currently applicable to IBD. We still do not have any evidence that a unique gene or sets of genes are predominantly expressed in the majority of IBD patients. As far as gene products whose function makes sense in IBD pathophysiology the list is too long and hypothetical to meaningfully pursue a candidate gene approach. The main reason for these limitations is that both CD and UC fall in the category of complex genetic (polygenic) disorders, which are frothed with biological, logistic and technical difficulties in the identification of complex and likely multiple gene variations (Table 1)[5-7]. In addition to these difficulties, others exist which include:

1. A variation in completely different genes may lead to the same functional phenotype (disease).
2. The same functional phenotype may be due to entirely different variations in different genes.
3. A single disease manifestation is commonly associated with multiple genes.
4. Most diseases involve multiple genes: many in the general population, fewer in a single patient, and various genes in different patients

Thus, it appears that the fundamental problem in linking genes to immune abnormalities in IBD is the apparent multiplicity of genes involved in its causation. Usually there is an inverse relationship between rare and common diseases in regard to identification of responsible genes. Diseases transmitted through simple dominant (e.g. achondroplasia) or simple recessive (e.g. haemophilia, Hirschsprung's disease, retinitis pigmentosa) inheritance are rare and have a very high frequency of affected sibs in the population, while those transmitted through multifactorial inheritance, such as diabetes, psoriasis, multiple sclerosis, epilepsy and coeliac disease, are more common but the frequency of affected sibs is lower[8]. IBD clearly falls in the second category.

Another essentially unexplored aspect of IBD genetics is whether spontaneous mutations might be responsible for the progressive increase in the incidence of IBD worldwide[9]. Not only is IBD on the increase but the disease appears at an increasingly lower age in children[10], and an increasingly larger proportion of children make up the entire IBD population (Figure 3). A decade ago, 10% of the entire CD population was younger than 10 years of age[11], whereas now this percentage has almost doubled (18%)[12]. The frequency of spontaneous mutations is 10^{-9} base pair per year multiplied by the number of cells in the

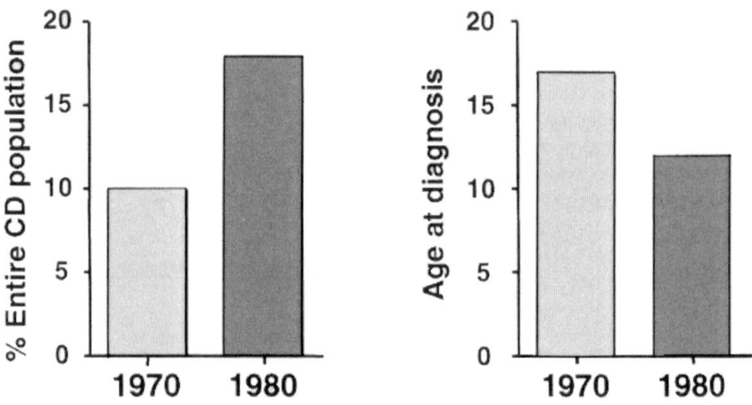

Figure 3   Changes in frequency and age in paediatric inflammatory bowel disease

body. Based on this formula the number of mutations in one generation is rather low and cannot explain the sharp increase in IBD during the past two generations. Moreover, most mutations have no functional consequence until an environmental factor causes the new mutation to become functionally important. This latter event is dramatically illustrated by the protective effect of chemokine receptor variants in HIV disease[13], or the prothrombotic effect of oral contraceptives in patients who are carriers of a particular prothrombin gene mutation[14]. This highlights the still cloudy but crucial relationship of genetic and environmental factors in IBD. There is little doubt that environmental factors represent major contributors to IBD and its growing incidence[15], but how one impacts on the other is unclear at the moment.

Thus, at least for the time being, we are challenged by the tremendous task of defining the multiple genes that are involved in IBD in face of the ultimate paradox in human genetics: if each individual is genetically unique (as proven by forensic studies), why should we expect that in different individuals the same genes cause the same disease through the same mechanisms? (A. Chakravarti, personal communication).

GENETIC AND IMMUNE MARKERS IN IBD: MULTIPLICITY, HETEROGENEITY AND INCONSISTENCY

As discussed earlier in this chapter, the multiplicity of genes apparently involved in IBD represents a major reason for the heterogeneity of both the immune response and clinical manifestations. One well-established way to facilitate the identification of genes of interest is to limit genetic analyses to strictly defined and well-characterized patient groups, ideally represented by twins, where concordance for the incidence of the disease is particularly high[16]. This approach has helped to identify a series of genetic and immunological markers that are significantly more common in these highly selected subgroups of affected individuals (Table 2)[17–25]. While useful, this approach provides information on

Table 2 Genetic, immunological and biochemical markers in IBD: association with selected clinical subgroups

Marker	Type	Patient subgroup	Reference
DR2	UC	ANCA +	17
DRB1*1502, DRw11	UC	Intractability	18
ICAM-1/R241	UC	ANCA –	19
TNFa2b1c2d4e1	CD		20
TNF-α/–308	UC		21
DR3 DQ2	UC	Female, distal disease	22
	IBD	Female, male, extensive	
4q	IBD	Mixed families	23
ecNOS polymorphism	UC	Early onset	24
NFκB1	CD		25

only a tiny proportion of the entire IBD population, raising serious concerns about the applicability of the findings to the majority of patients suffering from CD or UC, and the importance of these observations to the understanding of IBD immunopathogenesis. Another substantial concern is the observation that linkages with certain selected loci described in some populations at one particular location are not always confirmed in other populations with a different geographical or ethnic distribution[26]. In addition, depending on selection and methodology, the number of potential susceptibility loci continues to expand even in previously analysed populations[27], broadening rather than restricting the spectrum of genetic heterogeneity. This brings into question the degree of impact of genetic influences versus that of ethnic or environmental influences in regulating the immune response responsible for gut inflammation.

Most of the markers that have been associated with IBD are the same or linked to markers investigated in many other immune-mediated or autoimmune diseases[7,28,29] (Table 3). This suggests that there is shared genetic susceptibility to diseases primarily mediated through an immune effector function[30], and that similar effector systems are active in several diseases. This certainly facilitates the search for genes linked to altered immune function, but still leaves to the investigator the daunting task of identifying the sets of genes that are crucial to the development of each non-organ and organ-specific disease such as IBD. As stressed above, the extent of the heterogeneity of genetic and immune markers is an issue of practical importance when trying to identify IBD-predisposing genes. This notion has to be kept in mind when assumptions or conclusions are made based on data from experimental models of IBD. The list of 'IBD' animal models is quite large and it seems that any number of independent variations in genes related or unrelated to immune or intestinal functions may result in a model of experimental colitis[31]. This raises two issues. One is that of the discordance between animal models and human disease[6], and reminds us that, simply because of similar phenotypic manifestations, not all events occurring in the animal reflect events relevant to human disease. The second is that the diversity of gene variants that induce IBD in animals seems

Table 3 Putative susceptibility loci associated with autoimmune diseases

Locus	IDMM	Grave's	Myasthenia	Addison's	MS	SLE	JCA	Psoriasis	RA	IBD
HLA	+	+	+	+	+	+	+	+	+	+
TAP	+				+		+	+	+	
LMP	+						+			
INS	+									
IDDMI-10	+									
CTL-4	+	+								
T-cell receptor			+				+		+	
IL-1ra		+			+					
IL-1							+			
TNF						+			+	
Ig genes			+		+					
Thyrotropin receptor		+								
Acetylcholine receptor			+							
Steroid 21-hydroxylase				+						
Myelin basic protein					+					
Proteolipid protein					+					
Complement						+				
Heat shock proteins						+				

Adapted from ref. 30.

unlimited, raising the frightening prospect that immune abnormalities in humans with IBD are as varied and numerous as those inducing experimental IBD.

GENETICS AND IMMUNE FUNCTION IN IBD: TOO MANY CHOICES,TOO FEW DATA

Based on current knowledge one should seriously question whether it is presently possible to even begin to establish a cause-and-effect correlation between genetics of IBD and immune function. The number of chromosomes in which some type of putative linkage has been reported is at least 12 (Figure 4). The types of immune abnormalities described in CD or UC involve all components of the immune response, including antibody and autoantibody production, altered T-cell response, unregulated immunoregulatory and proinflammatory cytokine secretion, Th1/Th2 imbalance, abnormal production of growth factors, eicosanoids, reactive oxygen and nitrogen metabolites, overexpression of adhesion molecules, and a series of non-immune cell and extracellular matrix abnormalities[1,32]. The sheer number of putative loci and immune abnormalities renders unfeasible the performance of step-by-step screenings of what genes are expressed on what chromosome trying to establish a functional relationship that explains a reported immune defect. Furthermore, even if a relationship is established, it still remains to be proven that a particular relationship has causative effects in the initiation or perpetuation of gut inflammation and is actually relevant to the majority of patients. What makes matters even more problematic is that the genetic and immune correlations described so far are not necessarily strong. If we analyse, for example, the association of HLA molecules to IBD, some consistency exists for UC, but not for CD, and this depends on the population studied. Cytokines are considered of key importance

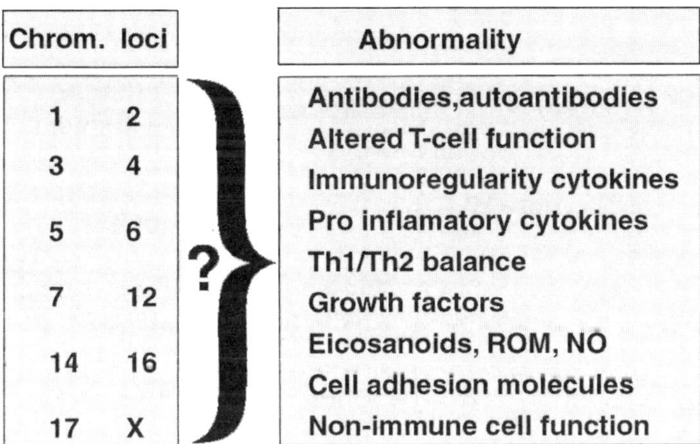

Figure 4 Genetic correlations and immune abnormalities in inflammatory bowel disease. ROM, reactive oxygen metabolites; NO, nitric oxide

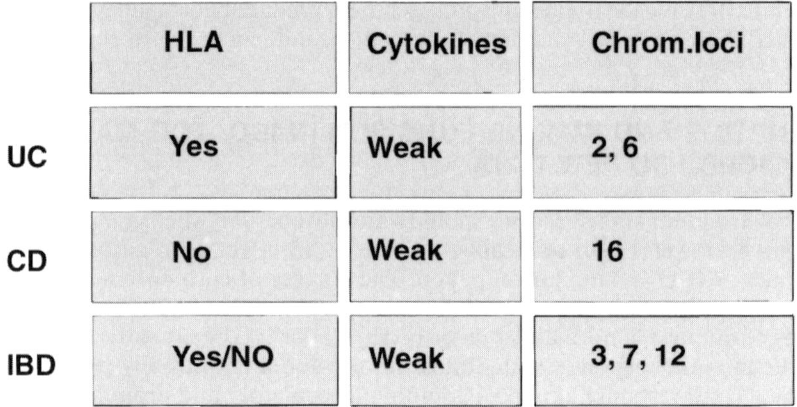

	HLA	Cytokines	Chrom.loci
UC	Yes	Weak	2, 6
CD	No	Weak	16
IBD	Yes/NO	Weak	3, 7, 12

Figure 5 Genetic and immune correlations in inflammatory bowel disease

to IBD pathogenesis, but even in this regard the association of cytokine genes to IBD is weak at best (Figure 5)[33].

In view of our multiple limitations it is also reasonable to ask whether the genetics of IBD are particularly complex or difficult to interpret, or whether these difficulties are common to other clinical conditions. In other words, how do genetics of IBD stack up against genetics of diseases with related immune-mediated pathophysiology? An excellent example is provided by gluten-sensitive enteropathy, or coeliac disease, a condition not only affecting the intestinal tract, but also unquestionably mediated by an inappropriately activated mucosal immune system (Figure 6)[34]. In regard to genetic linkages, coeliac disease has a very strong association with HLA class II molecules, particularly DQ2 and DQ8, with more than 90% of patients having the DQ2 heterodimer encoded

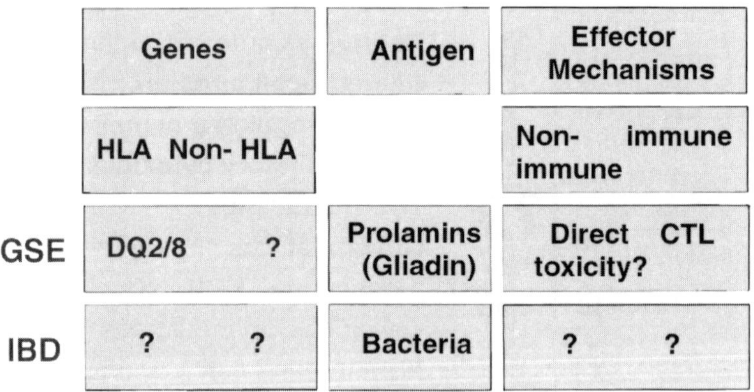

	Genes		Antigen	Effector Mechanisms	
	HLA	Non- HLA		Non-immune	immune
GSE	DQ2/8	?	Prolamins (Gliadin)	Direct	CTL toxicity?
IBD	?	?	Bacteria	?	?

Figure 6 Comparative pathogenic pathways in gluten-sensitive enteropathy (GSE) and inflammatory bowel disease

by A1*0501, B1*0201[35]. In IBD, HLA is associated only with UC, and strongly only in Japanese patients[36]. In coeliac disease the antigen inducing a pathogenic immune response is known, being represented by gliadin, a well-defined wheat-derived protein. Not only the antigen is known, but the presence of gliadin-specific HLA DQ restricted T cells has been irrefutably demonstrated in the small intestinal mucosa of coeliac disease patients[37]. Moreover, a highly specific enzymatic digestion that modifies gliadin and exposes the antigenic moieties specifically recognized by antigen-specific gut T cells has recently been elucidated[38]. In IBD the antigen(s) is unknown and may be multiple, and antigen-specific reactivity of direct pathogenic relevance has yet to be demonstrated in CD or UC patients. The possibility that components of the normal flora are the source of relevant antigens is only now being considered. Thus, this direct comparison indicates that IBD lags behind coeliac disease in regard to understanding the basic phenomena connecting genes to immune function. In spite of the more advanced knowledge existing in coeliac disease, the genes actually conditioning gluten-sensitive enteropathy remain unknown and, as a meagre consolation for IBD investigators, there is ample discordance on the results of genome-wide screening as far as pinning down potential susceptibility loci[39].

SUMMARY AND CONCLUSIONS

'The advent of recombinant DNA methods in the 1970s has allowed a revolution in human genetics whereby human traits and diseases could be analyzed at the level of a single gene. A second revolution is now underway which, with the anticipated completion of the entire DNA sequence of the human genome, will allow the molecular dissection of the common diseases and traits caused by multiple genes and an understanding of the role of the environment. However, the human genome is not one sequence but varies among all individuals. One can appreciate a third revolution in which this sequence diversity will be appreciated, understood and applied to humans'[40]. Until then, a realistic view of our current understanding of the impact of genetic on immune function in IBD can be summarized as follows:

1. The impact of IBD genetics on immune function must be interpreted in the context of genetic, immune and clinical heterogeneity.
2. In the absence of definitive genetic markers or immune abnormalities, it is presently impossible to accurately evaluate the impact of genetics on IBD immunopathogenesis.
3. Future studies must include the role of environmental factors on the impact of genetics on the effector mechanisms of IBD.

References

1. Fiocchi C. Inflammatory bowel disease: etiology and pathogenesis. Gastroenterology 1998;115:182–205.
2. Duerr RH. Genetics of inflammatory bowel disease. Inflamm Bowel Dis 1996;2:48–60.
3. Weyand CM, McCarthy TG, Goronzy JJ. Correlation between disease phenotype and genetic heterogeneity. J Clin Invest 1995;95:2120–6.

4. Cohen MB, Seidman E, Winter H *et al.* Controversies in pediatric inflammatory bowel disease. Inflam Bowel Dis 1998;4:203–27.
5. Lander ES, Schork NJ. Genetic dissection of complex traits. Science 1994;265:2037–48.
6. Weissman SM. Genetic bases for common polygenic disease. Proc Natl Acad Sci USA 1995;92:8543–4.
7. Sacks DB, McDonald JM. The pathogenesis of type II diabetes mellitus. A polygenic disease. Am J Clin Pathol 1996;105:149–56.
8. Todd JA. Genetic analysis of type 1 diabetes using whole genome approaches. Proc Natl Acad Sci USA 1995;92:8560–5.
9. Logan RFA. Inflammatory bowel disease incidence: up, down or unchanged? Gut 1998;42:309–11.
10. Olafsdottir EJ, Fluge G, Haug K. Chronic inflammatory bowel disease in children in western Norway. J Pediatr Gastroenterol Nutr 1989;8:454–8.
11. Gryboski JD, Spiro HM. Prognosis in children with Crohn's disease. Gastroenterology 1978;74:807–17.
12. Gryboski JD. Crohn's disease in children 10 years old or younger: comparison with ulcerative colitis. J Pediatr Gastroenterol Nutr 1994;18:174–82.
13. Garzino-Demo A, DeVico AL, Cocchi F, Gallo RC. β-Chemokines and protection from HIV type 1 disease. AIDS Res Hum Retroviruses 1998;14:S177–84.
14. Martinelli I, Sacchi E, Landi G, Taioli E, Duca F, Mannucci PM. High risk of cerebral-vein thrombosis in carriers of a prothrombin-gene mutation and in users of oral contraceptives. N Engl J Med 1998;338:1793–7.
15. Koutrobakis I, Manousos ON, Mewwissen SGM, Pena AS. Environmental risk factors in inflammatory bowel disease. Hepato-Gastroenterology 1996;43:381–93.
16. Tysk C, Lindberg E, Jarnerot G, Floderus-Myrhed B. Ulcerative colitis and Crohn's disease in unselected population of monozygotic and dizygotic twins: a study of heritability and the influence of smoking. Gut 1988;29:990–6.
17. Yang H, Rotter JI, Toyoda H *et al.* Ulcerative colitis: a genetically heterogeneous disorder defined by genetic (HLA class II) and subclinical (antineutrophil cytoplasmic antibodies) markers. J Clin Invest 1993;92:1080–4.
18. Masuda H, Nakamura Y, Tanaka T, Hayakawa S. Distinct relationship between HLA-DR genes and intractability of ulcerative colitis. Am J Gastroenterol 1994;89:1957–62.
19. Yang H, Vora DK, Targan SR, Toyoda H, Beaudet AL, Rotter JI. Intercellular adhesion molecule 1 gene associations with immunologic subsets of inflammatory bowel disease. Gastroenterology 1995;109:440–8.
20. Plevy SE, Targan SR, Yang H, Fernandez D, Rotter JI, Toyoda H. Tumor necrosis factor microsatellites define a Crohn's disease-associated haplotype on chromososme 6. Gastroenterology 1996;110:1053–60.
21. Bouma G, Xia B, Crusius JBA *et al.* Distribution of four polymorphisms in the tumour necrosis factor (TNF) genes in patients with inflammatory bowel disease. Clin Exp Immunol 1996;103:391–6.
22. Satsangi J, Welsh KI, Bunce M *et al.* Contribution of genes of the major histocompatibility complex to susceptibility and disease phenotype in inflammatory bowel disease. Lancet 1996;347:1212–17.
23. Cho JH, Nicolae DL, Fields CT *et al.* Identification of novel susceptibility loci for inflammatory bowel disease on chromosomes 1p, 3q, and 4q: Evidence for epistasis between 1p and IBD1. Proc Natl Acad Sci USA 1998;95:7502–7.
24. Furuse M, Kimura A, Esaki M *et al.* A polymorphism in the endothelial nitric oxide synthase (ECNOS) gene is associated with early onset of ulcerative colitis in Japanese. Gastroenterology 1999;115:A720.
25. Nosti-Escanilla MP, Gille JJP, Garcia-Gonzales MA, Pals G, Pena AS. Three NFKB1 gene polymorphisms in a Dutch population. Gastroenterology 1999;115:A786.
26. Rioux JD, Daly MJ, Green T *et al.* Absence of linkage between inflammatory bowel disease and selected loci on chromosomes 3, 7, 12, and 16. Gastroenterology 1998;115:1062–5.
27. Yang H, Ma Y, Ohmen JD *et al.* A genome-wide search identifies potential new susceptibility loci for Crohn's disease. Gastroenterology 1999;115:A848.
28. Barnes KC, Marsh DG. The genetics and complexity of allergy and asthma. Immunol Today 1998;19:325–32.

29. Bhalerao J, Bowcock AM. The genetics of psoriasis: a complex disorder of the skin and immune system. Hum Mol Genet 1998;7:1537–45.
30. Heward J, Gough SCL. Genetic susceptibility to the development of autoimmune disease. Clin Sci 1997;93:479–91.
31. Elson CO, Sartor RB, Tennyson GS, Riddell RH. Experimental models of inflammatory bowel disease. Gastroenterology 1995;109:1344–67.
32. Fiocchi C. Intestinal inflammation: a complex interplay of immune-non immune cell interactions. Am J Physiol 1997;273:G769–75.
33. Satsangi J, Parkes M, Jewell DP, Bell JI. Genetics of inflammatory bowel disease. Clin Sci 1998;94:473–8.
34. Godkin A, Jewell D. The pathogenesis of celiac disease. Gastroenterology 1998;115:206–10.
35. Sollid LM, Thorsby E. HLA susceptibility genes in celiac disease: genetic mapping and role in pathogenesis. Gastroenterology 1993;105:910–22.
36. Asakura H, Tsuchiya M, Aiso S *et al*. Association of the human lymphocyte-DR2 antigen with Japanese ulcerative colitis. Gastroenterology 1982;82:413–18.
37. Lundin KEA, Scott H, Hansen T *et al*. Gliadin-specific HLA-DQ(a1*0501,b1*0201) restricted T cells isolated from the small intestinal mucosa of celiac disease patients. J Exp Med 1993;178:187–96.
38. Molberg O, Macadam SN, Korner R *et al*. Tissue transglutaminase selectively modifies gliadin peptides that are recognized by gut-derived T cells in celiac disease. Nature Med 1998;4:713–17.
39. Yiannakou JY, King L, Brett P, Biagi F, Rosen-Bronson S, Ciclitira PJ. Complete genome screen for celiac disease using extended family linkage analysis. Gastroenterology 1999;115:A947.
40. Chakravarti A. Human genetics and genomics: to infinity and beyond. Award lecture at Case Western Reserve University School of Medicine, Cleveland, USA, 3 May 1999.

Section II
Pathogenesis

Moderator: **J. L. Wallace,** Calgary

4
Bacterial factors in inflammatory bowel disease pathogenesis

W. F. DOE

ABSTRACT

Intestinal bacteria and their products appear to contribute significantly to the pathogenesis of inflammatory bowel disease (IBD). Both commensal bacterial products, including lipopolysaccharides (LPS) and lipoteichoic acids, and potential pathogens may be implicated. Lamina propria cells in the intestinal mucosa are exposed to luminal LPS especially in the colon and distal ileum. CD14, the receptor for LPS–LPS binding protein complex, is expressed on blood monocytes recently recruited to the IBD mucosa. Activation of CD14 positive mononuclear phagocytes occurs at pg/ml concentrations of LPS resulting in protean biological effects, including secretion of proinflammatory cytokines, especially TNF-α, chemokines, proteases, and reactive oxygen and nitrogen species. Neutrophils recruited to the lesion of acute colitis induced in mice by oral dextran sulphate sodium similarly express CD14. The phenotype of inflammatory cells in the lesions of IBD therefore suggests a mechanism for persisting mucosal inflammation.

Recent insights into the importance of innate immunity as a front-line, early-detection antimicrobial defence system may be relevant to IBD pathogenesis. Innate immunity detects unique bacterial carbohydrate or lipid molecules using cell surface receptors, especially those on macrophages. Activation of these receptors initiates a discrete IL-12, interferon gamma pathway essential to macrophage killing of mycobacteria and some enteric bacterial pathogens. Inherited deficiency of peptides or their receptors in the IL-12–interferon gamma pathway results in susceptibility to mycobacterial and *Salmonella* infections as well as affecting granuloma formation in tissue. These recent findings suggest new avenues for exploring possible susceptibility factors in IBD.

INTRODUCTION

Bacterial factors appear central to the pathogenesis of the chronic mucosal lesion of the inflammatory bowel diseases (IBD) The intestinal epithelium is

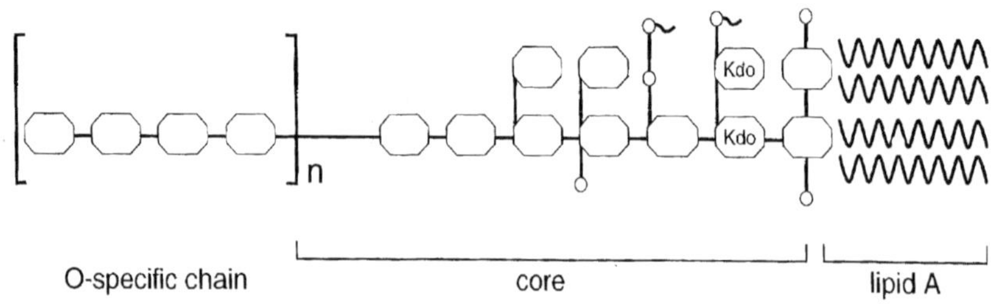

O-specific chain   core   lipid A

Kdo

Kdo

n

Figure 1 Structure of LPS showing the lipid A moiety responsible for nearly all biological responses, the core polysaccharide comprises 2-keto-3-deoxyoctulosonate (Kdo) and the O-specific chain consisting of complex repeating polysaccharides

exposed to the commensal bowel flora at concentrations of 1×10^8–10^{10} per ml of faecal fluid in the terminal ileum and colon. The flora comprise coliforms, Gram-positive anaerobes and a wide variety of flora derived from the oropharynx. The envelope structure of these bacteria is made up of an outer membrane that displays biologically active amphipathic molecules such as lipopolysaccharides (LPS or endotoxin) in Gram-negative bacteria[1] and lipoteichoic acids (LTA)[2] in Gram-positive bacteria. Furthermore, the envelope structure contains lipoproteins and peptidoglycans (PGN) which can also contribute to the induction or maintenance of inflammation[3]. Foremost among these bacterial cell wall constituents is LPS, which is not only a constituent of the bacterial outer membrane but is also secreted into the surrounding intestinal milieu. The structure of LPS comprises three elements (Figure 1). The lipid A moiety that is common to all Gram-negative bacteria is the most biologically active part of the molecule. Lipid A is attached to a carbohydrate core that is genus-specific and links to the third element, the O polysaccharide chains that determine strain specificity. LPS is a potent bacterial product that is in active picogram per milliliter concentrations[1]. It is not surprising therefore that mammals have developed protective systems for handling this noxious agent and similar bacterial products.

PROTECTIVE MECHANISMS AGAINST LPS

The molecular basis for the mechanisms that protect mammals against the threat of these highly reactive microbial cell wall materials and their proinflammatory potential has recently been elucidated. A plasma binding protein, lipid A binding protein (LBP) is a 60 kDa acute-phase protein synthesized principally by hepatocytes, that binds LPS in serum and in extracellular fluids to form LBP–LPS complexes, thereby reducing the threat posed by LPS to the host. A homologue of other plasma-binding proteins, LBP appears to act as a lipid transferase similar to cholesterol ester transfer protein. LBP promotes delivery of LPS to cells by disaggregating LPS complexes in plasma and transferring LPS molecules to receptors present on the surface of myeloid cells which bind the LBP–LPS complexes[4]. This mechanism confers greatly enhanced sensitivity to LPS, enabling activation of responder cells at up to 1000-fold lower LPS concentrations than the LPS levels required to activate receptor-negative cells[5]. But how does LPS bound to LBP exert its proinflammatory effect? The interaction between LPS and responsive cells is mediated through a series of receptors that has recently been characterized. CD14 is a pattern recognition receptor, expressed on the surface of macrophage[6,7] and neutrophil[8] populations, that binds LBP complexed to a range of biologically active bacterial molecules including LPS, LTA, PGN and a range of other Gram-negative and Gram-positive bacterial cell wall components. The expression of CD14 confers exquisite sensitivity reducing the amount of LPS required to activate cells by up to 10 000-fold[9]. But the CD14 receptor is not a transmembrane protein, and recent evidence suggests that a family of transmembrane protein receptors, homologues of the Toll receptors that regulate antifungal responses in the fruitfly *Drosophila melanogaster*, are implicated[10].

When LBP, acting as a lipid transferase, transfers deaggregated LPS to the CD14 receptor on the surface of some macrophage and neutrophil populations, the occupied CD14 receptor combines with Toll receptors to initiate transmembrane signal transduction via protein kinase cascades, to protein kinase C and activation of transcription factor NF-κB, resulting in transcription of proinflammatory cytokine genes. The intracellular domain of Toll receptors resembles the mammalian IL-1 receptors and defines a Toll/1L-1R receptor family[11]. It is thought that the function of LBP and CD14 is to present disaggregated LPS to Toll receptors, resulting in dimerization of Toll receptors and initiation of the intracellular signalling transduction pathways. Biologically active molecules from Gram-positive bacteria, including soluble PGN and LTA, also form complexes with LBP that bind to CD14 and induce transduction of intracellular signalling pathways, resulting in transcription of cytokine genes[12]. These studies elucidate mechanisms which appear to be triggered by biologically active components of all Gram-negative and Gram-positive bacteria to induce the release of proinflammatory cytokines and inflammatory mediators including chemokines, reactive oxygen and nitrogen species and neutral proteases (Figure 2).

IMPLICATIONS OF BACTERIAL CELL WALL PRODUCTS IN IBD PATHOGENESIS

Given the association between high concentrations of luminal commensal bacteria and the preferred sites for mucosal inflammation in IBD, the question arises as to whether bacterial cell wall molecules such as LPS, PGN or LTA are implicated in the pathogenesis of the lesion of IBD. The accumulated evidence suggests that they are. First, immunochemical staining for CD14 protein shows dense expression in IBD-affected mucosa, but not in histologically normal intestinal mucosa[13]. Moreover, fluorescence activated cell sorting (FACS) analysis of lamina propria mononuclear cells (LPMC) harvested from IBD-affected and normal intestine revealed a substantial population of CD14-positive cells that was not found in LPMC from normal colon[13]. Similarly, proinflammatory cytokine and chemokine expression in inflamed intestinal

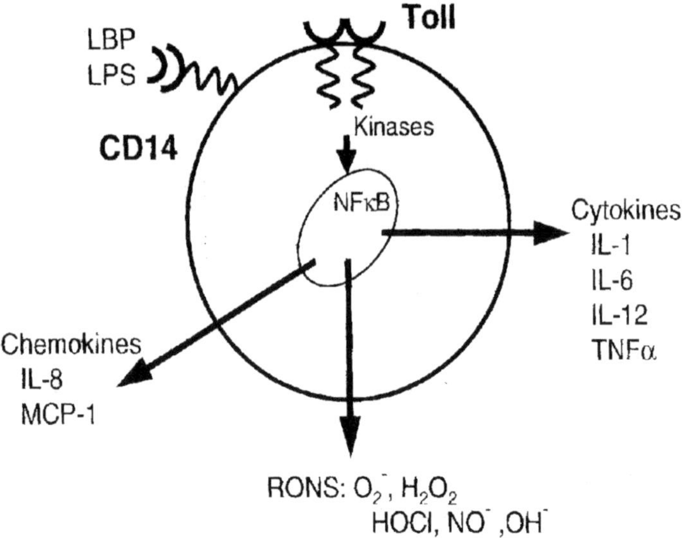

Figure 2 Diagram showing LBP–LPS complexes binding to the CD14 pattern recognition receptor and causing dimerization of transmembrane Toll receptors which transduce an intracellular signal to induce transcription of proinflammatory mediator genes and secretion of their products. RONS, reactive oxygen and nitrogen species

tissue[14], the clinical and histological response of refractory IBD patients to infused hybrid mouse/human anti-TNF-α[15] antibody and the finding of oxidized mucosal proteins in IBD-affected but not in normal mucosa[16], support the view that bacterial products are implicated in IBD pathogenesis.

Furthermore, animal models of chronic intestinal inflammation have been created experimentally using intramucosal PGN to induce a Crohn's-like lesion in rat terminal ileum[17] by producing 'knockout' mice and mice deficient in one cytokine such as TNF-α or IL-10, or in T cell receptors. These mice, however, develop chronic intestinal inflammation only when they are exposed to the normal environment. When raised under germ-free conditions, however, no chronic intestinal inflammation occurs, suggesting that population of the intestine by commensal bacteria is central to the pathogenesis of the intestinal inflammation[18].

INNATE IMMUNE SYSTEMS

How does the immune system respond to the serious threat of inflammatory injury from bacterial cell surface molecules? There are two immune systems. The acquired immune system comprises infinitely adaptable T and B lymphocytes. B cell receptors recognize native antigen conformation and chemical groups whilst T cell receptors principally recognize peptides bound to MHC cell surface proteins. Moreover, the generation of 'memory' T lymphocytes allows enhanced immune responses to infectious agents after re-exposure to the same antigens. This is characterized by exquisite sensitivity through somatic rearrangement of V, D and J elements of immunoglobulin and T cell receptor genes that can create up to 10^{11} lymphocyte clones expressing distinct antigen receptors. But this well-described form of immunity has two important defects: its response to infectious agents not previously experienced is delayed by the several days it takes for the clonal selection process to generate increasingly specific antibody- or cell-mediated immune responses. Secondly, adaptive immune responses lack the ability to distinguish potential microbial threats from innocuous foreign substances[19,20].

Relevant to IBD, however, is the more phylogenetically ancient, innate immune system. By contrast to acquired immunity, innate immune responses divide the environment into innocuous and potentially noxious agents by their capacity to detect microbial carbohydrate or lipid epitopes using cell surface receptors on macrophages, natural killer cells and neutrophil T cells that recognize carbohydrate or lipid antigens present in microorganisms, but not in mammals, to identify potentially threatening exposure to bacteria[21]. The innate immune response therefore is rapid, inflexible, and of limited specificity, but it is 'hard-wired' in contrast to the delayed, adaptive, highly specific response that characterizes acquired immunity. However, the two immune systems appear to be linked. The cellular and soluble elements of innate immunity appear to instruct the acquired immune response to select appropriate antigens and elimination strategies[19,20].

The innate immune system therefore responds quickly to new threats posed by microorganisms through a large number of recognition molecules. Some examples are listed in Table 1. Each of these detects microbial lipid, carbohydrate or protein molecules that are not found in mammals, and triggers a protective

Table 1 Innate immune system recognition molecules

Molecule	*Structure*	*Ligands*	*Function*
CRP	Pentraxin; Ca^{2+}-dependent lectin	Microbial polysaccharides	Activates C ↑phagocytosis
LBP	Lipid transferase	Catalyses LPS–CD14 transfer	↑LPS sensitivity inactivation LPS
S CD14	Leucine-rich protein	LPS, microbial cell wall components	↑LPS sensitivity with LPS binds to endothelial, MØ, PMN R
C3	Disulphide-linked dimer	Ester linkages, CHO, protein OH-groups	Ligand R attachment
MØ mannose R	8 CHO recognition domains	Multiple CHOs	Targets ags to class II-loading compartment
CD14	Lipid-anchored glycoprotein	LPS, microbial cell wall components	LPS sensitivity, microbe clearance, cytokine induction

C, complement; C3, third component of complement; CHO, carbohydrate; S CD14, soluble CD14 receptor protein; MØ, macrophages; PMN,neutrophils; R, receptor. Table modified from ref. 19, p. 51.

response. LBP, the recognition molecule for LPS and probably PGN and LTA, effectively enhances sensitivity to LPS some 1000-fold, as do both the cell-bound and soluble forms of CD14 receptors. Other recognition molecules such as the mannose receptor on macrophages and C reactive protein recognize bacterial carbohydrates and initiate opsonization of bacteria.

INNATE IMMUNITY AND INTESTINAL DISEASE

Experiments of nature suggest the importance of disordered innate immunity to intestinal disease. Studies of children suffering from persisting opportunistic mycobacterial infections showed lack of mature granuloma formation and multibacilliary mycobacterial lesions in draining lymph nodes as well as dysentery usually due to *Salmonella*. Conventional immune tests of T and B cell function were, however, normal. In many of the families there was evidence of consanguinity. These findings led to the discovery that the affected children were deficient for one of the constituents of the innate immune response pathway, interferon gamma receptors[22] or interleukin (IL)-12[23] or the IL-12 receptor[24] due to deletions or point mutations in genes coding for these molecules. Some of the infections were effectively treated by parenteral interferon gamma, establishing the importance of the innate immune system to protective immunity against mycobacterial and some enteric bacteria.

In the context of the intense research into susceptibility genes for Crohn's disease and ulcerative colitis, polymorphisms linked to the innate immune system may be of importance in understanding, and then preventing, the continuing inflammatory response that characterizes IBD. Polymorphisms for CD14, for example, have been found in myocardial infarction, in which one identified allele associated with reduced CD14 expression on macrophages has been linked to susceptibility to heart disease[25]. The molecular dissection of the bacterial factors and the innate immune pathway, together with the emerging data on gene polymorphisms for key molecules in the innate immune system, offers the prospect of new insights into understanding the pathogenesis of IBD.

References

1. Ulevitch RJ. Recognition of bacterial endotoxin by receptor-dependent mechanisms. Adv Immunol 1993;53:267–89.
2. Cleveland MG, Gorham JD, Murphy TL, Tuomanen E, Murphy KM. Lipoteichoic aid preparations of Gram-positive bacteria induce interleukin-12 through a CD14-dependent pathway. Infect Immun 1996;64:1906–12.
3. Gupta D, Kirkland TN, Viriyakosol S, Dziarski R. CD14 is a cell-activating receptor for bacterial peptidoglycan. J Biol Chem 1996;271:23310–6.
4. Mathison JC, Tobias PS, Wolfson E, Ulevitch RJ. Plasma lipopolysaccharide (LPS)-binding protein. J Immunol 1992;149:200–6.
5. Martin TR, Mathison JC, Tobias PS *et al.* Lipopolysaccharide binding protein enhances the responsiveness of alveolar macrophages to bacterial lipopolysaccharide. J Clin Invest 1992;90:2209–19.
6. Wright SD, Ramos RA, Tobias PS, Ulevitch RJ, Mathison JC. CD14 serves as the cellular receptor for complexes of lipopolysaccharide with lipopolysaccharide binding protein. Science 1990;249:1431–3.
7. Martin TR, Mongovin SM, Tobias PS *et al.* The CD14 differentiation antigen mediates the

development of endotoxin responsiveness during differentiation of mononuclear phagocytes. J Leuk Biol 1994;56:1–9.

8. Wright SD, Ramos RA, Hermanowski-Vosatka A, Rockwell P, Detmers PA. Activation of the adhesive capacity of CR3 on neutrophils by endotoxin: dependence on lipopolysaccharide binding protein and CD14. J Exp Med 1991;173:1281.

9. Lee JD, Kato K, Tobias PS, Kirkland TN, Ulevitch RJ. Transfection of CD14 into 70Z/3 cells dramatically enhances the sensitivity to complexes of lipopolysaccharide (LPS) and LPS binding protein. J Exp Med 1992;175:1697–1705.

10. Medzhitov R, Preston-Hurlburt P, Janeway CA Jr. A human homologue of the *Drosophila* Toll protein signals activation of adaptive immunity. Nature 1997;388:394–7.

11. Yang RB, Mark MR, Gray A *et al*. Toll-like receptor-2 mediates lipopolysaccharide-induced cellular signalling. Nature 1998;395:284–8.

12. Yoshimura A, Lien E, Ingalls RR, Tuomanen E, Dziarski R, Golenbock D. Recognition of Gram-positive bacterial cell wall components by the innate immune system occurs via Toll-like receptor 2. J Immunol 1999;163:1–5.

13. Grimm MC, Pavli P, Van de Pol E, Doe WF. Evidence for a CD14+ population of monocytes in inflammatory bowel disease mucosa – implications for pathogenesis. Clin Exp Immunol 1995;100:291–7.

14. Grimm MC, Elsbury SK, Pavli P, Doe WF. Enhanced expression and production of monocyte chemoattractant protein-1 in inflammatory bowel disease mucosa. J Leuk Biol 1996;56:804–2.

15. Targan SR, Hanauer SB, Van Deventer SJH *et al*. for the Crohn's Disease cA2 Study Group. A short term study of chimeric monoclonal antibody cA2 to tumor necrosis factor. N Engl J Med 1997;337:1029–35.

16. McKenzie SJ, Baker MS, Buffinton GD, Doe WF. Evidence of oxidant-induced injury to epithelial cells during inflammatory bowel disease. J Clin Invest 1996;98:136–41.

17. Sartor RB, Cromartie WJ, Powell DW *et al*. Granulomatous enterocolitis induced in rats by purified bacterial cell wall fragments. Gastroenterology 1985;89:587–95.

18. Elson Co, Sartor RB, Tennyson GS, Riddell RH. Experimental models of inflammatory bowel disease. Gastroenterology 1995;109:1344–67.

19. Fearon DT, Locksley RM. The instructive role of innate immunity in the acquired immune response. Science 1996;272:50–4.

20. Medzhitov R, Janeway CA Jr. Innate immune recognition and control of adaptive immune responses. Semin Immunol 1998;10:351–3.

21. Hoffman JA, Kafatos FC, Janeway CA, Ezekowitz RA. Phylogenetic perspectives in innate immunity. Science 1999;284:1313–18.

22. Jouanguy E, Lamhamedi-Cherradi S, Lammas D *et al*. A human IFNGR1 small deletion hotspot associated with dominant susceptibility to mycobacterial infection. Nature Genet 1999;21:1–9.

23. Altare F, Lammas D, Revy R *et al*. Inherited Interleukin 12 deficiency in a child with Bacille Calmette-Guerin and *Salmonella enteritidis* disseminated infection. J Clin Invest 1998;102:2035–40.

24. Altare F, Durandy A, Lammas D *et al*. Impairment of mycobacterial immunity in human interleukin-12 receptor deficiency. Science 1998;280:1432–5.

25. Hubacek JA, Pit'ha J, Skodova Z, Stanek V, Poledne R. C(–260) – T polymorphism in the promoter of the CD14 monocyte receptor gene as a risk factor for myocardial infarction. Circulation 1999;99:3218–20.

5
Inflammatory bowel disease: autoimmunity or chronic inflammation?

L. MAYER

ABSTRACT

The current concepts of autoimmunity have gone beyond the initial descriptions of autoantibodies. The nature of an autoreactive immune response must result in an organ-specific inflammatory reaction – e.g. pathogenic autoantibodies or autoreactive T cells. Many chronic inflammatory diseases have been called autoimmune by virtue of the presence of autoantibodies in the serum. However, when tested under appropriate conditions, transfer of these antibodies (Abs) into naive recipients has not resulted in reproduction of the disease. A classic example of a true autoimmune disorder is myasthenia gravis. Here antibodies to the acetylcholine receptor are responsible for the disease. Similarly, autoimmune haemolytic anaemia and thrombocytopenia appear to be directly autoantibody-mediated. This is in contrast to the autoimmune disease systemic lupus erythematosus. Antibodies to nuclear antigens (Ags) are not likely to induce primary disease but accelerated apoptosis with exposure of these 'hidden' Ags allows for Ag/Ab complex formation and complement activation. Within specific tissues this leads to active inflammation (e.g. lupus nephritis). The autoantigen is also involved in the pathology here.

What is the evidence for autoimmunity in inflammatory bowel disease (IBD)? In ulcerative colitis (UC) there are well-described autoantibodies (pANCA, anti-tropomyosin) but there is little evidence that they contribute to the inflammatory process. In Crohn's disease (CD) there are fewer examples of autoreactivity, especially related to the intestine. Is there autoreactivity on the T cell side, then? This is more difficult to document in humans. There is no evidence of enhanced autoreactive cytotoxic T cell activity (for example against epithelium). In mouse models of colitis the disease can be transferred by T cells but this is not direct proof that these are autoreactive; rather that they may be dysregulated. This leaves the alternative hypothesis that both UC and CD may be exaggerated immune responses against non-specific antigens (e.g. luminal contents). There is growing evidence for such a concept. Recent data suggest that there is T cell reactivity to colonic flora and that, in some settings, these T cells can transfer disease to a naive mouse. While it is unclear whether any of these models are truly CD-like or UC-like, the process appears to be interchangeable. The bottom line is that the initial inflammatory response in these models is Ag driven, not autoantigen-driven. A role for autoimmunity is less and less apparent.

INTRODUCTION

The goal of the systemic immune system is to recognize pathogens and mount a specific and focused immune response resulting in eradication of that pathogen. The adaptive immune system is characterized by its specificity and memory resulting from the clonal expansion of antigen-reactive T and B lymphocytes. These cells define foreignness in the context of 'self', initially deleting self-reactive cells and subsequently paralysing or anergizing self-reactive cells which escape deletion in the thymus or bone marrow. Deletion and anergy are two mechanisms of tolerance induction, preventing autoreactivity and potential autoimmune disease[1-7]. Yet despite these safeguards autoimmunity does occur, and it is the breakdown of normal tolerance mechanisms which accounts for disease.

MECHANISMS INVOLVED IN THE EXPRESSION OF AUTOREACTIVITY

Two scenarios exist to explain the development of autoimmunity: polyclonal activation[8-11] and breakdown of tolerance due to exposure to a crossreactive Ag[12-18]. While the role that each of these processes plays in the development of autoimmune disease has been the subject of continued debate, it is clear that both can account for some form of autoimmunity. We all have autoreactive cells circulating in our bloodstream or residing in local lymph nodes. Polyclonal activators of B cells result in autoantibody production *in vitro* (e.g. Epstein–Barr virus or pokeweed mitogen stimulation resulting in rheumatoid factor production)[19,20]. These findings would suggest that such self-reactive cells, while present, are tightly regulated, and that only strong T-independent activation can allow these cells to mature and secrete autoantibodies. From these findings one might postulate that autoimmunity can follow any polyclonal activation stimulus that an individual might be exposed to. It would also explain the panhypergammaglobulinaemia associated with a number of autoimmune diseases. On the other hand, polyclonal activation does not explain the selectivity of autoantibodies in specific disorders (e.g. anti-acetylcholine receptor in myasthenia gravis, anti-thyroglobulin Abs in Hashimoto's thyroiditis, etc.). If polyclonal activation were the only explanation for the development of autoimmunity, one would expect multiple autoantibodies in different diseases

For this reason the concept arose of crossreactive Ags leading to a break in self-tolerance. Some viral sequences share homology with self Ags and, in the process of generating an anti-viral response, an anti-self response evolves[21,22]. The true mechanisms involved in autoimmunity probably lie somewhere in the middle, taking into account poly-autoreactivity with some degree of selection. There are clearly multiple layers of regulation and selection which occur in a genetically susceptible host (which also plays a role) in order for an autoimmune disease to be manifest. The goals of current research efforts are to define susceptibility genes, to define potential crossreacting Ags and to define regulatory mechanisms which have gone awry.

Autoreactivity comes in two forms: T and B cell-mediated. B cell autoreactivity is easier to detect by the presence of autoantibodies in the serum. T cell autoreactivity is more difficult because the read-out, cytokines and T cell proliferation, is less specific. Cytotoxicity might exist but the nature of the Ag is less easily determined. However, one concept which has evolved over the past decade is that the majority of autoimmune disease are T cell-mediated and interruption of T cell activation pathways (i.e. interfering with CD40:CD40L interactions)[23–25] inhibit the development of disease (concept derived from animal models). Another emerging area is the role that apoptosis plays in the development of autoimmunity[26–29]. As suggested earlier, deletion or the induction of anergy in autoreactive cells might result in programmed cell death. One paradigm has developed which defines autoimmunity as a defect in this process. This concept is supported by the finding of defects in fas and fas ligand (apoptosis-inducing surface molecules) in lupus-prone MLR/1pr and gld mice, respectively[30–32]. In these models, failure to induce apoptosis of activated autoreactive cells results in the expansion of cell populations (adenopathy) and the emergence of autoreactive clones. Evidence for similar defects in human disease has been lacking. More recently several investigators have suggested that diseases such as systemic lupus erythematosus (SLE) may in fact relate to accelerated apoptosis (e.g. from sun-exposure in photosensitive individuals) exposing a number of previously hidden nuclear and cytoplasmic Ags. The resultant Ag load would result in the activation of anti-DNA, RNA, centromere etc, reactive B cells and autoantibody production. Once again, the reality may be somewhere in the middle.

This latter point raises the issue of the type of autoantigen in autoimmune diseases. Two forms of Ag exist: those that are exposed and readily available for complex formation (e.g. on the surface of a cell) and those that are normally hidden (e.g. DNA). The concept of pathogenic versus non-pathogenic autoantibodies has been critical to understanding these antigenic forms. A pathogenic autoantibody is one which is directly involved in disease pathogenesis. Examples include the anti-acetylcholine receptor Ab in myasthenia, Ab to the TSH receptor in Grave's disease or Abs to RBC or platelets in autoimmune haemolytic anaemia and immune thrombocytopenic purpura. In these diseases the autoantibody interacts directly with the affected organ or cell type and either blocks or stimulates activity or facilitates the destruction of the cell. Pathogenic autoantibodies which contribute to the disease but are not organ-specific include anti-DNA Abs in SLE which deposit in the glomerulus of the kidney, activate the complement cascade and promote local inflammation and tissue destruction. It is important to note that this form of pathogenic autoantibody is not too dissimilar in activity from soluble Ag/Ab immune complexes composed of viral or bacterial Ags. Such complexes can deposit in the kidney, joints and skin, causing a classic serum sickness reaction which involves complement activation and the induction of inflammation. Such might be the case in polyarteritis nodosa where complexes of HbSAg and anti-HbSAg deposit in the endothelium of medium-sized vessels and result in arteritis or inflammation within the blood vessel wall[33,34].

These pathogenic autoantibodies must be distinguished from those which are not pathogenic. For example, there is little evidence that rheumatoid factor (anti-IgG Abs) has any role in the development of rheumatoid arthritis. In this case autoantibodies serve as markers of disease. Furthermore, some anti-DNA Abs may result in renal disease while others are well tolerated. The ability to bind to or deposit in tissue (or form soluble complexes) may dictate pathogenicity. Many individuals have detectable autoantibodies in their serum without any evidence of disease. In this case their presence might indicate the existence of polyclonal activation. For example antinuclear antibodies are frequently found in patients with subacute bacterial endocarditis (chronic immune activation with bacterial Ags) but no disease results from their presence[35].

Thus autoantibodies can cause disease, be markers of disease or just innocent bystanders reflecting an active inflammatory or immune state.

AUTOIMMUNITY AND IBD

What is the evidence for or against autoimmunity in IBD? Perlmann and Broberger first reported the presence of Abs to intestinal epithelium in patients with UC. They suggested that these Abs crossreacted with *E. coli* Ags and that they potentially were responsible for the epithelial cell destruction seen in UC. However, subsequent studies failed to confirm this hypothesis, and transfer of Abs into other species failed to produce colitis. Several animal models of acute inflammation were reported to be associated with the presence of 'anti-colon Abs'. These too failed to transfer disease and fell from favour. As studies broadened, the anti-epithelial cell Abs were also detected in patients with self-limited intestinal inflammatory diseases, suggesting that they were the result rather than the cause of the inflammation.

Several investigators pursued this area, however. Roche *et al.*[36,37] defined an anti-epithelial cell autoantibody ECAC whose titres not only rose and fell with disease activity, but it was also present in a large percentage of first-degree relatives. This Ag was never molecularly defined. Around the same time Das and co-workers described an anti-epithelial cell Ab obtained from colonic washes in UC patients. This IgG Ab recognized a 40 kDa surface membrane molecule which was subsequently identified as a member of the tropomyosin family[38–42]. Titers of this Ab also appear to correlate with disease activity and its expression could be co-localized with terminal complement components. The anti-40 kDa Ab was specific for UC as it was not detected in inflammatory controls or patients with CD, although by itself it was not cytotoxic. Interestingly two animal models of UC develop the anti-40 kDa Ab, the cottontop tamarin and the TcR-α knockout. Similar to the human experience, these Abs do not appear to be responsible for disease development.

The autoantibody in UC which has received considerable attention is pANCA (perinuclear antineutrophil cytoplasmic Ab)[38–48]. This, auto-Ab is related to the Wegener's autoantibody, cANCA, which recognizes myeloperoxidase within the cell. The difference is the staining pattern, pANCA giving a perinuclear pattern while cANCA recognizes cytoplasmic vesicles. pANCA titres do not appear to correlate with disease activity; in fact pANCA in the serum persists post-colectomy. There is also more evidence of pANCA positivity in first-degree relatives although, as alluded to earlier, this does not correlate with disease in these family members. It may either reflect a genetic predisposition or some form of immune dysregulation. The exact nature of the Ag recognized by this autoantibody has not been completely characterized although recent data suggest that it might crossreact with luminal bacteria. Initial studies suggested that it was histone H1.

UC patients appear to express more autoantibodies than do patients with CD. This may relate to the often-quoted Th2 dominance of this disease. However, this concept has recently been called into question. Ag/Ab complex deposition in the tissue would enhance complement activation, chemotaxis of inflammatory cells and local production of inflammatory mediators. CD is associated with fewer if any auto-Abs. There are Abs against bacterial products and yeast; for example anti-*Saccharomyces cerevisiae* Ab, in CD[49–51].

Are these autoantibodies critical for the disease process? Two clinical examples suggest that this is not the case. Colitis can still be induced in cytokine gene targeted deletions in mice in the absence of B cells. Furthermore, the CD45RB[hi] T cell transfer into SCID mouse model develops colitis without any B cells (and without any CD8$^+$ cytotoxic T cells)[52]. A significant percentage of patients with common variable immunodeficiency (hypo- or agammaglobulinaemia) develop a CD-like non-infectious segmental colitis[53]. These clinical observations point the process in the direction of the T cell. As discussed above, T cells can be autoreactive, and due to the nature of the TcR/MHC/peptide interaction (i.e. low affinity) there is a higher likelihood of autoreactivity. Are there autoreactive T cells in IBD? The answer to this question is not clear. There is little evidence for the existence of cytotoxic T cells in the lamina propria of patients with IBD. Thus, in their absence, they are unlikely to play any role in the disease process. In animal models of IBD, T cells transfer disease[54–58]; however, there is little evidence that they are autoreactive. Rather the evidence points towards dysregulated immunity (T cell reactivity) to account for the development of disease. While the inductive phase of helper T cells is antigen-specific, the effector phase (cytokine) is not. After activation, T cells can secrete cytokines which promote an inflammatory response in the tissue. This might explain why therapies directed against T cells (anti-CD4, lymphapheresis, cyclosporin, etc.) are effective in these diseases. Thus it appears that heightened (dysregulated) T cell activation results in mucosal disease. Failure of T cell regulation might account for uncontrolled immunity and inflammation. T cells recognizing caecal bacterial Ags can transfer disease in the C3H/HeBir mouse[59]. This is not autoreactivity; merely mucosal reactivity.

SUMMARY

Many chronic inflammatory diseases such as asthma, multiple sclerosis and rheumatoid arthritis pose similar problems. The availability of mouse models has moved us forward but we are left with partial answers. It is likely that T cells initiate the disease process and that the reactivity is to luminal Ags. The perpetuation of inflammation may be a combination of persistent Ag and the development (or expansion) of autoreactive cells, as a result of either crossreactivity or polyclonal activation. The data to date would not support autoreactivity as a primary event in IBD (CD > UC). However, as our ability to dissect out human models improves, we should be able to ascertain the specific contribution of each aspect of this aberrant immune response and potentially develop novel therapeutic approaches.

Acknowledgement

This work was supported by PHS grants AI 23504 and AI 24671.

References

1. Cruse JM, Lewis, Jr, RE. The immune system victorious: selective preservation of self. Immunol Res 1993;12:101–14.
2. Goodnow CC. Balancing immunity and tolerance: deleting and tuning lymphocyte repertoires. Proc Natl Acad Sci USA 1996;93:2264–71.
3. Johnson JG, Jenkins MK. The role of anergy in peripheral T cell unresponsiveness. Life Sci 1994;55:1767–80.
4. Kroemer G, Martinez C. Clonal deletion, anergy and immunosuppression are connected in series to guarantee self-tolerance. Res Immunol 1992;143.335–40.
5. Malvey EN, Telander DG, Vanasek TL, Mueller DL. The role of clonal anergy in the avoidance of autoimmunity: inactivation of autocrine growth without loss of effector function. Immunol Rev 1998;165:301–18.
6. Streilein JW, Takeuchi M, Taylor AW. Immune privilege, T-cell tolerance, and tissue-restricted autoimmunity. Hum Immunol 1997;52.138–43.
7. Weigle WO. Immunologic tolerance: development and disruption [comment]. Hosp Pract (Off Ed) 1995;30:81–4,89–92.
8. Klinman DM. Polyclonal B cell activation in lupus-prone mice precedes and predicts the development of autoimmune disease. J Clin Invest 1990;86:1249–54.
9. Hamilton KJ, Satoh M, Swartz J, Richards HB, Reeves WH. Influence of microbial stimulation on hypergammaglobulinemia and autoantibody production in pristane-induced lupus. Clin Immunol Immunopathol 1998;86:271–9.
10. Suzuki H, Kundig TM, Furlonger C et al. Deregulated T cell activation and autoimmunity in mice lacking interleukin-2 receptor beta. Science 1995;268:1472–6.
11. Faxvaag A, Moen T, Dalen AB. Polyclonal activation of B-lymphocytes and induction of autoimmunity in retrovirus infected NMRI mice. Scand J Immunol 1993;38:459–62.
12. Gran B, Hemmer B, Martin R. Molecular mimicry and multiple sclerosis – a possible role for degenerate T cell recognition in the induction of autoimmune responses. J Neural Transm Suppl 1999;55:19–31.
13. Banki K, Colombo E, Sia F et al. Oligodendrocyte-specific expression and autoantigenicity of transaldolase in multiple sclerosis. J Exp Med 1994;180:1649–63.
14. Heyma P, Harrison LC, Robins-Browne R. Thyrotrophin (TSH) binding sites on Yersinia enterocolitica recognized by immunoglobulins from humans with Graves' disease. Clin Exp Immunol 1986;64:249–54.
15. Vandenbroucke-Grauls CM, Appelmelk BJ. Helicobacter pylori LPS: molecular mimicry with the host and role in autoimmunity. Ital J Gastroenterol Hepatol 1998;30(suppl. 3):S259–60.
16. Kammer AR, van der Burg SH, Grabscheid B et al. Molecular mimicry of human cytochrome P450 by hepatitis C virus at the level of cytotoxic T cell recognition. J Exp Med 1999;190:169–76

17. Abu-Shakra M, Buskila D, Shoenfeld Y. Molecular mimicry between host and pathogen: examples from parasites and implication. Immunol Lett 1999;67:147–52.
18. Ring GH, Lakkis FG. Breakdown of self-tolerance and the pathogenesis of autoimmunity. Semin Nephrol 1999;19:25–33.
19. Pisko EJ, Panetti M, Foster SL, Turner RA. Human rheumatoid factor-producing cell induction by 2-mercaptoethanol: immunomodulation by a simple thiol compound. Int J Immunopharmacol 1983;5:163–71.
20. Levinson AI, Tar L. *In vitro* IgM rheumatoid-factor production induced by tetanus toxoid. J Allergy Clin Immunol. 1988;81:730–6.
21. Horwitz MS, Sarvetnick N Viruses, host responses, and autoimmunity [In Process Citation]. Immunol Rev 1999;169:241–53.
22. von Herrath MG, Oldstone MB. Virus-induced autoimmune disease. Curr Opin Immunol 1996;8:878–85.
23. Grewal IS, Foellmer HG, Grewal KD *et al*. Requirement for CD40 ligand in costimulation induction, T cell activation, and experimental allergic encephalomyelitis. Science 1996;273:1864–7.
24. van Kooten C, Banchereau J. Functional role of CD40 and its ligand. Int Arch Allergy Immunol 1997;113:393–9.
25. Noelle RJ, Mackey M, Foy T, Buhlmann J, Burns C. CD40 and its ligand in autoimmunity. Am NY Acad Sci 1997;815:384–91.
26. Humphreys-Beher MG, Peck AB, Dang H, Talal N. The role of apoptosis in the initiation of the autoimmune response in Sjogren's syndrome. Clin Exp Immunol 1999;116:383–7.
27. Mauricio D, Mandrup-Poulsen T. Apoptosis and the pathogenesis of IDDM: a question of life and death. Diabetes 1998;47:1537–43.
28. Brunner T, Mueller C. Is autoimmunity coming to a Fas(t) end? [news; comment]. Nat Med 1999;5:19–20.
29. Levine JS, Koh JS. The role of apoptosis in autoimmunity: immunogen, antigen, and accelerant. Semin Nephrol 1999;19:34–47.
30. Rifkin IR, Channavajhala PL, Kiefer HL *et al*. Acceleration of lpr lymphoproliferative and autoimmune disease by transgenic protein kinase CK2 alpha. J Immunol 1998;161:5164–70.
31. Kimura M, Matsuzawa A. Autoimmunity in mice bearing lprcg: a novel mutant gene. Int Rev Immunol 1994;11:193–210.
32. Yasutomo K, Maeda K, Nagata S *et al*. Defective T cells from gld mice play a pivotal role in development of Thy-1.2+B220+ cells and autoimmunity. J Immunol 1994;153:5855–64.
33. Guillevin L, Lhote F, Cohen P *et al*. Polyarteritis nodosa related to hepatitis B virus. A prospective study with long-term observation of 41 patients. Medicine (Baltimore) 1995;74:238–53.
34. Johnson RJ, Couser WG. Hepatitis B infection and renal disease: clinical, immunopathogenetic and therapeutic considerations. Kidney Int 1990;37:663–76.
35. Bacon PA, Davidson C, Smith B. Antibodies to candida and autoantibodies in sub-acute bacterial endocarditis. Q J Med 1974;43:537–50.
36. Roche JK, Fiocchi C, Youngman K. Sensitization to epithelial antigens in chronic mucosal inflammatory disease. Characterization of human intestinal mucosa-derived mononuclear cells reactive with purified epithelial cell-associated components *in vitro*. J Clin Invest 1985;75:522–30.
37. Fiocchi C, Roche JK, Michener WM. High prevalence of antibodies to intestinal epithelial antigens in patients with inflammatory bowel disease and their relatives [see comments]. Ann Intern Med. 1989;110:786–94.
38. Hamilton MI, Bradley NJ, Srai SK, Thrasivoulou C, Pounder RE, Wakefield AJ. Autoimmunity in ulcerative colitis: tropomyosin is not the major antigenic determinant of the Das monoclonal antibody, 7E12H12. Clin Exp Immunol 1995;99:404–11.
39. Halstensen TS. [Anders Jahre Prize for young researchers 1994. Chronic intestinal inflammation studies with multi-colored immunohistochemistry]. Nord Med 1995;110:56–9.
40. Geng X, Biancone L, Dai HH, *et al*. Tropomyosin isoforms in intestinal mucosa: production of autoantibodies to tropomyosin isoforms in ulcerative colitis. Gastroenterology 1998;114:912–22.
41. Biancone L, Monteleone G, Marasco R, Pallone F. Autoimmunity to tropomyosin isoforms in ulcerative colitis (UC) patients and unaffected relatives. Clin Exp Immunol 1998;113:198–205.

42. Biancone L, Mandal A, Yang H *et al*. Production of immunoglobulin G and G1 antibodies to cytoskeletal protein by lamina propria cells in ulcerative colitis [see comments]. Gastroenterology 1995;109:3–12.
43. Hauschild S, Schmitt WH, Csernok E, Flesch BK, Rautmann A, Gross WL. ANCA in systemic vasculitides, collagen vascular diseases, rheumatic disorders and inflammatory bowel diseases. Adv Exp Med Biol 1993;336:245–51.
44. Pokorny CS, Norton ID, McCaughan GW, Selby WS. Anti-neutrophil cytoplasmic antibody: a prognostic indicator in primary sclerosing cholangitis. J Gastroenterol Hepatol 1994;9:40–4.
45. Patel RT, Stokes R, Birch D, Ibbotson J, Keighley MR. Influence of total colectomy on serum antineutrophil cytoplasmic antibodies in inflammatory bowel disease. Br J Surg 1994;81:724–6.
46. Seibold F, Slametschka D, Gregor M, Weber P. Neutrophil autoantibodies: a genetic marker in primary sclerosing cholangitis and ulcerative colitis [see comments]. Gastroenterology 1994;107:532–6.
47. Targan SR, Landers C, Vidrich A, Czaja AJ. High-titer antineutrophil cytoplasmic antibodies in type-1 autoimmune hepatitis [see comments]. Gastroenterology 1995;108:1159–66.
48. Targan SR, Landers CJ, Cobb L, MacDermott RP, Vidrich A. Perinuclear anti-neutrophil cytoplasmic antibodies are spontaneously produced by mucosal B cells of ulcerative colitis patients. J Immunol 1995;155:3262–7.
49. Hoffenberg EJ, Fidanza S, Sauaia A. Serologic testing for inflammatory bowel disease. J Pediatr 1999;134:447–52.
50. Sendid B, Quinton JF, Charrier G, *et al*. Anti-*Saccharomyces cerevisiae* mannan antibodies in familial Crohn's disease. Am J Gastroenterol 1998;93:1306–10.
51. Quinton JF, Sendid B, Reumaux D, *et al*. Anti-*Saccharomyces cerevisiae* mannan antibodies combined with antineutrophil cytoplasmic autoantibodies in inflammatory bowel disease: prevalence and diagnostic role. Gut 1998;42:788–91.
52. Powrie F, Leach MW, Mauze S, Menon S, Caddle LB, Coffman RL. Inhibition of Th1 responses prevents inflammatory bowel disease in scid mice reconstituted with CD45RBhi CD4+ T cells. Immunity 1994;1:553–62.
53. Cunningham-Rundles C. Clinical and immunologic studies of common variable immunodeficiency. Curr Opin Pediatr 1994;6:676–81.
54. Onderdonk AB, Steeves RM, Cisneros RL, Bronson RT. Adoptive transfer of immune enhancement of experimental ulcerative colitis. Infect Immun 1984;46:84–7.
55. Ito H, Fathman CG. CD45RBhigh CD4+ T cells from IFN-gamma knockout mice do not induce wasting disease. J Autoimmun 1997;10:455–9.
56. Simpson SJ, Shah S, Comiskey M *et al*. T-cell-mediated pathology in two models of experimental colitis depends predominantly on the interleukin 12/Signal transducer and activator of transcription (Stat)-4 pathway, but is not conditional on interferon gamma expression by T cells. J Exp Med 1998;187:1225–34.
57. Koh WP, Chan E, Scott K *et al*. TCR-mediated involvement of CD4+ transgenic T cells in spontaneous inflammatory bowel disease in lymphopenic mice. J Immunol 1999;162:7208–16.
58. De Winter H, Cheroutre H, Kronenberg M. Mucosal immunity and inflammation. II. The yin and yang of T cells in intestinal inflammation: pathogenic and protective roles in a mouse colitis model. Am J Physiol 1999;276:G1317–21.
59. Cong Y, Brandwein SL, McCabe RP *et al*. CD4+ T cells reactive to enteric bacterial antigens in spontaneously colitic C3H/HeJBir mice: increased T helper cell type 1 response and ability to transfer disease. J Exp Med 1998;187:855–64.

6
Neutrophil–epithelial interactions, and efforts to down-regulate them, in inflammatory bowel disease

A. T. GEWIRTZ AND J. L. MADARA

ABSTRACT

The histopathological hallmark of the active flares of inflammatory bowel disease (IBD) is the transepithelial migration of neutrophils (so-called crypt abscess). The fact that such active intestinal inflammation correlates with patient symptoms suggests a major role for neutrophil transmigration in causing the epithelial dysfunction characteristic of IBD. Transmigrating neutrophils disrupt epithelial barrier function exposing subepithelial cells to the noxious milieu of the intestinal lumen. Further, these neutrophils can directly induce the intestinal epithelia to secrete chloride ions into the lumen – an event which serves as the basis for secretory diarrhoea. It has recently become clear that intestinal epithelial cells may play an active role in orchestrating neutrophil movement to the lumen. Since the event of neutrophil transepithelial migration characteristic of active IBD is identical to that seen in response to epithelial surface colonization by pathogens, it is likely that one can gain insight into the former event by better understanding the latter circumstance. We have used the model of *Salmonella typhimurium*–intestinal epithelial interaction for this purpose. We have shown that, in response to detection of *S. typhimurium*, epithelia secrete chemokines in a polarized manner such that neutrophils are directed through the lamina propria and subsequently across the epithelia. *S. typhimurium* activates these epithelial cell proinflammatory signalling pathways by inducing an increase in cytoplasmic $[Ca^{2+}]$ that leads to activation of the transcription factor NF-κB. Since such evolutionarily conserved defence mechanisms might be aberrantly triggered to result in the same cellular responses in the absence of pathogens (for example in IBD) we are now defining mechanisms to down-regulate these proinflammatory signals that direct intestinal inflammation. The arachidonate metabolite lipoxin A_4 (LXA_4) is an endogenously biosynthesized anti-inflammatory eicosanoid. Receptors for LXA_4 are expressed on both intestinal epithelial cells and neutrophils. Further, we find LXA_4 and its analogues down-regulate the above molecular events which define intestinal inflammation in *in-vitro* models. Thus, it is possible that activating anti-inflammatory signalling pathways with analogues of LXA_4 may prove to be a successful therapeutic strategy for treating IBD.

ROLE OF NEUTROPHIL–EPITHELIAL INTERACTIONS IN IBD

The histopathology of the active flares of chronic inflammatory intestinal diseases (i.e. Crohn's disease and ulcerative colitis – collectively IBD) is very similar to that observed in response to disease induced by enteric pathogens. In either case the hallmark of active disease is the presence of polymorphonuclear leucocytes (neutrophils) which have migrated to and across the intestinal epithelium into the lumen forming a crypt abscess. This neutrophil movement is thought to be not merely the defining indicator of active intestinal inflammation, it also appears to play a major role in causing the sequelae associated with this disease state. Neutrophils that have transmigrated to the intestinal lumen can induce the epithelial cells lining the intestine to secrete chloride ions into the lumen[1-4]. This chloride secretion drives the water movement that is the basis for the secretory diarrhoea which accompanies intestinal inflammation. Further, transmigrating neutrophils impale epithelial tight junctions, thus disrupting this tissue's barrier function[5,6], allowing access of the luminal contents to subepithelial cells that are not used to bathing in this noxious milieu[6]. The responses of these cells (especially lamina propria macrophages) to exposure to the toxins and microbes of the intestinal lumen will result in further promotion of the inflammatory state (for review see ref. 7). Additionally, infiltrating neutrophils secrete oxidants and proteases that can further damage the epithelia as well as induce secretion of cytokines/chemokines that will also exacerbate the inflammatory state. It is likely this immune inflammatory response plays a role in host defence against some luminal pathogens. Indeed, it seems fairly effective, since pathogens that elicit intestinal inflammation do not usually cause systemic illness. However, neutrophil–epithelial interactions very similar to this occur in the absence of any known pathogens in persons afflicted with IBD, and thus may play a role in such disorders.

MOLECULAR BASIS OF INTESTINAL MUCOSAL INFLAMMATORY RESPONSE

While enteric pathogens are clearly able to trigger activation of a mucosal inflammatory response in healthy individuals, a provoking agonist(s) which initiates the active flares in IDD patients has not yet been identified. It has been suggested that normal gut microflora or their metabolites might serve as a trigger since, in mouse models of IBD, development of disease is dependent upon the presence of such organisms (reviewed in ref. 8). To gain insight into how, in IBD, normal gut microflora might induce intestinal inflammation, we have studied how pathogens induce intestinal inflammation.

The primary host interface with, and barrier against, enteric microorganisms are the epithelial cells which line the intestinal tract. Recent studies have shown that the intestinal epithelium is not a passive barrier but plays an active role in orchestrating the immune inflammatory response. In response to enteric pathogens the epithelium secretes cytokines/chemokines that recruit and activate immune cells. Cytokines secreted by epithelial cells include pleiotropic proinflammatory cytokines such as TNF-α and IL-1β[9] that can act on neighbouring epithelial cells as well as underlying immune cells. Furthermore, the intestinal epithelia can secrete polymorphonuclear neutrophil leucocyte (PMN) chemoattractants in a polarized manner such that PMN are recruited to, and directed to migrate across, the intestinal epithelia. Specifically, in response to the pathogen *Salmonella typhimurium*, model intestinal epithelia secrete interleukin-8 (IL-8) basolaterally[10,11] and pathogen-elicited epithelial chemoattractant (PEEC) apically[12]. The IL-8 secretion serves to recruit PMN to a subepithelial compartment and PEEC secretion drives the final step of PMN movement to the intestinal lumen. The fact that expression of these cytokines/chemokines is elevated in the intestinal mucosa of IBD patients[13–16] suggests that they are also involved in directing the movement of immune cells in these disorders.

To investigate how epithelial cell chemokine expression might be inappropriately regulated in IBD, we are examining how epithelial cell chemokine expression is normally appropriately regulated in response to enteric pathogens. Using cultured model intestinal epithelia and the enteric pathogen *S. typhimurium* we observed that, although this pathogen is invasive, epithelial chemokine secretion results not from bacterial entry[17], but rather via bacterial activation of host proinflammatory signalling pathways. Specifically, *S. typhimurium* induces an increase in host intracellular $[Ca^{2+}]$ (and probably other signals) that leads to activation of the proinflammatory transcription factor NF-κB resulting in expression of IL-8 and probably other inflammatory cytokines[18]. Epithelial cell PEEC secretion is regulated by a distinct but yet to be elucidated mechanism[17]. Activation of epithelial cell proinflammatory signalling pathways requires bacterial metabolic activity rather than mere adherence, suggesting that *S. typhimurium* metabolites that are known to be injected into epithelial cells may be involved.

As seems to normally be the case in humans, we have found that in our model system non-pathogenic intestinal *Escherichia coli* strains do not induce these proinflammatory events, thus raising the question how such pathways might become activated, seemingly in the absence of pathogens in IBD. Several possibilities exist. It is possible that IBD results from as-yet-unrecognized pathogens. Although considerable efforts have yet to reveal such organisms, it seems premature to rule out their existence. Expanded efforts using new approaches to finding such organisms are currently under way[19]. Additionally, there is the possibility that the gut epithelia of IBD patients responds to 'normal' microflora as if enteric pathogens had been detected. Another possibility is that epithelial cells respond to signals derived from subepithelial cells (abberrantly stimulated or genetically hyperresponsive) in a way that mimics the evolved response to pathogens. This could perhaps result from an epithelial defect or an altered cytokine environment. Defining whether these or other events occur in IBD and, if so, what are their underlying causes, is important to understanding the pathogenesis of this disorder.

DOWN-REGULATING INTESTINAL INFLAMMATION VIA THE ENDOGENOUS ANTI-INFLAMMATORY PATHWAY

Because neutrophil–epithelial interactions may play a role in IBD, we have sought to define mechanisms to down-regulate these interactions. Active inflammation in the intestine, and elsewhere, is normally self-limiting. However, there is no known mechanism inherent in proinflammatory pathways that explains why this is the case. For example, considering the positive feedback loops underlying inflammation, this process would be driven towards amplification naturally (i.e. cytokine secretion leading to immune cell recruitment and more cytokine secretion, etc.) regardless of whether or not the infection (or other provoking agonist) was cleared. Thus, it has been postulated that anti-inflammatory pathways must also exist, although they have only recently begun to be recognized. One class of metabolites that appears to be such endogenous anti-inflammatory mediators are the lipoxins (for review see ref. 20). Lipoxins (LX) are lipoxygenase (LO) interaction products of arachidonic acid. Their biosynthesis proceeds via the actions of two distinct LO that are not expressed in any single cell type. Rather, LX are made by the actions of more than one cell type on an individual molecule of arachidonic acid. For example, epithelial cells contain 15-LO and neutrophils contain 5-LO. The actions of these enzymes enable neutrophils and epithelial cells that are in close proximity to cooperate to make LO. A variety of other pathways convert the LO interaction product into one or more of several possible species of LX. The requirement of cell cooperation for LX biosynthesis restricts LX production to already-inflamed sites and is thus one factor making these eicosanoids a good candidate to play a role in limiting inflammation.

In contrast to most other arachidonate metabolites which have bioactivities that promote inflammation, LX have an array of bioactivites (see below) that strongly suggest their in-vivo role is that of counter-regulator to proinflammatory molecules. The best-characterized LX, both in terms of its bioactivity and mechanism of action, is lipoxin A_4 (LXA$_4$). This lipid mediator acts via a specific high-affinity ($k_d \approx 1$ nM) seven-transmembrane α-helix G-protein coupled receptor (termed LXA$_4$R)[21]. Synthetic stable analogues of LXA$_4$ which are more resistant to degradation than the native eicosanoid yet retain ability to specifically ligate the LXA$_4$R exhibit greater anti-inflammatory activity than LXA$_4$ (see ref. 22). One compound which behaves as an LXA$_4$ stable analogue in that it competes for the LXA$_4$ receptor, is resistant to enzymatic degradation, and has anti-inflammatory bioactivity is the 15-epimer of LXA$_4$ (15-epi-LXA$_4$)[23]. Interestingly, 15-epi- LXA$_4$ may be biosynthesized *in vivo* by a pathway involving cyclooxygenase that has been acetylated by aspirin[23]. Thus, some of the bioactions from aspirin may come from activation of counter-regulatory pathways via the LXA$_4$R

In an *In-vitro* model of intestinal inflammation, stable analogues of LXA$_4$ down-regulated events which define and may cause intestinal inflammation. This bioaction was due to LXA$_4$ analogues acting both on the intestinal epithelia and on neutrophils, both of which express the LXA$_4$R[24,25]. LXA$_4$, and its analogues, reduce neutrophil movement[26] and transepithelial migration[27] to exogenous chemotactic gradients. Additionally, LXA$_4$ analogues down-regulate epithelial cell secretion of chemokines that direct neutrophil movement. Specifically, LXA_4 analogues reduce epithelial cell IL-8 secretion (by up to 80%) in response to either the proinflammatory cytokine TNF-α or the gastroenteritis-eliciting pathogen *S. typhimurium*[25,28]. Furthermore, LXA_4 analogues down-regulate epithelial secretion of PEEC by about 60%[28]. This down-regulation of epithelial chemokine secretion reduces neutrophil movement through the underlying matrix as well as across model intestinal epithelia. If, in this model system, we expose both the neutrophils and the epithelia to LXA_4 analogues, we observe nearly complete attenuation of neutrophil transepithelial movement (Gewirtz and Madara, unpublished observation). Since the flares of active disease in IBD patients may result from bacterial–epithelial–neutrophil interactions, this is a particularly encouraging observation. LXA_4 analogue down-regulation of neutrophil movement is probably mediated by the LXA_4R as the abilities of various LXA_4 analogues to exhibit this bioactivity correlate strictly with their ability to specifically ligate the LXA_4R. Consistent with the k_d of the LXA_4R, LXA_4 and its analogues exhibit these bioactions at subnanomolar–nanomolar concentrations. The specific signalling mechanism by which LXA_4 analogues down-regulate these proinflammatory functional events has not yet been defined, but appears to be mediated via down-regulation of NF-κB (our unpublished results), a central switch in many proinflammatory pathways.

Not only are the symptoms of active IBD attributable, at least in part, to neutrophil influx, but the products these neutrophils secrete are probably responsible for much of the damage that results to host tissue during active intestinal inflammation. Specifically, both the reactive oxygen metabolites and granule proteases that activated neutrophils secrete can damage host tissue, as well as further promoting the inflammatory state. LXA_4 stable analogues down-regulate neutrophil release of these proteases, thus representing another potential mechanism by which these lipid mediators can be therapeutic for diseases characterized by active inflammation[29]. Importantly, such down-regulation of neutrophil degranulation is observed in response to immune complexes similar to those found in abundance in several chronic inflammatory diseases including IBD, adult respiratory distress syndrome, and glomerulonephritis. Like the above-described anti-inflammatory bioactions of LXA_4 analogues, LXA_4 analogue down-regulation of neutrophil degranulation is also mediated by the LXA_4R.

It is possible that LXA_4 analogues will also be able to down-regulate intestinal inflammation *in vivo* and thus be potentially therapeutic for IBD. LXA_4, and its analogues, potently down-regulate inflammation in well-defined animal models such as the hamster cheek pouch and the mouse ear[30,31]. The anti-inflammatory bioactivity exhibited by LXA_4 analogues in this *in-vivo* assay was more potent than that exhibited by equimolar concentrations of dexamethasone. Encouragingly, it has recently been shown that human sections of colonic mucosa exhibit a down-regulation of chemokine secretion (both IL-8 and macrophage chemotactic protein [MCP]-1) in response to LXA_4 stable analogues[32], supporting the notion that these analogues will act in the intestine as they do in other tissues and cell culture. In both this *ex-vivo* system, and the *in-vitro* model described above, chemokine secretion was down-regulated via treating with LXA_4 analogues prior to the addition of a provoking agonist. Thus, we speculate that these compounds may be able to down-regulate the initiation of the active flares of IBD. Importantly, unlike non-steroidal anti-inflammatory drugs (NSAID), LXA_4 analogues are unlikely to inhibit the biosynthesis of cytoprotective prostaglandins because LXA_4 analogues do not inhibit the cyclooxygenase enzymes that mediate the formation of such prostaglandins. While one NSAID, aspirin, leads to generation of stable ligands (15-epi-LX) for the LXA_4R, like other NSAID it still blocks prostaglandin biosynthesis, probably accounting for its negative effects in the intestine. Therefore, direct administration of LXA_4 stable analogues may provide anti-inflammatory bioactivity without the negative effects associated with NSAID. We are currently investigating this question in mouse *in-vivo* models.

References

1. Nash S, Parkos CA, Nusrat A, Delp C, Madara JL. *In vitro* model of intestinal crypt abscess: a novel neutrophil-derived secretagogue activity. J Clin Invest 1991;87:1474–7.
2. Madara JL, Patapoff TW, Gillece-Castro B *et al*. 5'-Adenosine monophosphate is the neutrophil-derived paracrine factor that elicits chloride secretion from T84 intestinal epithelial cells. J Clin Invest 1993;91:2320–5.
3. Madara JL, Parkos CA, Colgan SP *et al*. Cl⁻ secretion in a model intestinal epithelium induced by a neutrophil-derived secretagogue. J Clin Invest 1992;89:1938–44.
4. Madara JL, Nash S, Parkos C. Neutrophil–Epithelial Cell Interactions in the Intestine. New York: Plenum Press 1991
5. Nash S, Stafford J, Madara JL. Effects of polymorphonuclear leukocyte transmigration on barrier function of cultured intestinal epithelial monolayers. J Clin Invest 1987;80:1104–13.
6. Madara J. Loosening TJs. Lessons from the intestine. J Clin Invest. 1989;83:1089–94.
7. McCormick B, Gewirtz A, Madara JL. Epithelial crosstalk with bacteria and immune cells. Curr Opin Gastroenter. 1998;14:492–7.
8. Baumgart DC, McVay LD, Carding SR. Mechanisms of immune cell-mediated tissue injury in inflammatory bowel disease. Int J Mol Med 1998;1:315–32.
9. Jung HC, Eckmann L, Yang S-K *et al*. A distinct array of proinflammatory cytokines is expressed in human colon epithelial cells in response to bacterial invasion. J Clin Invest 1995;95:55–65.
10. McCormick BA, Colgan SP, Archer CD, Miller SI, Madara JL. *Salmonella typhimurium* attachment to human intestinal epithelial monolayers: transcellular signalling to subepithelial neutrophils. J Cell Biol 1993;123:895–907.
11. McCormick B, Hofman P, Kim J, Carnes D, Miller S, Madara J. Surface attachment of *Salmonella typhimurium* to intestinal epithelia imprints the subepithelial matrix with gradients chemotactic for neutorphils. J Cell Biol 1995;131:1599–608.
12. McCormick BA, Parkos CA, Colgan SP, Carnes DK, Madara JL. Apical secretion of a pathogen-elicited epithelial chemoattractant (PEEC) activity in response to surface colonization of intestinal epithelia by *Salmonella typhimurium*. J Immunol 1998;160:455–6.
13. Daig R, Andus T, Aschenbrenner E, Falk W, Scholmerich J, Gross V. Increased interleukin 8 expression in the colon mucosa of patients with inflammatory bowel disease. Gut 1996;38:216–22.
14. Funakoshi K, Sugimura K, Sasakawa T *et al*. Study of cytokines in ulcerative colitis. J Gastroenterol 1995;30(Suppl 8):61–3
15. Mazzucchelli L, Hauser C, Zgraggen K *et al*. Expression of interleukin-8 gene in inflammatory bowel disease is related to the histological grade of active inflammation. Am J Pathol 1994;144:997–1007
16. Nielsen OH, Rudiger N, Gaustadnes M, Horn T. Intestinal interleukin-8 concentration and gene expression in inflammatory bowel disease. Scand J Gastroenterol 1997;32:1028–34.
17. Gewirtz AT, Siber AM, Madara JL, McCormick BA. Orchestration of neutrophil movement by intestinal epithelial cells in response to *Salmonella typhimurium* can be uncoupled from bacterial internalization [In Process Citation]. Infect Immun 1999;67:608–17.

18. Gewirtz AT, Rao AN, Simon P, Carnes D, Madara JL, Neish AS. *S. typhimurium*-induced IL-8 secretion is mediated by Ca++ dependent NFkb activation. (Manuscript Submitted for publication)
19. Relman DA. The search for unrecognized pathogens. Science 1999;284:1308–10.
20. Serhan CN. Lipoxins and novel aspirin-triggered 15-epi-lipoxins (ATL): a jungle of cell–cell interactions or a therapeutic opportunity? Prostaglandins 1997;53:107–37.
21. Fiore S, Maddox JF, Perez HD, Serhan CN. Identification of a human cDNA encoding a functional high affinity lipoxin A4 receptor. J Exp Med 1994;180:253–60.
22. Serhan CN, Maddox JF, Petasis NA *et al.* Design of lipoxin A4 stable analogs that block transmigration and adhesion of human neutrophils. Biochemistry 1995;34:14609–15.
23. Claria J, Serhan CN. Aspirin triggers previously undescribed bioactive eicosanoids by human endothelial cell–leukocyte interactions. Proc Natl Acad Sci USA 1995;92:9475–9.
24. Fiore S, Romano M, Reardon E, Serhan CN. Induction of functional lipoxin A4 receptors in HL-60 cells. Blood 1993;81:3395–403.
25. Gronert KG, Gewirtz AT, Madara JL, Serhan CN. Identification of a human enterocyte lipoxin A4 receptor that is regulated by IL-13 and INF-γ that inhibits TNF-α-induced IL-8 release. J Exp Med 1998;187:1285–94.
26. Lee TH, Horton CE, Kyan-Aung U, Haskard D, Crea AE, Spur BW. Lipoxin A4 and lipoxin B4 inhibit chemotactic responses of human neutrophils stimulated by leukotriene B4 and *N*-formyl-L-methionyl-L-leucyl-L-phenylalanine. Clin Sci 1989;77:195–203.
27. Colgan SP, Serhan CN, Parkos CA, Delp-Archer C. Madara JL. Lipoxin A4 modulates transmigration of human neutrophils across intestinal epithelial monolayers. J Clin Invest 1993;92:75–82.
28. Gewirtz AT, McCormick B, Neish AS *et al.* Pathogen-induced chemokine secretion from model intestinal epithelium is inhibited by lipoxin A4 analogs. J Clin Invest 1998;101:1860–9.
29. Gewirtz AT, Fokin VV, Petasis NA, Serhan CN, Madara JL. LXA$_4$, aspirin-triggered 15-epi LXA$_4$, and their stable analogs electively down-regulate PMN azurophilic degranulation. Am J Phys (Cell) 1999;276 (In press).
30. Raud J, Palmertz U, Dahlen SE, Hedqvist P. Lipoxins inhibit microvascular inflammatory actions of leukotriene B4. Adv Exp Med Biol 1991;314:185–92.
31. Takano T, Fiore S, Maddox JF, Brady HR, Petasis NA, Serhan CN. Aspirin-triggered 15-epi-lipoxin A4 and LXA4 stable analogs are potent inhibitors of accute inflammation: evidence for anti-inflammatory receptors. J Exp Med 1997;185:1693–704.
32. Goh J, Baird AW, Goodson C. Stable lipoxin analogs attenuate chemokine release from cytokine activated human colonic epithelium. Gastroenterology 1999;116:A724.

7
Understanding inflammatory bowel disease at the millennium: tentative answers and future questions

D. K. PODOLSKY

ABSTRACT

Considerable progress has been made in recent years in the delineation of important factors that contribute to the development of inflammatory bowel disease (IBD), as well as the wide spectrum of key mediators. This progress enables a more focused assessment of the goals necessary to arrive at an understanding of the processes initiating IBD. Identification of specific disease-associated genes building on recent progress achieved through genomic screening with microsatellite markers is a key priority. Already concerted efforts are focused in areas identified by initial screening of multiply-affected kindreds. It remains to be determined whether identification of these genes will make insights into disease mechanisms self-evident, or whether these same factors are also important in the vast majority of patients who have no family history.

The identification of specific genes associated with IBD may serve primarily to enable more focused inquiry into host–environment interaction. It is already clear that genes are insufficient to cause IBD. However, the key factors in the environment which are essential to initiate and sustain inflammation are yet to be identified, or at least validated.

T cell populations associated with Crohn's disease responding to specific antigens may well be central. These should meet the criteria of being sufficient in a susceptible host to confer disease, and cloning of these T cells should allow delineation of their antigen specificity. Verification of key constituents of the microflora that participate in either initiation or perpetuation of inflammatory activity represents a third goal. This will undoubtedly require refined animal models which enable the assessment of identified candidate microbial species. The mechanisms of microbial interaction with the mucosa need to be defined, whether this reflects direct interaction with the epithelium or penetration of antigen or other proinflammatory bacterial products through the mucosa. Finally, the nature and function of the intestinal barrier should be defined. Reliable means for assessing the structure and function of the epithelial barrier *in vivo* will be essential to resolving the relative importance of the barrier function in either preventing or enabling IBD.

The significant progress in identifying a wide variety of mediators, most notably cytokines, that contribute to immunoinflammatory responses provides a framework for setting additional priorities in the next 10 years. Beyond identification of all of the regulatory peptides that are present in the mucosa in the setting of IBD, the relative hierarchy, as well as temporal sequence of expression and biological activity, of these mediators must be defined. This will be essential not only for understanding the evolution of inflammation but in guiding targeted blockade or expression of various peptide mediators. The same will also apply to non-cytokine mediators. Delineation of the cell signalling mechanisms through which the inflammatory mediators elicit cellular responses is another important priority. Characterization of these pathways within specific cell populations will also provide a rational basis for focusing translational efforts to develop effective therapeutic interventions. Finally, basic understanding of the mechanisms which ultimately down-regulate inflammatory responses, and most importantly enable healing of the mucosa to re-establish normal homeostasis, are essential goals of future research.

While it is apparent that considerable further work is necessary, progress in recent years has suggested future research directions and the suitability of tools to achieve those goals.

INTRODUCTION

Over recent years significant progress has been made in the definition of factors which play an important role in the development of inflammatory bowel disease (IBD). This progress has made possible better understanding, at least in a broad sense, of factors that contribute to initiation of disease, as well as many of the processes which are important in amplifying inflammatory processes that ultimately result in the clinical manifestation of disease. Yet understanding of specific processes of disease initiation and progression remains significantly incomplete. In order to define the goals and requirements for achieving a comprehensive understanding of IBD pathogenesis it is helpful first to summarize the current understanding of disease mechanisms. A survey of the most important recent advances helps frame more formal questions and future research priorities.

New approaches to the identification of genes associated with susceptibility to IBD are among the most important developments in the past few years. Given the consistent demonstration of increased disease frequency among first-degree relatives of a proband, and the disproportionate increase in monozygotic versus dizygotic twins, the genetic hypothesis (i.e. that genes confer risk of IBD) is the most solidly based premise of IBD disease mechanism. Despite considerable efforts the candidate gene approach has produced only modest advances in our understanding of IBD. This approach requires prior insight into disease processes. Emphasis on assessment of candidate genes has been overtaken by genomic screening using anonymous microsatellite markers. This methodological approach obviates the inherent limitations of candidate marker studies which are, by definition, hampered because of our highly fragmented and incomplete understanding of disease processes, and thus of which genes may be relevant. Use of genomic screening allows assessment of genetic associations without prior bias about the nature of the disease-related genes. While it is reasonable to suppose 'IBD gene(s)' include those encoding proteins related directly to the immune system as discussed below, it is also plausible that genes important for maintaining an adequate epithelial barrier may be central to determining predisposition to IBD. However, the breadth of genes which could functionally modulate either immune response of the mucosal barrier is enormous, providing an inherent challenge to achieving success through the candidate gene approach. Although considerable effort will be needed before eventual success in identifying specific disease-associated genes (and an indeterminable amount of subsequent study to define the mechanisms through which the encoded proteins effect this predisposition), initial screening can provide some important insight into basic features of IBD which have been sorely needed to address long-running controversies. The latter include whether these disorders are indeed distinct (i.e. are regions of genomic association identical?), whether the clinically defined disorders are pathogenetically homogeneous (i.e. are genomic associations consistent among individuals with varying disease phenotype within each of the major forms, ulcerative colitis (UC) and Crohn's disease (CD)), and finally, is susceptibility monogenic or multigenic (i.e. are there one or more disease-dominant genes; are there modifier genes?).

It is important to note that the relevance of loci identified in patients from multiplex families to mechanisms of disease in the great majority of patients who do not have a family history remains as yet uncertain. Thus it is premature to exclude the possibility that the subset of individuals with a family history who necessarily are the subjects encompassed by microsatellite marker linkage studies are not representative of the majority of patients. However, precedents from the study of other diseases make it likely that study of these 'exceptions' will identify critical common disease elements. Nonetheless, the possibility that patients within a multiplex family may be distinguished by a genetic contribution not relevant to the majority of patients, underscores the importance, as discussed below, of association studies of gene associations identified in linkage studies.

These genomic screening approaches are already providing answers. The presence of a locus on chromosome 16 in CD to the exclusion of UC has now been validated in a number of centres. Other loci, including sites on chromosomes 3, 4, 6 and 11, have been identified, though confirmation for these additional loci has been variable. Some loci are common to both major forms of IBD, and some disease specific loci have been reported but need to be validated in other populations. Already, available findings support the assumption that UC and CD are distinct but share common elements. As a corollary, these findings indicate that multiple genetic factors may determine disease phenotype, including basic disease category, possibly site of disease and disease severity.

In conjunction with the new focus on identification of IBD-associated loci enabled by genomic screening, development of mutant murine lines by transgenic and targeted gene deletion techniques has been a major force in refining current concepts of IBD pathogenesis. Following the nearly simultaneous recognition of 'spontaneous' colitis in murine lines rendered deficient in α/β TCR bearing lymphocytes, IL-2 or IL-10 expression by targeted deletion of the respective gene (and a generalized gastrointestinal inflammatory diathesis in rats coexpressing HLA-B27 and human β2-microglobulin), numerous murine lines with either gain-of-function or functional inactivation of a variety of gene targets have been established and characterized. Many mutant lines possessing altered function of a wide variety of genes have been found to develop colitis. However, many other mutant lines do not (spontaneously) develop IBD. An axiomatic insight provided by these animals is the proof that a genetic alteration can be sufficient to lead to colitis, without other further specific exogenous experimental manipulation. Importantly, continued characterization studies of a number of these genetic models have demonstrated that the phenotypic expression of disease (e.g. age of onset and severity) may vary widely when the same genetic mutation is crossed onto different strains, underscoring the ability of other genetic loci to act as modifier genes. This observation provides a ready context for the emerging valuable perspective on the results of linkage analysis described above, by underscoring that distinctions between forms of IBD as either a single disorder with divergent manifestations, two diseases or several, may in fact be more subtle. It is also self-evident that more than one genetic factor could predispose to IBD.

Among the important lessons that have already been learned from study of these mutant rodent lines, it is evident that colitis may result from alteration of many different genes. However, it is possible to broadly classify these genes into two categories: those involved in immune function and those that contribute to the epithelial barrier. It should be noted that modulation of barrier integrity as the functional effect resulting from many of the genes that yield colitis is still only presumptive, e.g. mdr1, Gi2α, keratin 8, transforming growth factor (TGF) β_1 (which also profoundly affects immune response). However, in others the relationship seems clear, e.g. chimaeras expressing a dominant-negative transgene that blockades N-cadherin and ITF deficiency that predisposes to chronic colitis after an otherwise self-limited colitis due to impaired epithelial healing. Moreover, this paradigm of dual pathways that can predispose to colitis may be easily applied to the many earlier models of IBD that were developed through the administration of exogenous agents, e.g. trinitrobenzene sulphonic acid as an 'immune model' and DSS as a 'barrier model'.

Comparative analysis of mutant rodent lines, which develop IBD, has already provided a number of additional important insights. First, comparative analysis of the residual immune system in mutant lines in which a gene presumptively involved in immune response has been modulated suggests that a select subpopulation of CD4$^+$ lymphocytes is necessary for colitis. This is validated by transfer of comparable CD4$^+$ subsets into SCID mice with resultant development of colitis. The latter have also enabled demonstration that the pro-colitis-inducing CD4$^+$ lymphocytes, which appear to be present in all animals, are counterbalanced by other lymphocyte subsets, which presumably exert 'suppressive' effects. This implies that colitis may be as much the result of removal of an active 'brake' on mucosal immune responses as it is the result of active 'inappropriate' immune response. If this model is relevant to humans it suggests that even normal individuals contain specific T-lymphocyte populations which promote IBD. This inference would imply that loss of the counterbalancing suppressor lymphocytes or response to the latter's suppressive effects could result in colitis. The latter is also reinforced by the absence of any colitis in many profoundly immunodeficient animals, indicating that the innate immune system (i.e. lacking a capability for specific immune recognition) is sufficient in conjunction with the normal mucosal barrier to prevent infection from luminal flora.

Study of the mutant murine lines and the characterization of exogenous rodent models have also reinforced concepts of the key role of specific lymphocyte subsets in defining the phenotypic features of discrete forms of IBD. Thus established Crohn's disease in humans and many of the murine models reflects a dominant role of Th1 lamina propria lymphocytes. Activation of these lymphocytes leads to production of interferon gamma (1FN-γ) and interleukin-2 (IL-2) which drive monocyte/macrophage activation. The latter then produce IL-12 (and probably IL-18) which feed back to reinforce Th1 activation, concurrent with production of cytokines (e.g. tumour necrosis factor (TNF) and IL-1) which lead to broad amplification of non-specific inflammatory pathways. In contrast UC and a limited number of animal models (including the T-cell antigen receptor-α (TCR-α) deficient animal) are characterized by a predominance of Th2 lymphocytes, though in the human disease they may not produce the full spectrum of cytokines usually found as products of Th2 lymphocytes. The production of IL-4 may well be responsible via activation of B cells for the altered production of immunoglobulin by UC mucosa that has long been recognized. However, an essential uncertainty is whether this dichotomy of typical lymphocyte subsets is present at the time of initial disease onset. Even more important as a question of overriding importance is whether the predominant lymphocyte phenotype reflects response to a specific limited number of bacteria and/or other luminal antigens. Conversely it remains to be determined whether broad suppression of these lymphocytes can be achieved by the bystander action observed in murine models of so-called Th3 or Tr1 lymphocytes.

Further observations obtained from study of mutant mice underscore the potential importance of cooperative interaction between genetically determined host susceptibility and environmental factors. The importance of the luminal flora as a key disease determinant is evident from the virtual absence of colitis seen in susceptible mutant lines when maintained in a germ-free state. The emergence of colitis in mutant animals reconstituted with elements of normal flora indicates that bacterial populations contribute to the development of IBD through mechanisms distinct from those typical of infectious disorders, i.e. in the absence of either known toxin production or tissue invasion. The requirement for a luminal flora may explain the preponderance of colitis to the virtual exclusion of small-bowel disease (with some exceptions including the HLA-B27 transgenic rat, TGF-β-deficient, glial fibrillary acidic protein targeted ablation of enteric glia and perhaps IL-10- deficient mice) in the mutant lines. It remains unclear whether this feature implies mechanisms more relevant to UC than

CD. These findings may be relevant to the observed clinical benefit of antibiotic treatment in some IBD patients, though ironically this is most evident in CD patients, and often with antibiotics distinct from those that might be anticipated if predicated on the particular importance of specific species implicated in experimental studies.

The general potential relationship between genetic and environmental factors is apparent from the increased susceptibility of some mutant lines to induced colitis. Although no 'spontaneous' colitis appears to develop in some mutant lines, they have a propensity for severe injury and ongoing disease when exposed to challenge with an exogenous agent. This is exemplified by intestinal trefoil family factor-deficient mice. As noted above, despite normal mucosal architecture, administration of standard doses of DSS over a limited period leads to severe ongoing colitis, presumably due to failure of healing mechanisms to re-establish epithelial continuity. Cooperative interaction which leads from 'normal' mucosa to ongoing colitis may arguably be more closely analogous to IBD in humans than mutant models in which disease occurs uniformly.

In addition to advances in genetic studies and the development of so-called genetic models which should shed new light on mechanisms underlying the initiation of IBD, significant progress has been made in identifying key immune and inflammatory mediators that contribute to disease perpetuation and amplification. Most importantly, these mediators are the more proximate factors that produce clinical manifestations of disease. Although a comprehensive summary of mediators is beyond the scope of this overview, it is clear that they include key cytokines, chemokines, products of arachidonic acid metabolism, neuropeptides, growth factors and reactive oxygen metabolites. In addition, adhesion molecules and their counter-receptors which participate in recruitment of inflammatory cells, most especially neutrophils and homing lymphocytes, to sites of disease are critical in sustaining activity. It is important to emphasize that expression, activation and inactivation of various mediators and cell populations, are intricately inter-regulated by the various mediators. Most importantly, these mediators offer targets for pharmacological intervention.

Alterations in the expression of many cytokines and chemokines have been found in IBD patients, although in most the alterations have not been consistently observed. Among the more than 25 regulatory peptides that have been assessed, several may be especially important. These include a combination of interleukins, which suggest a Th1 dominant profile, at least in CD patients (see above). The broadly proinflammatory cytokines are critical, perhaps most especially TNF-α, while the chemokines IL-8 and ENA78 and MCP-1 may respectively have a significant role in recruiting neutrophils and macrophages in conjunction with leukotrienes.

Despite the substantial progress that has been made, critical and fundamental issues still require resolution. Nonetheless the achievements of these past few years have made possible more focused questions that permit setting priorities for future research efforts. On the basis of our current understanding of pathophysiological processes, the goals for basis research studies of IBD in the future include the following seven areas.

1. Identification and characterization of IBD-associated genes

As indicated above, rapid progress is being made in identifying regions of the genome likely to possess IBD genes in family linkage studies. Beyond initial validation by confirmation in separate kindred collections, more refined localization will be the next priority through development of markers that will allow ever-finer mapping within these regions. Ultimately the relevance of genes identified through linkage studies should be further confirmed by association studies using DNA obtained from individuals with non-familial IBD and suitable controls. As important as the daunting sequencing and informatics needed to achieve technical success in these undertakings, progress will be substantially facilitated by cooperative sharing of information among groups utilizing different genomic DNA banks to rapidly confirm proposed disease linkage of loci.

Until actual IBD genes are identified the further challenges to understanding their contribution to IBD cannot be accurately gauged. If specific germline mutations are identified (as opposed to simple restriction fragment length polymorphisms) in appropriate members of kindreds, the genes may be directly implicated. Given what has already been learned from animal models, these genes may encode any of a wide range of targets. Indeed those studies are at best an underestimate of the variety of these genes, e.g. conceptually genes involved in the signalling pathways for each of the factors already implicated could result in a similar phenotype. While the functional importance of the gene products may be self-evident, substantial work may be needed to understand the mechanisms through which these genes promote the development of IBD.

2. Definition of IBD-associated bacteria and bacterial products.

A necessary albeit not-sufficient role for luminal bacteria in colitis is strongly supported by recent studies in murine models and generally supported by clinical observation. However, it is clear that efforts focusing on identification of bacteria or other flora which are pathogenic through conventional mechanisms may not be sufficient. Specific flora and their products which promote the development of colitis need to be identified using the murine models. It remains to be determined whether the bacteria that promote colitis are common to the various models. Confirmation of the relevance of these species or alternative counterparts in humans remains an overriding priority. This will probably require refinement of *in-vitro* experimental systems utilizing human tissues or cell populations, as well as human clinical trials to test the critical role of these bacteria and/or products through therapeutic intervention.

3. Isolation of IBD-associated T cell subsets

Evidence that T cell subsets are central to the pathogenesis of IBD in murine models seems incontrovertible. Circumstantial data support the probable relevance of these observations in humans. Future research must encompass a comprehensive catalogue of mucosal T cells in IBD and identification of specific populations associated with these disorders. It should be noted that the latter may actually include *loss* of some T cell populations as much as induction of T cell subsets. This will necessitate full phenotypic characterization of all T cells present in the intestine and molecular characterization of their receptors. While the latter has been carried out on a limited number of specimens, and revealed the oligoclonality of these cells, more extensive study is needed, including comparison of populations from affected and unaffected bowel as well as comparisons during disease activity and remission, and between disease and suitable controls. Finally, the actual antigen specificity of any disease-associated T cells needs to be established. This will require cloning of these T cells and determination of the processed antigen bound by the T cell receptors as a prelude to evaluation of their functional role in promoting IBD.

Assessing the importance of putative disease-associated T cells will remain a challenge and suitable experimental models are needed. However, these may be achieved through the application of described techniques for *in-vivo* culture of fetal intestine after subcutaneous implantation in mice or alternatively reconstituted SCID mice. These systems may allow for assessment of the ability of T cells isolated from IBD patients and controls to induce or suppress IBD.

4. Delineation of mucosal–cell interactions

It is clear that the immune (and inflammatory) state of the mucosa reflects the aggregate of the polymorphic interactions among diverse mucosal cell populations. While many specific facets of discrete interactions between pairs of different cell populations have been defined, as yet there is no coherent and comprehensive understanding of the multiple oscillating and multiply-reinforcing network of cell interactions which reflect the ambient states of mucosal function. Application of neural network theory may ultimately inform an understanding of both normal and inflamed intestinal mucosa.

5. Definitive assessment of mucosal barrier function

Despite extensive study, results of efforts to assess the integrity of mucosal barrier function in patients with IBD have not yet yielded definitive results. This may reflect the choice of methods that are inadequate to define alterations or the possibility that alterations in the barrier do not play a primary role in human IBD despite the conceptual plausibility raised by animal studies. It is also possible that impaired reconstitution of normal barrier function may be more important than intrinsic defects in the steady state when disease is inactive (see below). In order to determine the role, if any, of altered barrier function in IBD, a more complete understanding of the structural components forming the mucosal barrier is needed, including details of the premucosal mucous gel, the constituents of tight junctions and their regulation and intestinal transport mechanisms. While substantial progress has been made in characterizing each of these components, understanding remains incomplete, limiting the ability to definitively assess alterations in IBD. In addition, more definitive approaches to assessment of overall barrier function are needed. Ideally these should include techniques for determination of mucosal resistance *in vivo* as well as in mucosal cultures *in vitro*.

6. Delineation of mechanisms of mucosal repair and healing

In addition to basic studies of intrinsic barrier function and its potential alteration in IBD, progress is needed in basic understanding of the mechanisms by which healing is accomplished and normal mucosal architecture re-established after initial injury. It is likely that these mechanisms are also common to other forms of mucosal injury. Re-establishing continuity of the surface epithelium through the combined effects of migration (restitution) and proliferation is essential to ultimate down-regulation of inflammation. The mechanisms through which inflammation is down-regulated may ultimately be as important as initial activation of these processes in IBD. Indeed studies of the ITF-deficient mouse have illustrated the ability of impaired repair function to result in ongoing colitis. Further understanding of the basic mechanisms through which inflammation is down-regulated and healing accomplished may also facilitate development of new therapeutic interventions.

7. Determination of the role of soluble mediators

The appreciation of the enormous number and variety of soluble mediators, both peptide and non-peptide, that may play a role in mucosal immune and inflammatory responses prompts key priorities for future research. While continued consideration of alterations in additional mediators in IBD, as they are identified (e.g. IL-18) is necessary, determination of the functional hierarchy among mediators is essential. Thus the relative importance of different cytokines and chemokines is needed to achieve a coherent understanding of pathophysiological processes in IBD. Importantly, understanding of any hierarchy among mediators will be critical in establishing priorities for the development of targeted therapeutic interventions; the enormous number of potential targets makes this a necessity. Achieving consensus about the role of specific mediators within the complex mixture present in association with IBD will depend on the availability of suitable agonists and antagonists. While many are available, robust techniques for specific modulation of the numerous regulatory peptides that may play a role in IBD are needed. The latter may include antisense as well as transgenic and gene knockout techniques. However, methods for selective modulation of mediator content and function in the context of existing models of IBD are also essential.

Finally, more complete understanding of the mechanisms of action of the IBD-associated mediators is needed. This includes determination of the target cell populations and their functional responses, but also the signalling pathways through which these responses are effected. An understanding of signalling may enable design of strategies to modulate mediator responses more effectively than targeting of the mediators themselves.

In summary, many questions remain to be answered before a complete understanding of the pathogenesis of IBD is achieved. These include delineation of fundamental mucosal processes and disease-specific dynamics. However, recent studies have provided more sharply focused research questions, and permit the ability to set priorities for the application of increasingly more powerful research tools.

Section III
Clinical challenges in inflammatory bowel disease

Moderators: **D. Taullard,** Montevideo
D. G. Gall, Calgary

8
Diagnosis of inflammatory bowel disease: an update

M. ROBINSON

ABSTRACT

Idiopathic inflammatory bowel disease (IBD) is now a well-recognized class designation for two overlapping 'lower' gastrointestinal disorders, more or less neatly divided into mucosal ulcerative colitis (UC) and Crohn's disease (CD). Although IBD pathogenesis remains obscure and subject to aggressive investigation, evidence is accumulating for the hypothesis that both UC and CD are syndromes with multiple aetiologies. Differentiation of UC from CD, though not based on pathogenic mechanisms, permits description of disease patterns, prediction of outcomes based on natural history, and may point towards the most appropriate treatment strategies. The unknown pathogeneses and varied manifestations of these disorders present a diagnostic challenge to physicians. Genetic, environmental and immune factors are all involved in determining susceptibility to IBD. How then should 'IBD diagnosis' be approached for this heterogeneous group of illnesses with varying causes?

Diagnosis of IBD has relied largely on patient history and physical examination, radiographic and endoscopic findings, and standard laboratory parameters. In general, UC is characterized by diffuse and relatively superficial mucosal inflammation with bloody diarrhoea as its cardinal clinical manifestation. CD involves focal and transmural inflammatory changes, often causing systemic manifestations in addition to pain and tenderness and diarrhoea. Technological and scientific advances have been brought to bear in diagnosis and assessment of these disorders, particularly in terms of newer serological markers of inflammation. Antibody to *Saccharomyces cerevisiae* (ASCA) has been demonstrated in up to 79% of the sera of CD patients. Antineutrophil cytoplasmic antibodies (ANCA), autoantibodies directed against intracellular components of neutrophils, are present in the sera of 60–80% of patients with UC. ANCA antibodies have also been detected in a clinically distinct subpopulation of patients with CD. Analysis of these markers provides evidence of clinical, genetic and immunological heterogeneity, and implies distinct types of mucosal inflammation. As more is understood about the pathogenesis of IBD, it seems likely that therapy can be refined to interfere at specific points in the disease process, depending upon the specific dysregulation identified. Diagnosis and therapy thus can merge.

INTRODUCTION

The term idiopathic inflammatory bowel disease (IBD) includes both ulcerative colitis (UC) and Crohn's disease (CD). Crohn and co-workers published a joint paper in 1932[1], which along with a follow-up paper in 1933 by Crohn's two colleagues established the basis for much of our current perception of CD. If idiopathic IBD existed before the twentieth century it was not yet differentiated from infectious colitides, although several descriptions of possible idiopathic IBD may exist in earlier medical literature[2]. To date, IBD aetiology remains uncertain, and is the subject of aggressive investigation (including infectious agents, immune reactivity, genetic predisposition, abnormal intestinal permeability, and many other avenues). Evidence is accumulating in support of the hypothesis that both UC and CD are disorders with multiple aetiologies.

The unknown pathogeneses and varied manifestations of UC and CD present a diagnostic challenge to physicians. Practical issues of clinical diagnosis demand differentiation of therapeutically distinct subgroups. Diagnostic precision will advance in parallel with research-based knowledge of pathophysiology and pathogenesis. In general, differential diagnostic distinctions should have clear therapeutic implications. Until quite recently, treatments for various subgroups of IBD have been non-specific and overlapping, and therapeutic decisions have not varied with exact diagnosis or disease location. However, with the advent of several ostensibly more disease-specific therapies, differentiation of UC from CD, as well as the assortment of disease subgroups, has been much more clinically relevant.

In the past the diagnosis of IBD has relied largely on patient history and physical examination, radiographic and endoscopic findings, and standard laboratory parameters.

Some of these diagnostic tools may be costly, can be invasive, and sometimes pose significant risks. For many patients the process of refining a diagnosis can span months or years, sometimes with many of these uncomfortable tests frequently repeated. Fortunately there have been some significant advances in diagnosis and treatment of IBD, including experienced endoscopists, histopathologists, and the new serological markers of inflammation.

CROHN'S DISEASE

Based on epidemiological data a young Caucasian North American or Western European patient presenting with diarrhoea, anorexia, weight loss, abdominal pain, fever, and an abdominal mass would be quite likely to have CD. If such a patient were female, other suggestive findings could include infertility and/or menstrual irregularities. Unlike the situation in mucosal UC, gross bleeding is much less common in CD (although it can sometimes occur). Prominent abdominal pain is more likely to occur in CD than in UC. CD is a remitting and relapsing disorder with a wide range of clinical manifestations. In approximately 40% of patients with CD the disease is limited to the small intestine[3]. From 10% to 30% of patients will have disease affecting the colon exclusively[3]. This latter group of patients often presents the greatest diagnostic challenge in terms of differentiating CD from UC. Disease behaviour in CD can be characterized as fibrostenotic, penetrating, inflammatory and/or 'ulcerative colitis-like'. In ileal disease, unless very deep ulcers are present, visible haematochezia is uncommon. As suggested above, the epidemiology of presentation is quite important. CD tends to affect younger patients, although it can appear at any age. It is much more common in certain ethnic groups, e.g. patients of Jewish background. It has been identified less frequently in Asians, Africans, and African Americans, although the incidence of IBD in these groups seems to be on the rise.

Overall, CD is diagnosed using clinical signs and symptoms, by endoscopic findings, by X-rays, and by the judicious use of pathology from endoscopic biopsies and from resected intestinal segments. Physical examination can be most helpful in the diagnosis of CD, beginning with general evaluation for signs of ill-health and wasting. Careful perianal examination may identify potentially diagnostic indolent fissures, succulent violaceous tags, and fistulas that are so characteristic of this disease.

In CD the types of lesions, as well as the location(s) of disease involvement, may affect clinical presentation, diagnostic approach and treatments prescribed. Lesions may be classified as diffuse, focal or segmental, and each can be associated with a range of complications. Diffuse inflammation can produce fissures, deep ulcerations and pseudopolyps, and can produce a 'cobblestone' appearance. Pseudopolyps rarely can be sufficiently large to cause partial obstructions and bleeding. Diffuse lesions can thicken the bowel wall, disturb motility, and occasionally result in toxic dilation. Focal lesions may progress to the development of sinus and fistulous tracts, as well as abscesses. Segmental lesions may lead to luminal narrowing, stricture formation and perforation.

Endoscopy can be extremely useful in the diagnosis of CD. Tiny aphthoid lesions may be the earliest manifestation of disease, often surrounded by a red halo[4]. Later in the course of the disease, ulceration is the dominant finding in CD. Ulcers may range from tiny to extensive, and they may be serpiginous and have nodular borders. Radiological signs of CD are many and varied. Some important radiographic findings include strictures, internal fistulas, and the X-ray counterparts of the ulcerations seen at endoscopy[5].

Biopsies taken in suspected CD should be multiple and from areas of normal mucosal appearance, as well as maximally abnormal mucosa. Granulomas can be helpful if present, and other important findings include transmural extension of inflammation and discontinuity of the inflammatory infiltrate[6]. Ischaemia and CD need to be differentiated, but ischaemia usually involves a single segment of intestine, commonly the splenic flexure. Ischaemic bowel disease frequently can be diagnosed by the characteristic history of sudden pain followed by bloody diarrhoea and by unique endoscopic and radiological features.

Since CD was initially perceived to be a disorder of the terminal ileum, and since this is the segment typically involved and often resected if surgical intervention is required, diagnosis of ileal CD is quite important. High-pressure peristaltic contractions predominate in the normal ileum, in irritable bowel syndrome sufferers, and presumably in CD[7]. Such contractions may have some role in CD pathophysiology, possibly directly related to the pathogenesis of typical cramping abdominal pain. Ileal absorptive function is also important, and loss of ileal reabsorption of bile acids contributes to diarrhoea characteristic of small intestinal CD. Unfortunately there is little apparent correlation between the gross (or endoscopic) appearance of the ileum and the nature or extent of symptoms[8]. Nevertheless, both symptoms and morphology have important roles in the diagnosis of IBD, including CD.

Scintigraphy using ^{99m}Tc-HMPAO, ^{111}In-labelled human polyclonal immunoglobulin G (^{111}In-IgG) and other tags have been studied in attempts to localize inflammation using relatively non-invasive technologies. Some results have been promising versus the more invasive procedures traditionally employed in IBD diagnosis[9]. Positron emission tomography (PET) using fluorine-18-fluoro-deoxyglucose (FDG) has also been evaluated as an alternative to conventional studies in identification and localization of active intestinal inflammation. While PET scanning and scintigraphy are unlikely to replace conventional studies, they may be useful when endoscopy is not feasible[10].

The Crohn's Disease Activity Index (CDAI)[11] has sometimes been a component of CD assessment, particularly in clinical trials. However, the CDAI is more useful in following disease course than in initial diagnostic evaluation. It is now widely acknowledged that this empirically derived index is flawed as a measure of disease state, and it is even less well suited to providing differential diagnostic information. However, it does focus on some of the common signs and symptoms in CD. Such features include abdominal pain and tenderness (usually in the right iliac fossa), the presence of an abdominal mass, perianal disease (especially fistulas), diarrhoea (as measured by the use of antidiarrhoeal medications), and fever. Other aspects of the CDAI include anaemia, weight loss, and loss of general well-being. Thus, although there seems to be no role for the general use of the CDAI in clinical practice, familiarity with its components can be helpful as a guide to the clinician evaluating CD patients. Many other clinical observations can point towards the diagnosis and staging of CD. Borborygmi and/or abdominal distension may be present, more likely in advanced disease with small bowel obstructive elements. Extraintestinal IBD manifestations may provide very important clues to the diagnosis of CD. Dermatological lesions, arthropathies, ophthalmic conditions and hepatobiliary diseases are common in association with CD. Haematological, thrombotic and neurological disorders sometimes accompany CD.

Traditionally, the diagnosis of CD has relied on clinical characteristics and disease behaviour. New serological tests, however, are now available which potentially might facilitate and expedite the diagnostic process. While there has been some variation in reports of the diagnostic value of these tests, differences in detection methodology and population characteristics are presumably responsible for reported dissimilarities. Recently, serum immune markers have been used in clinical settings to characterize subgroups of patients with UC and CD.

Antibody to *Saccharomyces cerevisiae* (ASCA) has been found in sera of up to 79% of CD patients[12]. The specificity of the ASCA response versus other antigen markers such as *Candida albicans* antibodies is strong evidence against generalized enhanced permeability as an explanation for the presence of this antibody in CD. Sendid *et al.* demonstrated that yeast cell wall phosphopeptidomannans were the epitopes responsible for the antigenic reactivity demonstrated by ASCA[+] CD sera[13]. Mannans are believed to be the major antigenic component of yeast cell walls and are an important antigenic constituent of mycobacteria and other microorganisms[14]. The clinical significance of ASCA expression in CD is not thoroughly defined; however, recently published reports suggest potential relationships to disease pathogenesis. Darroch *et al.* demonstrated that soluble preparations of *S. cerevisiae* can induce *in-vitro* lymphoproliferative responses, similar to known recall antigens[15]. Taylor *et al.* described association of ASCA with the tumour necrosis factor (TNF) microsatellite haplotype, a11b4c1d3e3, in IBD patients. It is thought that a gene related to ASCA expression resides on chromosome 6 within the MHC, in the vicinity of this TNF haplotype, and that a mutation located on the haplotype contributes to ASCA expression[16]. Combined, these findings suggest that serum ASCA expression reflects a specific mucosal immune-mediated response.

There are some definite clinical correlations between ASCA status and CD. For example, the presence of ASCA, particularly high levels of ASCA, seems to be a marker for early age of disease onset, longer disease duration, and the combination of small bowel and colonic CD involvement[17]. Distinct disease behaviours have also been associated, such as the development of fibrostenosis and penetrating inflammation. In addition, ASCA expression seems to predict the requirement for more frequent surgery episodes among patients with CD.

ASCA-expressing CD patients can be further subdivided by immunoglobulin isotype status, i.e. IgA or IgG. The type of ASCA, as well as the amount expressed, is associated with specific disease manifestations. For example, both IgG and IgA ASCA at high levels, in individuals that do *not* express antineutrophil cytoplasmic antibodies (ANCA), are associated with a more aggressive form of CD. Other potentially important pairings of disease manifestations and serum markers have also been postulated, including prediction of response to specific immunomodulatory therapies.

ANCA, autoantibodies directed against intracellular components of neutrophils, are present in the sera of most patients with UC (see below) and ANCA antibodies have also been detected in a clinically distinct subpopulation of patients with CD. CD patients expressing pANCA have clinical features of left-sided colitis associated with endoscopic and/or histopathological features typical of UC[18]. This 'ulcerative colitis-like' phenotype has been confirmed in several CD populations[19-21]. Additionally, the serum immunoglobulin G (IgG) subclass profile of pANCA[+] CD is similar to that seen in UC[22]. Thus, in CD, the presence of serum pANCA suggests a mucosal inflammatory process similar to pANCA[+] subgroups of UC. Although incompletely defined, there may be significant therapeutic implications for serological differentiation including ASCA and ANCA and other markers, particularly with refinement of the therapeutic armamentarium in the new century ahead.

ULCERATIVE COLITIS

UC, like CD, is a disease of completely unknown aetiology that affects varying segments of the colonic mucosa. Similar to CD, UC is most likely to start in adolescence, although onset can be at any age. UC is found predominantly in Western, industrialized countries. Although genetic predisposition may have more influence in CD, familial patterns are present in both. Principal UC symptoms include diarrhoea with frequent small-volume stools, tenesmus, faecal incontinence, and gross rectal bleeding. Although less commonly than in CD, some UC patients will demonstrate abdominal pain, anorexia, and weight loss. Symptom severity may correlate with the length and intensity of colonic inflammation. UC nomenclature is based on the proximal extent of visibly inflamed colonic mucosa; e.g. proctitis, left-sided colitis, and pancolitis. Systemic symptoms complicating UC include fever, tachycardia and fatigue, along with immune-mediated extraintestinal manifestations including arthritis, pyoderma gangrenosum, erythema nodosum, iritis, and sclerosing cholangitis. Genetic predilection may immunologically prime patients to disease activation by one or more environmental stimuli.

UC often emerges acutely, but a more subtle and gradual onset can also occur. Recurrent symptomatic flares frequently characterize this illness. Commonest manifestations are diarrhoea, rectal bleeding, and tenesmus. Rectal bleeding is a cardinal characteristic of UC (although not universally present). With disease progression, bloody stools often intensify and may involve purulent exudate intermixed with faeces. Tenesmus is extremely common in UC, often coexisting with incontinence. Rectal symptoms as well as other symptoms of UC often persist following endoscopic remission. If onset of UC is more subtle and insidious, vague discomfort and diarrhoea may gradually progress until the disease becomes overt with passage of grossly bloody stools. Within 1 month of symptom onset, 40% of patients will manifest maximally severe disease. Although severity of symptoms partially depends on the extent of active colitis, it is difficult to be certain of the mucosal distribution of disease at onset unless complete endoscopic assessment is undertaken.

Severe adverse clinical outcomes include disability, hospitalization, immediate surgery or death, and these still cannot dependably be predicted in patients presenting with IBD. Symptomatic and laboratory findings can suggest outcome, and these parameters often correlate with the gastrointestinal and systemic physiological changes of mucosal inflammation. In most instances endoscopy to the splenic flexure should be sufficient to determine disease severity since the great majority of patients with severe endoscopic colitis have maximally abnormal endoscopic findings in the descending colon or more distally. Although classical dogma described maximal UC severity in the distal colon, it is now known that some patients have more intense inflammation proximally. Proximal severity seems particularly likely in recipients of rectal therapy that favourably modifies distal disease while more proximal mucosal abnormalities persist. If more than 10% of the colonic mucosal surface is involved with active colitis, clinical course may be more severe than with lesser involvement. Regardless of disease extent, systemic symptoms of abdominal pain, fever and severe malaise undoubtedly are directly related to quantitative cytokine release[23].

Sigmoidoscopy is the most useful initial test in the assessment of suspected UC, and granularity and friability are the hallmarks of this disease[24]. Other common endoscopic findings include blunted or absent valve edges and signs of diffuse symmetric and continuous inflammation with rectal involvement[25]. As noted in sections below, there can be striking exceptions to most of the formerly unquestioned 'rules' regarding rectal activity and patchiness of inflammatory changes. Biopsies taken from suspected cases of UC should be sampled from involved and uninvolved areas, and the most typical histological finding is the crypt abscess and the presence of irregularly shaped and branched crypt distortion[26].

Classically, estimation of clinical disease severity has been based on symptoms and selected laboratory tests, defined by Truelove and Witts[27]. A subsequent Oxford modification of this scale uses the number of bowel motions and one or more laboratory parameters to provide improved disease categorization versus the five original criteria[28]. Several of the nuances of IBD pathophysiology must be considered in this definition of disease severity. Bloody diarrhoea presumably correlates closely with degree of mucosal injury, and bleeding is usually the central feature for estimation of disease severity. Fever and tachycardia may accompany cytokine release from colonic inflammation and/or associated systemic infection, a complication that increases morbidity and mortality in UC. Diarrhoea in UC rarely causes dehydration solely based on intestinal fluid loss, but UC patients may become dehydrated due to the combination of anorexia and fever-driven fluid loss with their diarrhoea. Anaemia develops as a result of acute and chronic blood loss, along with suppressed haematopoiesis of chronic illness. Erythrocyte sedimentation rates beyond 30 mm/h indicate a systemic response to colonic inflammation. Hypoalbuminaemia, often seen in advanced IBD, is a multifactorial laboratory finding highly predictive of serious disease. Intestinal albumin loss correlates with the severity of colonic inflammation, and albumin synthesis can be suppressed as evinced by prealbumin decrements with severe disease[29].

Radiological evidence for severe disease includes dilation of the colonic lumen to more than 5 cm in diameter and/or irregularity of the mucosal surface outlined by gas on a plain abdominal film[30]. Double-contrast barium enema was the original classical technique for diagnosis of UC, now largely supplanted by endoscopy. When performed, contrast radiology is now primarily used to attempt to differentiate UC from CD[31]. Carbonnel et al.[23] described endoscopic criteria for severity including extensive deep ulcerations, mucosal detachment on the edge of these ulcerations, well-like ulcerations and extensive mucosal abrasions. Severe radiographic and/or endoscopic changes may predict the need for surgical intervention.

UC epidemiology and therapeutic responses may have shifted over time, as seen with data from three studies performed over different decades. Jalan et al.[32] described 399 UC patients, 180 assessed at initial disease presentation. Of these, 35% had severe colitis, and 30% underwent colectomy. Gross mortality improved over time, even within these decades of 1950–67. Sinclair et al.[33] described 537 patients seen between 1967 and 1976. Only 33 of these patients had severe colitis, and there was a 29% colectomy rate. Travis et al.[34] summarized courses of 49 patients during 1992–93, all severe and 16 during their initial attack. This series had a 19% colectomy rate. Even today, patients with aggressive and severe UC are likely to require hospitalization and/or surgical intervention. This includes early colectomy, particularly in patients with pancolitis early in their disease course. Despite study design variances over the years, it appears that 20–30% of patients with an initial acute, severe presentation will ultimately require colectomy. Dramatic improvement in mortality has occurred with advances in overall medical management. Disease progression has been summarized in several studies[34–39]. While >20% of patients have only one episode of colitis, <8% have unremitting disease. It seems likely that many patients with a single episode of colitis may actually have had some unrecognized infectious colitis. Langholz *et al.*[39] described patients with initial active disease, fever, and weight loss who responded to medical management with resulting sustained remission. These results do not agree with our concept of UC as a chronic and invariably relapsing disease.

Many prospective studies of UC report frequent disease extension such as the evolution of proctitis or left-sided colitis to pancolitis. However, historical limitations in diagnostic technology may have blurred the differentiation of distal and more proximal disease. Farmer *et al.*[36] published the most detailed epidemiological study specifically addressing disease extension, postulating that at least 20% of UC patients would have an extension of colon involvement at some time during their illness. This study demonstrated an adjusted odds ratio of 14.8 for extension of mucosal involvement in severe left-sided colitis or proctitis. Forty-six per cent of patients with proctitis had disease extension, and 70% with left-sided colitis extended their disease. Direct visualization using modern endoscopic techniques should further clarify issues related to initial localization of disease in UC and to the progression of disease extent[39].

The natural course of UC fluctuates between relapses and exacerbations. The need for maintenance therapy to prevent relapse was established as early as 1965[40]. A study of 112 patients with long-term access to maintenance medication found that 39% had more than one relapse a year, 53% had only one relapse a year, and only 8% were in remission for the entire 7-year study period[41]. Chronicity of disease is a central diagnostic feature.

In ulcerative proctitis, visible inflammation is limited to the rectum. Thirty per cent of patients with UC present with ulcerative proctitis, and such individuals usually have a relatively benign disease course. Proctitis usually produces limited systemic symptoms, but there are certainly many 'local' complaints related to inflamed rectal mucosa. Typical proctitis commonly causes vague lower abdominal or pelvic pain, a feeling of rectal discomfort, tenesmus and tenderness with rectal examination. Abnormal laboratory tests such as those found with extensive intestinal inflammation are unusual in proctitis, and the finding of such indices suggests that disease has extended more proximally. Differences in initial presentation, clinical course and related divergences in response to treatment indicate that ulcerative proctitis may represent a different disease entity than more extensive UC.

A positive family history for IBD is a very helpful historical clue for initially diagnosing IBD in a patient presenting for the first time with chronic diarrhoea. Exogenous factors known to precipitate IBD are also risk factors for relapses[42]. Aspirin and non-steroidal anti-inflammatory drugs (NSAID) may produce an

IBD-like illness and/or induce IBD relapse[43–46]. NSAID exacerbation of IBD occurs as a result of: (1) decreased prostaglandin production, (2) inhibition of oxidative phosphorylation, (3) selective inhibition of fatty oxidation in colonocytes, (4) direct chemical mucosal injury throughout the gastrointestinal tract, and/or (5) production of increased intestinal permeability and consequent exposure to luminal antigens. Changes in intestinal permeability may be the most important aspect of NSAID in IBD pathogenesis, since increased permeability allows induction of the immunoregulatory processes known to be abnormal in IBD. Non-enteric infections, including respiratory infections, have been related to activation of colitis. Up-regulation of the immune system in response to systemic infections may also activate the gastrointestinal immune system, thus exacerbating UC. Enteric infections induce gastrointestinal immune function in order to eradicate the offending organism, but there can also be unwanted amplification of immune response and consequent exacerbation of UC[47]. Antibiotics have also been associated with symptomatic relapses of UC, presumably by unfavourably altering gut flora and antigenic stimulation. Smoking cessation is another relatively recently recognized environmental association with UC flares[48].

Gender differences in IBD have not been recognized in large epidemiological studies[33,36,39]. However, oral contraceptive use has been proposed as a possible risk factor for both UC and CD. For many years psychological stress has been thought to represent an important contributing factor to disease symptoms. Resurgent interest in the 'molecular' role of stress in IBD has followed recognition of the importance of the enteric nervous system in gastrointestinal immunology[49].

Diagnostic tests to identify treatable infectious diseases that mimic IBD should always be performed initially. Although most enteric infections have definite acute-onset and clinical courses, some intestinal infections can last for weeks to months. In acute IBD and with relapses, faecal leucocytes, eosinophils, and Charcot–Leyden crystals can be assessed, and their presence may correlate with colonic inflammation. Urinalysis may provide a marker for dehydration due to diarrhoea, fever, and impaired fluid intake. Blood tests including complete blood counts, chemistries and indices of inflammation (e.g., erythrocyte sedimentation rate, C-reactive protein) can be useful in delineating disease severity and for differentiation of IBD from functional bowel disorders. Recently, more sophisticated serological tests have been developed that can provide useful data regarding the diagnosis and characteristics of UC.

As presented above, serum immune markers seem to differentiate subgroups of patients with UC and CD. ANCA autoantibodies directed against intracellular components of neutrophils are present in the sera of most patients with UC. ANCA expression in UC permits stratification at the mucosal, clinical, and genetic levels, and has been associated with distinct clinical subgroups[50–57]. UC-associated ANCA exhibits perinuclear highlighting (pANCA) on indirect immunofluorescent (IIF) microscopy. Vidrich et al. have demonstrated that the pANCA of UC is DNAase-sensitive; i.e. neutrophils lose the characteristic perinuclear IIF staining pattern when pretreated with DNAase[58]. *Serum* pANCA is thought to reflect *mucosal* pANCA production, presumably involving disease-related recognition of mucosal antigen(s) and local production of pANCA[50]. Clinically, pANCA in UC appears to be associated with: (1) treatment-resistant left-sided disease[51]; (2) an aggressive disease course[52,53]; (3) surgery early in the course of disease[54]; and (4) the development of pouchitis following ileal pouch–anal anastomosis (IPAA)[55–57]. Genetic studies have demonstrated that ANCA expression allows stratification of subpopulations of UC along with the presence of specific HLA markers[59–61].

Histological evaluation of endoscopic biopsies is important in distinguishing UC from CD and in identifying other causes of inflammation. For example, rectal CD must be distinguished from solitary rectal ulcer syndrome. *Clostridium difficile* leads to acute and severe colitis in patients with or without IBD. Typical *C. difficile* colitis histology includes 'volcanic'-appearing eruption of inflammatory cells from the mucosa. Because *C. difficile* may be an important cause of colitis, recognition of the histological characteristics of *C. difficile* selects patients for treatment with metronidazole or vancomycin. Identification of ischaemia is also important in the management of patients with suspected IBD, particularly in elderly patients who present with acute colitis. This can be accomplished with judicious use of clinical, radiographic, and histological data. Unlike UC and CD, acute self-limiting colitis does not cause crypt distortion that is typical in chronic IBD. Dense eosinophilic infiltration can be a prominent feature of IBD histology. Less frequently seen, but very important in the assessment of IBD biopsy histopathology, is dysplasia, best sought in the absence of active inflammation. When present in the setting of chronic IBD, dysplasia should lead to prophylactic colectomy in order to avert development of advanced colon malignancy.

DIFFERENTIAL DIAGNOSIS IN IBD

It is essential that UC should be distinguished from infective colitis, and it seems philosophically appropriate to attempt to separate UC from CD. UC ordinarily presents with a history of disease duration sufficient to eliminate most confounding infections. Despite this caution, infectious diseases ordinarily considered to have a short natural history may be prolonged. Several cases of *Campylobacter jejuni* epidemic diarrhoea have lasted weeks rather than the usual 3–7 days. Chronic *Clostridium difficile* and *Aeromonas hydrophilus* infections also rarely mimic UC. General principles for distinguishing infectious colitis from UC include the usual acute course of infectious colitis and the classical histological changes of distorted crypt architecture and basal plasmacytosis that favour UC[62]. Crohn's colitis occasionally may be quite difficult to differentiate from UC. Extraintestinal manifestations of IBD seem to occur more frequently in CD, but this is insufficient for a specific diagnosis. Endoscopically oedematous mucosa with typical linear ulceration may not be present early in the clinical course of CD. Crohn's proctitis is rare, but this presentation can occur, and it may sometimes be confused with solitary rectal ulcer syndrome or with conventional ulcerative proctitis. Biological markers such as pANCA or ASCA may help distinguish UC from CD, but current information is probably not yet adequate to support universal clinical application of these tests. Complications of IBD either may relate to the gut or may be systemic. Massive haemorrhage, toxic megacolon and perforation are extremely severe complications that may occur early in the course of UC or with acute relapses. Strictures, carcinoma of the colon, sclerosing cholangitis and cholangiocarcinoma are complications associated with chronic disease.

EVOLVING CLINICAL PATTERNS OF IBD

Although diagnostic separation of UC and CD was always considered important, the disorders have often seemed to merge in clinical practice. Improved diagnostic approaches at earlier stages of disease have changed our perceptions of the complex interrelationships between these similar illnesses. Until the colonoscopy era, Crohn's colitis was not always easily recognized. However, its incidence seems to be growing rapidly, perhaps in part because of the widened application of endoscopy and biopsy. More frequent colonoscopy examinations, often performed in the setting of clinical trials such as those related to the use of mesalamine in left-sided UC, led to the discovery of the 'caecal patch'. This was an area of overt inflammation in the caecum of patients who otherwise had proctitis or other left-sided colitis by all criteria. Such a pattern is now accepted as consistent with UC and an incidental patch of caecal inflammation. Previously such a finding might have been interpreted as a 'skip area' indicating Crohn's colitis. It is now well accepted that UC may be worse proximally, a view not accepted by gastrointestinal specialists in the recent past. Such non-homogeneous inflammation in UC has now been documented in numerous clinical trials. Future studies, particularly those employing newly available serological markers, are quite likely to provide better guidelines for defining prognostically important IBD subgroups.

Despite mounting evidence for the utility of ANCA and ASCA, the topic remains controversial, and many clinicians have not yet adopted use of these tests. Nevertheless, the concept that advanced serological testing should lead to improved therapy seems extremely attractive. To date, most studies in adult populations have been performed retrospectively, through chart review and analysis. To provide the most accurate assessment of the absolute diagnostic potential of these serum immune markers they merit carefully planned large prospective studies of new patients with UC and CD. With improved diagnostic accuracy, therapeutic success should parallel discrimination of important IBD subpopulations. Refinements in therapy will certainly continue to evolve. Ever-improving treatment options almost certainly will also lead to identification of large numbers of patients with 'subclinical' IBD. Such patients also may receive substantial benefits from the application of enhanced therapeutic modalities. Thus, IBD diagnosis will continue to be an area of challenges, rapid evolution, and clinical importance.

References

1. Crohn BB, Ginzburg G, Oppenheimer GD. Regional ileitis: a pathologic and clinical entity. J Am Med Assoc 1932;99:1323–9.
2. Nugent FW, Kolack PF. Differential diagnosis of chronic ulcerative colitis and Crohn's disease of the colon. In: Kirsner JB, Shorter RG, editors. Inflammatory Bowel Disease. Philadelphia, PA: Lea & Febiger; 1988:194 6.

3. Farmer RG, Hawk WA, Turnbull RB, Jr. Clinical patterns in Crohn's disease: a statistical study of 615 cases. Gastroenterology 1975;68:627–35.
4. Watier A, Devroede G, Perey B *et al.* Small erythematous mucosal plaques: an endoscopic sign of Crohn's disease. Gut 1984;21:835–9.
5. Lichtenstein JE. Radiologic pathologic correlation of inflammatory bowel disease. Radiol Clin N Am 1987;25:3–24.
6. Tytgat GNJ. Inflammatory bowel disease. Aspects of differential diagnosis. In: Rachmilewitz D, editor. Inflammatory Bowel Diseases 1986. Dordrecht: Martinus Nijhoff; 1986:105–14.
7. Philips SF, Quigley EE, Kumar D, Kamath PS. Motility and ileocolonic function. Gut 1980;29:390–406.
8. Rutgeerts P, Geboes G, Vantrappen G, Beyls J, Keiremans R, Hiele M. Predictability of the postoperative course of Crohn's disease. Gastroenterology 1990;99:956–63.
9. Bianconi L, Scopinaro F, Ierardi M *et al.* 99mTc-HMPAO granulocyte scintigraphy in the early detection of postoperative asymptomatic recurrence in Crohn's disease. Dig Dis Sci 1997;42:1549–56.
10. Jacobson K, Mernagh JR, Green T *et al.* Positron emission tomography in the investigation of pediatric inflammatory bowel disease. Gastroenterology 1999;116:G223.
11. Best WR, Bektel JM, Singleton JW, Kern F, Development of a Crohn's disease activity index: National Cooperative Crohn's Disease Study. Gastroenterology 1976;70:439–44.
12. Barclay GR, McKenzie H, Pennington J, Parratt D, Pennington CR. The effect of dietary yeast on the activity of stable chronic Crohn's disease. Scand J Gastroenterol Suppl 1992;27:196–200.
13. Sendid B, Colombel, JF, Jacquinot PM *et al.* Specific antibody response to oligomannosidic epitopes in Crohn's disease. Clin Diagn Lab Immunol 1996;3:219–26.
14. McKenzie H, Main J, Pennington CR, Parratt D. Antibody to selected strains of *Saccharomyces cerevisiae* (baker's and brewer's yeast) and *Candida albicans* in Crohn's disease. Gut 1990;31:536–8.
15. Darroch CJ, Christmas SE, Barnes RM. *In vitro* human lymphocyte proliferative responses to a glycoprotein of the yeast *Saccharomyces cerevisiae*. Immunology 1994;81:247–52.
16. Taylor KD, Li Z, Barry M *et al.* Tumor necrosis factor microsatellite haplotype A11B4C1D3E3 is associated with anti-*Saccharomyces cerevisiae* antibody (ASCA) across clinical forms of inflammatory bowel disease. Gastroenterology 1998;114:A1098.
17. Vasiliauska EA, Plevy SE, Targan SR. Stratification of Crohn's disease by antineutrophil cytoplasmic antibodies (ANCA) and anti-*Saccharomyces cerevisiae* antibody (ASCA) distinguishes phenotypic subgroups. Gastroenterology 1997;112:1112.
18. Vasiliauskas EA, Plevy SE, Landers CJ *et al.* Perinuclear antineutrophil cytoplasmic antibodies in patients with Crohn's disease define a clinical subgroup. Gastroenterology 1996;110:1810–19.
19. Satsangi J, Landers CJ, Welsh KI, Koss K, Targan SR, Jewell DP. The presence of anti-neutrophil antibodies reflects clinical and genetic heterogeneity within inflammatory bowel disease. Inflamm Bowel Dis 1998;4:18–26.
20. Ruemmele FM, Targan SR, Levy G, Dubinsky M, Braun J, Seidman EG. Diagnostic accuracy of novel serological assays in pediatric inflammatory bowel disease. Gastroenterology 1998;115:822–9.
21. Freeman HJ. Atypical perinuclear antineutrophil cytoplasmic antibodies (p-ANCA) in patients with Crohn's disease. Gastroenterology 1998;114:A979.
22. Plevy SE, Landers CJ, Vasiliauskas EA, Targan SR, Vidrich A. Alterations in serum immunoglobulin (Ig) G subclasses provide evidence for distinct immune responses in pANCA positive Crohn's disease patients. Gastroenterology 1996;110:A993.
23. Carbonnel F, Lavergne A, Lemann M *et al.* Colonoscopy in acute colitis: a safe and reliable tool for assessment of severity. Dig Dis Sci 1994;39:1550–7.
24. Hogan WJ, Hensley GJ, Geenen JE. Endoscopic evaluation of inflammatory bowel disease. Med Clin N Am 1980;64:1083–102.
25. Waye JD, Hunt RH. Colonoscopic diagnosis of inflammatory bowel disease. Surg Clin N Am 1982;62:905–13.
26. Goldman H. Acute vs. chronic colitis: how and when to distinguish by biopsy. Gastroenterology 1984;86:199–201.
27. Truelove SC, Witts LJ. Cortisone in ulcerative colitis: final report on a therapeutic trial. Br Med J 1955;2:1041–8.

28. Gallagher ND, Goulston SSM, Wyndham N, Morrow W. The management of fulminant ulcerative colitis. Gut 1962;3:306–11.
29. Buckell NA, Lennard-Jones JE, Hernandez MA, Kohn J, Riches PG, Wadsworth J. Measurement of serum proteins during attacks of ulcerative colitis as a guide to patient management. Gut 1979;20:22–7.
30. Buckell NA, Williams GT, Bartram CI, Lennard-Jones JE. Depth of ulceration in acute colitis: correlation with outcomes and clinical and radiologic features. Gastroenterology 1980;79:19–25.
31. Kelvin FM, Oddson TA, Rice RP *et al.* Double contrast barium enema in Crohn's disease and ulcerative colitis. Am J Roentgenol 1981;137:207–13.
32. Jalan KN, Prescott RJ, Sircus W *et al.* An experience of ulcerative colitis: II. Short term outcome. Gastroenterology 1970;59:589–609.
33. Sinclair TS, Brunt PW, Mowat NAG. Nonspecific proctocolitis in northeastern Scotland: a community study. Gastroenterology 1983;85:1–11.
34. Travis SPL, Farrant JM, Ricketts C *et al.* Predicting outcome in severe ulcerative colitis. Gut 1996;38:905–10.
35. Isgar B, Harman M, Kaye MD, Whorwell PJ. Symptoms of irritable bowel syndrome in ulcerative colitis in remission. Gut 1983;24:190–2.
36. Farmer RG, Easley KA, Rankin GB. Clinical patterns, natural history, and progression of ulcerative colitis: a long-term follow-up of 1116 patients. Dig Dis Sci 1993;38:1137–46.
37. Stonnington CM, Phillips SF, Sinsmeister AR, Melton LJ. Prognosis of chronic ulcerative colitis in a community. Gut 1987;28:1261–6.
38. Leijonmarck CE, Persson PG, Hellers G. Factors affecting colectomy rate in ulcerative colitis: an epidemiologic study. Gut 1990;31:329–33.
39. Langholz E, Munkholm P, Davidsen M, Binder V. Course of ulcerative colitis: analysis of changes in disease activity over years. Gastroenterology 1994;107:3–11.
40. Misiewicz JJ, Lennard-Jones JE, Connell AM, Baron JH, Avery Jones F. Controlled trial of sulphasalazine in maintenance therapy for ulcerative colitis. Lancet 1965;1:185–8.
41. Bresci G, Parisi G, Gambardella L *et al.* Evaluation of clinical patterns in ulcerative colitis: a long-term follow-up. Int J Clin Pharmacol Res 1997;17:17–22.
42. Riley SA, Mani V, Goodman MJ, Lucas S. Why do patients with ulcerative colitis relapse? Gut 1990;31:179–83.
43. Rampton DS, McNeil NI, Sarner M. Analgesic ingestion and other factors preceding relapse in ulcerative colitis. Gut 1983;24:187–9.
44. Evans JMM, McMahon AD, Murray FE, McDevitt, MacDonald TM. Non-steroidal anti-inflammatory drugs are associated with emergency admission to hospital for colitis due to inflammatory bowel disease. Gut 1997;40:619–22.
45. Roediger WEW, Millard S. Selective inhibition of fatty acid oxidation in colonocytes by ibuprofen: a cause of colitis? Gut 1995;36:55–9.
46. Kaufmann HJ, Taubin HL. Nonsteroidal anti-inflammatory drugs activate quiescent inflammatory bowel disease. Ann Intern Med 1987;107:513–16.
47. Newman A, Lambert JR. *Campylobacter jejuni* causing flare-up in inflammatory bowel disease. Lancet 1980;2:919.
48. Fraga XF, Vergara M, Medina C, Casellas F, Bermejo B, Malagelada JR. Effects of smoking on the presentation and clinical course of inflammatory bowel disease. Eur J Gastroenterol Hepatol 1997;9:683–7.
49. Levenstein S, Prantera C, Varvo V *et al.* Psychological stress and disease activity in ulcerative colitis: a multidimensional cross-sectional study. Am J Gastroenterol 1994;89:1219–25.
50. Targan SR, Landers CJ, Cobb L, MacDermott RP, Vidrich A. Perinuclear anti-neutrophil cytoplasmic antibodies are spontaneously produced by mucosal B cells of ulcerative colitis patients. J Immunol 1995;155:3262–7.
51. Sandborn WJ, Landers CJ, Tremaine WJ, Targan SR. Association of antineutrophil cytoplasmic antibodies with resistance to treatment of left sided ulcerative colitis: results of a pilot study. Mayo Clin Proc 1996;71:431–6.
52. Vecchi M, Bianchi MB, Sinico RA *et al.* Antibodies to neutrophil cytoplasm in Italian patients with ulcerative colitis: sensitivity, specificity and recognition of putative antigens. Digestion 1994;55:34–9.
53. Vecchi M, Bianchi MB, Calabresi G, Meucci G, Tatarella M, de Franchis R. Long-term

observation of the perinuclear anti-cytoplasmic antibody status in ulcerative colitis patients. Scand J Gastroenterol 1998;33:170–3.

54. Boerr LA, Sambuelli AM, Katz S *et al.* Clinical heterogeneity of ulcerative colitis in relation to frequency of pANCA reactivity. Gastroenterology 1995;108:A785.

55. Vecchi M, Gionchetti P, Bianchi MB *et al.* p-ANCA and development of pouchitis in ulcerative colitis patients after proctocolectomy and ileoanal pouch anastomosis. Lancet 1994;344:886–7.

56. Patel RT, Stokes R, Birch C, Ibbotson J, Keighley MRB. Influence of total colectomy on serum antineutrophil cytoplasmic antibodies in inflammatory bowel disease. Br J Surg 1994;81:724–6.

57. Sandborn WJ, Landers CJ, Tremaine WJ, Targan SR. Antineutrophil cytoplasmic antibody correlates with chronic pouchitis after ileal pouch–anal anastomosis. Am J Gastroenterol 1995;90:740–7.

58. Vidrich A, Lee J, James E, Cobb L, Targan S. Segregation of pANCA antigenic recognition by DNase treatment of neutrophils: ulcerative colitis, type 1 autoimmune hepatitis, and primary sclerosing cholangitis. J Clin Immunol 1995;15:293–9.

59. Toyoda H, Wang SJ, Yang HY *et al.* Distinct associations of HLA class II genes with inflammatory bowel disease. Gastroenterology 1993;104:741–8.

60. Yang HY, Rotter JI, Toyoda H *et al.* Ulcerative colitis: a genetically heterogeneous disorder defined by genetic (HLA class II) and subclinical (antineutrophil cytoplasmic antibodies) markers. J Clin Invest 1993;92:1080–4.

61. Satsangi J, Landers CJ, Welsh KI, Koss K, Targan SR, Jewell DP. The presence of anti-neutrophil antibodies reflects clinical and genetic heterogeneity within inflammatory bowel disease. Inflamm Bowel Dis 1998;4:18–26.

62. Schumacher G, Sandstedt B, Mollby R, Kollberg B. Clinical and histologic features differentiating non-relapsing colitis from first attacks of inflammatory bowel disease. Scand J Gastroenterol 1991;26:151–61.

9
Recent developments in the diagnosis and management of paediatric inflammatory bowel disease

E. G. SEIDMAN, M. DUBINSKY, H. PATRIQUIN,
G. MARX AND Y. THÉORÊT

ABSTRACT

Inflammatory bowel disease (IBD) in the paediatric age group presents many challenges to the health-care team. Research efforts by the Ste Justine Hospital IBD Center in Montreal have led to advances in three areas: (a) serological tests to screen for IBD and to distinguish between forms of colitis, (b) Doppler sonography to demonstrate disease activity, and (c) pharmacogenomics to optimize therapy with azathioprine and 6-mercaptopurine.

(a) In mild cases the non-specific symptoms of IBD may be mistaken for a functional bowel disorder, delaying the diagnosis. Recently, improved serological assays have allowed clinicians to screen for IBD with a high degree of disease specificity. Using a combination of assays to detect circulating perinuclear antineutrophil cytoplasmic antibodies (pANCA) and antibodies to the oligomannosidic epitopes of the dietary yeast *Saccharomyces cerevisiae* (ASCA); we have shown these tests to be highly specific for ulcerative colitis and Crohn's disease, respectively. Double positivity (IgA and IgG) for ASCA was found to be 100% specific for Crohn's disease. When combined with other normal routine laboratory test results (haemoglobin, platelet count, erythrocyte sedimentation rate, serum albumin and iron), negative pANCA and ASCA tests have a very high negative predictive value for IBD.

(b) Not uncommonly, children and adolescents with Crohn's disease manifest few symptoms yet present with anorexia and growth failure. The availability of a non-invasive imaging technique to demonstrate subclinical inflammation in such cases would be of benefit in their management. Intestinal wall vessel density was estimated using colour Doppler sonography. Among a group of 47 children who underwent 61 examinations, affected loops were thicker ($p<0.001$) and vessel density was more frequently moderate or high (2–4, and >5 vessels/cm^2, respectively) in active disease (CDAI >150) compared to quiescent disease. This method is simple to perform in young patients and has the potential for monitoring the course of the disease.

1. The cytotoxic and immunosuppressive properties of 6-mercaptopurine (6-MP) and its parent drug azathioprine (AZA) are mediated via their intracellular conversion to their metabolites: 6-thioguanine (6-TG) nucleotides and 6-methylmercaptopurine (6-MMP) ribonucleotides, the latter mediated via the genetically controlled thiopurine methyltransferase (TPMT) enzymatic pathway. 6-MP metabolite concentrations (pmol/8×10^8 red blood cells were periodically measured by high-performance liquid chromatography assay in 93 paediatric IBD patients receiving 6-MP or AZA for at least 4 months. Therapeutic response was determined by disease activity indices coincidentally with haematological, pancreatic and hepatic laboratory parameters. TPMT mutations were identified by allele-specific oligonucleotide hybridization. Clinical response correlated with erythrocyte 6-TG levels (<0.0001), but not with 6-MMP levels or 6-MP dose. The frequency of therapeutic response significantly increased at 6-TG levels >230 pmol/8×10^8 RBC ($p<0.001$). Hepatotoxicity correlated with high 6-MMP levels ($p<0.05$). Leukopenia was associated with higher 6-TG levels during remission ($p<0.04$). Eight of 93 patients heterozygous for the TPMT allele had higher 6-TG levels ($p<0.0001$), and all responded to therapy, 6-MP metabolite levels and TPMT molecular analysis thus provide clinicians with useful tools for optimizing therapeutic response to 6-MP/AZA and for identifying individuals at increased risk for drug-induced toxicity.

INTRODUCTION

IBD in the paediatric age group presents many challenges to the health-care team. In this report we review the recent clinical research efforts at the Ste Justine Hospital IBD Centre in Montreal, which have led to advances in several areas: (a) the use of serological tests to screen for IBD and to distinguish between forms of colitis; (b) the utilization of Doppler sonography to demonstrate disease activity; (c) the application of pharmacogenomics to optimize therapy with azathioprine and 6-mercaptopurine; and (d) the detection and treatment of osteopenia.

MISSED VERSUS MISDIAGNOSIS OF IBD: THE USE OF NOVEL SEROLOGICAL TESTS

In mild cases the non-specific symptoms of IBD (abdominal pain, diarrhoea, etc.) may be easily mistaken for a functional bowel disorder, thus delaying the diagnosis. This is particularly true for Crohn's disease (CD), in which growth failure, arthralgias, or fever may be the sole presenting complaint, at times in the absence of any gastrointestinal symptoms[1]. In contrast, in most cases of ulcerative colitis (UC), haematochezia generally leads to rapid consultation and a diagnostic colonoscopy. Patients with CD, on the other hand, may complain of insidious abdominal pain, without other more alarming symptoms or signs. The diagnosis of CD in the paediatric age group is thus more often delayed than for UC, not uncommonly for over a year. There is thus a clinical need for accurate non-invasive screening tests for IBD, much like what has been achieved for coeliac disease.

Recently, the clinical utility of novel serological assays in screening for IBD, as well as their ability to discriminate between types of IBD, has been the subject of considerable research[2]. Perinuclear antineutrophil cytoplasmic autoantibodies (pANCA) have become established as a marker of UC. More recently, antibodies to oligomannosidic epitopes of the yeast *Saccharomyces cerevisiae* (ASCA) have been the focus of much interest as a marker of CD. Using serological testing for both pANCA and ASCA (Table 1), we have shown that these tests are highly specific for UC and CD, respectively[3]. Double positivity (IgA and IgG) for ASCA was found to be 100% specific for paediatric CD in this series[3].

One of the beneficial uses of these tests is to assist the clinician in distinguishing between UC and CD when the disease is restricted to the colon. CD is usually readily diagnosed by routine clinical, endoscopic, radiological and histological criteria, when the involvement of the colon is non-homogeneous, or if the disease extends into the proximal gastrointestinal tract or small bowel. Diffuse or homogeneous colitis, on the other hand, while typical of UC, may be seen at times in patients with CD. The precise classification of these entities becomes clinically very relevant if surgery is being contemplated. CD patients with an

Table 1 Predictive value of serological tests for IBD in the paediatric age group

Test	Interpretation	
	Crohn's disease	*Ulcerative colitis*
ELISA-based		
ASCA		
positive	Possible*	N/A
negative	Not excluded	N/A
ANCA		
positive	Not excluded	Likely*
negative	N/A	Not excluded
Complete assays		
ASCA		
IgG positive	Likely	N/A
IgA positive	Likely	N/A
Both positive	Highly probable	N/A
pANCA		
positive	Not excluded	Highly probable

ASCA = Anti-*Saccharomyces cerevesiae* antibodies, ANCA = antineutrophil cytoplasmic antibodies, pANCA = perinuclear ANCA.
*ELISA-based tests, if positive, should be confirmed by complete assay testing.

'ulcerative colitis-like' presentation may also be pANCA-positive[2–4]. Therefore, only the presence of ASCA can truly be considered specific for CD. In a recent study by Quinton *et al.*, pANCA-negative/ASCA-positive results were 97% specific and had a 96% positive predictive value for CD, whereas pANCA-positive/ASCA-negative assays were 97% specific and were 92.5% predictive value-positive for UC[5]. In view of the disparate prognosis after colectomy in ulcerative versus Crohn's colitis, the reported data suggest that ASCA and pANCA testing should be carried out prior to elective 'curative' surgery for UC.

As noted above, in many cases the diagnosis of IBD is delayed in children and adolescents due to their non-specific presenting complaints. Reliable screening tests would be potentially helpful in these circumstances, expediting the diagnosis and treatment. Furthermore, a high negative predictive value of serological tests would potentially avoid unnecessary, more invasive and costly testing (colonoscopy, barium studies of the small bowel). A recent study in adults reported that the negative predictive value of ASCA for CD was 94.5%. In terms of paediatric patients we have found that pANCA and ASCA testing can also be useful in terms of screening for possible IBD in patients with non-specific symptoms and a normal physical examination. As illustrated in Figure 1, when combined in series with five other routine laboratory test results (haemoglobin, platelet count, erythrocyte sedimentation rate, serum albumin and iron), negative pANCA and ASCA tests can be useful adjunctive tests to screen for possible IBD. Our recent data using this combined approach[6] suggest that ELISA-based pANCA and ASCA testing can help clinicians 'rule out' IBD in patients with functional bowel disorders, without subjecting patients to more invasive testing, such as complete colonoscopy and barium studies of the upper gastrointestinal tract and small bowel. The incorporation of sequential non-invasive testing into such a diagnostic strategy (Figure 1) may thus avoid unnecessary and costly evaluations, and facilitate clinical decision-making when the diagnosis of IBD in children is initially uncertain.

DOPPLER SONOGRAPHY TO DETECT DISEASE ACTIVITY IN CD

Not uncommonly, children and adolescents with CD manifest few symptoms, yet are found to have anorexia and growth failure[1,7]. The availability of a non-invasive imaging technique to demonstrate subclinical inflammation in such cases would be of benefit in their management. Active CD is associated with neovascularization, perhaps in response to increased angiogenesis growth factor release. We carried out a study to estimate intestinal wall vessel density as a function of disease activity, using pulsed colour Doppler sonography[8]. Among the group of paediatric patients with CD, affected bowel loops were found to be thicker ($p<0.001$). Vessel density was more frequently moderate or high (2–4, and >5 vessels/cm^2, respectively) in active, compared to quiescent disease (Table 2).

This method is simple to perform in young patients and has the potential for non-invasive monitoring of the course of the disease. Doppler sonography

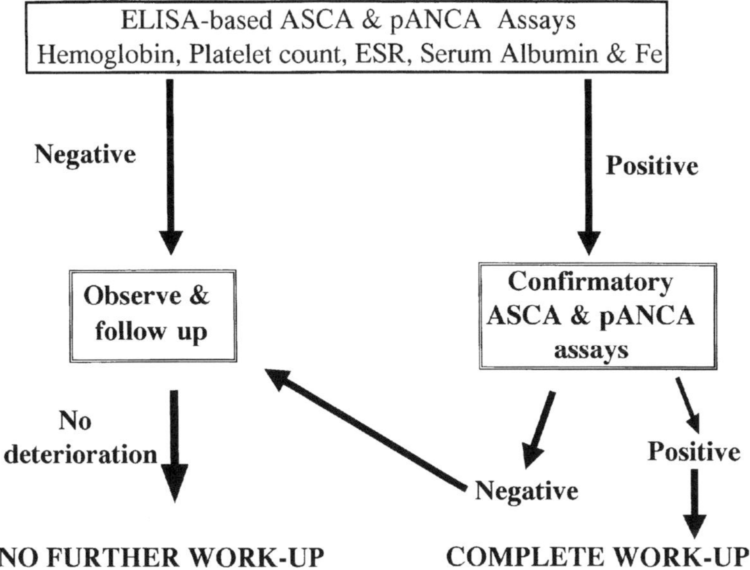

Figure 1 Proposed diagnostic strategy for children and adolescents suspected of having IBD, without physical signs suggestive of IBD. All patients are first screened using the modified ASCA/pANCA ELISA-based assays. Coincidentally, blood is drawn for other routine parameters to screen for IBD, including haemoglobin, platelet count, erythrocyte sedimentation rate (ESR), as well as serum iron and albumin. According to this strategy, patients who have a negative modified assay or negative diagnostic test sequence (modified or ELISA-based screen positive, followed by the traditional tests with immunofluorescence being negative) are observed in follow-up, without further work-up at that time. Positive ELISA-based assay results should be confirmed with the traditional ASCA/pANCA assays. Those patients with positive ELISA-based and traditional assays would then undergo a complete diagnostic investigation, including colonoscopy with biopsies, as well as barium upper gastrointestinal series and small-bowel follow-through. In a recent study[6], we found that had this test sequence been performed upon initial presentation, 93% (95% CI: 84–98%) of non-IBD controls would have been correctly diagnosed in the absence of further investigations

Table 2 Vessel density estimation by Doppler ultrasound reflects disease activity in paediatric Crohn's disease

Vessel density (no./cm²)	Crohn's disease activity*
Low (0–1)	Quiescent
Modest (2–4)	Active
High (≥5)	Active

*Based on a study in 47 children, the sensitivity of moderate or high vessel density for active disease was 93.5%, with a specificity of 73%; the positive and negative predictive values were 91.5% and 78.6%, respectively[9].

may prove to be a useful tool to objectively document response to therapy without resorting to more invasive endoscopic or radiological studies.

PHARMACOGENOMIC TESTING TO OPTIMIZE RESPONSE TO IMMUNOSUPPRESSIVE THERAPY

6-Mercaptopuine (6-MP) and its parent drug azathioprine (AZA) are highly effective immunosuppressive drugs for the long-term management of both CD and UC[9,10]. Their cytotoxic and immunosuppressive properties are mediated via their intracellular conversion to their principal metabolites (Figure 2), 6-thioguanine (6-TG) nucleotides and 6-methylmercaptopurine (6-MMP) ribonucleotides[11]. The latter pathway is mediated via the genetically controlled thiopurine methyltransferase (TPMT) enzymatic pathway[12]. Approximately 11% of individuals carry a mutation on one of their TPMT alleles, leading to intermediate enzyme activity, shunting more of the drug towards 6-TG production (Figure 2).

We have established[13] that the measurement of intracellular 6-MP metabolite

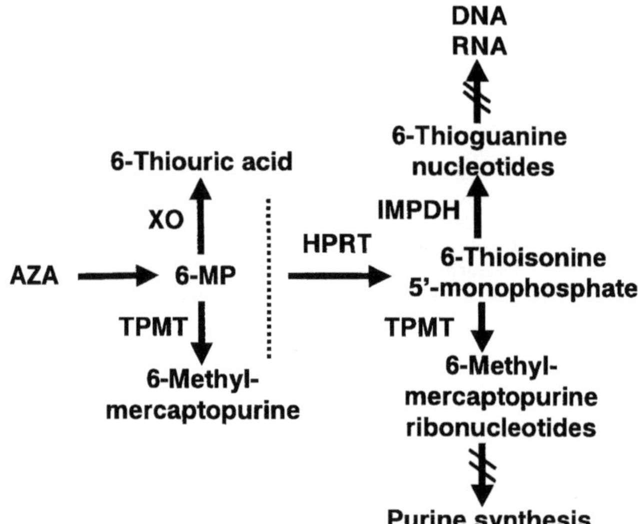

Figure 2   6-Mercaptopurine metabolism. Oral azathioprine (AZA) is rapidly converted to 6-MP by a non-enzymatic process. Initial 6-MP transformations occur along competing catabolic (XO: xanthine oxidase; TPMT: thiopurine methyltransferase) and anabolic (HPRT: hypoxanthine phosphoribosyltransferase) enzymatic pathways. The latter intracellular pathway (dashed line) leads to drug conversion into 6-thioguanine nucleotides (6-TGN), which have been shown to be the most important factor associated with treatment efficacy. TPMT converts the drug into 6-methyl-mercaptopurine ribonucleotides (6-MMP), which may interfere with purine metabolism. High erythrocyte 6-MMP levels have been associated with hepatotoxicity. Patients heterozygous for a mutant allele of TPMT will convert a higher proportion of the drug into 6-TG. This translates into a higher success rate, but with a greater chance of myelosuppression

Table 3 Interpretation of 6-mercaptopurine metabolite measurement

6-TG*		6-MMP*	Interpretation
Undetectable	or	Very low	Non-adherence to therapy
Low (<235)		Low (<2000)	Inadequate dose (if patient is a non-responder)
Low (<235)		Normal to high	Patient with preferential metabolism via TPMT pathway; consider increasing dose if liver enzymes normal
>235; <450		<5700	Ideal therapeutic range
<450		>5700	Potential hepatotoxicity
>450		<5700	Potential bone marrow toxicity
High		Low	Likely TPMT deficiency (heterozygote); potential bone marrow toxicity
High		Absent	Likely TPMT absence (homozygous mutation)

*pmol/8×10^8 erythrocytes.

concentrations by high-performance liquid chromatography assists in identifying why certain IBD patients do not respond to 6-MP or AZA therapy, as well as determining the cause of many of the adverse effects of these drugs (Table 3). Therapeutic response was determined by disease activity indices coincidentally with haematological, pancreatic and hepatic laboratory parameters. TPMT mutations were identified by allele-specific oligonucleotide hybridization. Clinical response correlated with erythrocyte 6-TG levels (<0.0001), but not with 6-MMP levels or 6-MP dose. The frequency of therapeutic response significantly increased at 6-TG levels greater than a cut-off of 235 pmol/8×10^8 red blood cells ($p<0.001$). On the other hand, hepatotoxicity correlated with high erythrocyte 6-MMP levels ($p<0.05$). Leukopenia was associated with higher 6-TG levels during remission ($p<0.04$).

Patients heterozygous for the TPMT allele shunt more of the drug towards the rate-limiting inosine monophosphate dehydrogenase pathway (Figure 2), and had higher 6-TG levels ($p<0.0001$). In our study all heterozygotes responded to therapy. However, identification of a TPMT mutation on one allele should alert the physician to prescribe a lower initial dose of 6-MP or AZA, because of the increased risk of bone marrow toxicity. 6-MP metabolite levels and TPMT molecular analysis thus provide clinicians with useful tools for optimizing therapeutic response to 6-MP/AZA and for identifying individuals at increased risk for drug-induced toxicity. Use of metabolite measurement to gauge drug dose can help prevent bone marrow toxicity from excessive 6-TG concentrations.

DETECTION AND TREATMENT OF BONE DISEASE IN PAEDIATRIC IBD

The lifelong prevention of osteoporosis is a goal that begins during childhood, a time of rapid bone growth and increasing density. The presence of osteoporosis carries a 30% increase for the risk of fracture. In order to prevent osteoporosis one must first identify patients at high risk. Children and adolescents with IBD may have multiple risk factors, including the presence of a chronic inflammatory disorder with the overproduction of inflammatory cytokines that lead to increased bone resorption. Other risk factors may include undernutrition, a sedentary lifestyle and glucocorticoid therapy. Therefore, bone mineral density (BMD) should be measured as part of the work-up of IBD patients in the paediatric age group. This is well accomplished by dual-energy X-ray absorptiometry (DEXA), provided that the results are interpreted in terms of bone or height age, rather than in terms of chronological age, as explained below[14].

In a recent study in 43 paediatric patients with quiescent CD, an abnormally low z score for BMD (below 2 standard deviations for chronological age) was observed in 44% of the cases[14]. However, 21% of patients had a delayed bone age, consistent with their growth failure and chronic malnutrition. When the BMD was interpreted in terms of the patients' bone age, rather than their chronological age, less than 30% of the childhood CD cases had true BMD deficits. Thus, correct BMD determination in paediatric IBD patients requires interpretation in terms of bone age, rather than chronological age.

Strategies to prevent and treat osteoporosis include modifying risk factors, such as correcting malnutrition, optimizing intake of calcium and vitamin D, encouraging physical exercise, and limiting glucocorticoid therapy when possible. Several of these goals can be accomplished if nutritional therapy is employed for the management of active disease, rather than conventional corticosteroids[15]. If there is no improvement in BMD, bisphosphonate therapy should be considered. These drugs can help maintain BMD even if corticosteroids are used because of their long skeletal half-life. Repeat DEXA should be carried out to confirm adequate response to therapy, since the absorption of these drugs is often problematic. If necessary, bisphosphonates can be administered intravenously.

Acknowledgements

This work was supported in part by funding from the Charles Bruneau Foundation (Y.T.) and the *Arc-en Ciel* Fund from the Sainte Justine Hospital Foundation (E.G.S.), by a Research Scholarship Award from the Fonds de la Recherche en Santé de Quebec (E.G.S.), and a Research Fellowship Award from the Crohn's and Colitis Foundation of America (M.D.). The authors thank Dr Steve Rose and his colleagues at Prometheus Laboratories for their technical support, as well as Danielle St Cyr Huot and Amanda Gillian Seidman for assistance with manuscript preparation.

References

1. Seidman E. Inflammatory bowel diseases. In: Roy C, Silverman A, Alagille D, editors. Pediatric Clinical Gastroenterology, 4th edn. St-Louis, MO: CV Mosby; 1995:417–93.
2. Seidman E. Are serological tests for IBD useful to clinicians? Inflamm Bowel Dis 1999;5:237.
3. Ruemmele FM, Targan S, Levy G, Dubinsky M, Braun, Seidman EG. Diagnostic accuracy of serological assays in pediatric inflammatory bowel disease. Gastroenterology 1998;115:822–9.

4. Vasiliauskas EA, Plevy PE, Landers CJ *et al.* Perinuclear antineutrophil cytoplasmic antibodies in patients with Crohn's disease define a clinical subgroup. Gastroenterology 1996;110:1810–19.
5. Quinton JF, Sendid B, Reumaux D *et al. Anti-Saccharomyces cerevisiae* mannan antibodies combined with antineutrophil cytoplasmic autoantibodies in inflammatory bowel disease: prevalence and diagnostic role. Gut 1998;42:788–91.
6. Dubinsky MC, Ofman J, Targan S, Ruemmele F, Seidman E. ASCA and ANCA testing: important tools for clinical decision making in pediatric IBD. Gastroenterology 1999;116:A702.
7. Seidman E, LeLeiko N, Ament M *et al.* Nutritional issues in pediatric inflammatory bowel disease. J Pediatr Gastroenterol Nutr 1991;12:424–38.
8. Spalinger JH, Patriquin H, Miron M-C, Dubois J, Herzog D, Seidman EG. Doppler sonography in pediatric Crohn's disease: vessel density in the diseased bowel reflects disease activity. Radiology (In press).
9. Pearson DC, May GR, Fick GH, Sutherland LR. Azathioprine and 6-mercaptopurine in Crohn's disease. A meta-analysis. Ann Intern Med 1995;123:132–42.
10. Hawthorne AB, Logan RF, Hawkey CJ *et al.* Randomized controlled trial of azathioprine withdrawal in ulcerative colitis. Br Med J 1992;305:20–2.
11. Cuffari C, Théorêt Y, Latour S, Seidman EG. 6-Mercaptopurine metabolism in Crohn's disease: correlation with efficacy and toxicity. Gut 1996;39:401–6.
12. Lennard L. Clinical implications of thiopurine methyltransferase – optimization of drug dosage and potential drug interactions. Ther Drug Monit 1998;20:527–31.
13. Dubinsky MC, Lamothe S, Yang HY *et al.* Pharmacogenomics and metabolite measurement for 6-mercaptopurine therapy in inflammatory bowel disease. Gastroenterology (In press).
14. Herzog D, Bishop N, Glorieux F, Seidman EG. Interpretation of bone mineral density values in pediatric Crohn's disease. Inflamm Bowel Dis 1998;4:261–7.
15. Seidman E. Nutritional therapy for Crohn's disease: lessons from the Ste-Justine Hospital experience. Inflamm Bowel Dis 1997;3:49–53.

10
Inflammatory bowel disease in the elderly

G. R. GREENBERG AND I. TAI

ABSTRACT

Inflammatory bowel disease (IBD) characteristically presents in early adulthood, but a second incidence peak is observed in the sixth to eighth decade of life. Ulcerative colitis (UC) presenting in older patients tends to show a predilection for distal involvement, with the initial attack often being more severe than in younger patients. The response to medical management, risk of extension and requirement for surgery, however, are similar to younger patients. The spectrum of medical management options is also similar, although the risk of complications related to prolonged steroid use, in particular hyperglycaemia, hypertension and osteoporosis, may be higher. The use of immunosuppressive agents may also be associated with a higher risk of infection. Although early studies suggested a higher complication rate and early mortality in elderly UC patients, more recent evaluations indicate the outcome is comparable to younger IBD patients. A small increase in mortality occurs postoperatively and seems more often related to co-morbid disease rather than to UC. The spectrum of clinical presentations for Crohn's disease (CD), including extraintestinal manifestations and perianal disease, is no different from a younger population, with the exception of a higher incidence of Crohn's colitis and a lower rate of surgery. However, in elderly Crohn's colitis patients who require surgery either due to disease severity or complications, postoperative mortality and complication rates related to surgery may be higher. The overall mortality rate in elderly patients with CD is, however, not different from the general population. The risk of recurrence after resection seems to be less in older patients with CD. Important differential or coexistent diagnoses in the evaluation of elderly patients with possible IBD include ischaemic colitis, diverticulitis, neoplasms, infectious causes including *Clostridium difficile* and *Escherichia coli* 0157:H7, and NSAID-related fibrotic strictures. Thus, with certain exceptions, the presentation, clinical course and response to therapy for elderly patients presenting with IBD tend to be comparable to a younger population.

INTRODUCTION

Ulcerative colitis (UC) and Crohn's disease (CD) characteristically present in early adulthood, although a second incidence peak is described in the sixth to eighth decade of life. With the proportional rise of an elderly population, physicians are more likely to be faced with the challenges surrounding the diagnosis and therapy of inflammatory bowel disease (IBD) in older individuals. It is therefore timely to highlight the clinical features and special considerations surrounding management issues of UC and CD in the elderly. Although there is no uniform consensus as to what constitutes an older population, this review has focused on an age of 60 years or greater.

EPIDEMIOLOGICAL CONSIDERATIONS

Certain epidemiological studies have indicated a bimodal distribution for the age of presentation of IBD. Whereas the first mode typically occurs in the third decade, a second peak is described between the ages of 50 and 80 years[1–5]. There is no clear explanation for this observation. Among the suggested possibilities are distinct disease entities, disease presentation modified by genetic haplotypes, or environmental factors modified by the ageing process, including ischaemia, altered immune regulation or the increased use of certain drugs, such as non-steroidal anti-inflammatory agents[6].

Investigations addressing the epidemiology of CD suggest that the highest or second-highest age-specific incidence occurs in subjects between 70 and 80 years of age[2,3]. Because not all studies have specifically described an age-specific incidence, a recent review[7] of 28 epidemiological studies conducted up to 1986 tabulated the proportion of patients with IBD whose disease developed after a median age of 60 years (range 40–70 years). In this age group the proportion of patients who developed CD averaged 16% (range 7–26%), while the proportion of patients who developed UC averaged 12% (range 8–12%). In the older IBD population the incidence of UC tends to be more common, ranging from one to three times that of CD. In part this variability is a reflection of whether proctosigmoiditis, a more frequent disease in the elderly, is considered an independent entity from panulcerative colitis[8,9]. When compared to ulcerative colitis there is, however, a more rapid rise in the incidence of CD in the elderly, as reported for the general population. Data from certain countries such as Scandinavia[10] tend to show that the higher incidence of UC in the elderly is restricted to males. On the other hand, certain studies have suggested a female preponderance of CD in the elderly[1,6], although other investigations[10] have not demonstrated any gender specificity.

ULCERATIVE COLITIS

Clinical characteristics

The clinical presentation of UC in the elderly parallels younger patients with the typical features of diarrhoea, rectal bleeding and urgency. The frequency and type of extraintestinal manifestations including joint and eye involvement also seems to parallel younger patients, although skin manifestations may be less frequent[11]. Weight loss may be disproportionately greater in the older population when compared to a younger group, perhaps due to co-morbid conditions. Upon initial presentation, elderly patients tend to have more aggressive and severe disease. In one study[12] the proportion of patients with severe disease was 45% in the elderly compared with 28% in the younger population. This finding is reflected in the higher incidence of complication rates. For example, in one early series[13], the frequency of toxic megacolon was reported to be 30% and was associated with a higher complication and mortality rate. Although a hypercoaguable state is associated with IBD, the incidence of mortality rates from cerebral or cardiac events is not increased in the elderly IBD population[14]. Infections caused by *Escherichia coli* 0157:H7[15] or *Clostridium difficile* and ischaemic colitis are important conditions that require differentiation from UC. Distinguishing features of ischaemic colitis include a history of vascular disease, focal involvement with rectal sparing and rapid resolution in about one-half of cases[16,17].

Distribution

In certain series a greater proportion of patients presenting with UC at an older age were found to have proctitis or proctosigmoiditis[11,18]. The proportion of patients with proctosigmoiditis ranged from 10% to 15% higher in the elderly, compared to a younger group. On the other hand, a large population-based study[10] showed no difference in the distribution of proctosigmoiditis, left-sided colitis or pancolitis between older and younger patients, perhaps reflecting the variability in population- and hospital-based investigations. Notwithstanding observations that a greater proportion of UC patients have disease limited to the rectum and sigmoid colon, the severity of the disease tends to be greater in elderly patients[9,12].

Clinical outcome

Early series from three decades ago reported a higher fatality rate in older patients presenting with UC. Mortality rates were described to be as high as 16.3% in elderly patients, compared with 5.9% in younger patients[12,19]. However, more recent studies described only marginally increased mortality rates of 2.4% in older patients compared with 1% in patients under 60 years of age[18], and other studies have reported no mortality regardless of age[20,21], probably reflecting improved management strategies.

Medical therapy

There is no uniform consensus on drug requirements and outcome in elderly patients with UC. Certain studies have noted that, when compared to a younger population, a higher proportion of elderly patients require hospital admission with the first attack and have a greater requirement for systemic administration of corticosteroids[20]. The proportion of patients achieving remission with medical therapy is no different compared with younger patients, but the time to response may be slower[11]. This notion is reflected by data suggesting that elderly patients who require hospital admission have an almost two-fold greater length of hospital stay with a mean of 22.5 days compared to 12.5 days in younger patients[22]. In elderly patients with proctosigmoiditis there also is a tendency towards a longer duration of activity and a shorter period of remission[11].

Complications of drug therapy

In general, patients over age 60 tend to show a two-fold greater incidence of drug-related adverse events[23]. In particular the frequency and severity of corticosteroid-related side-effects are increased in the elderly[24]. Notable adverse events include an increased risk of osteopenia and fracture, hyperglycaemia, eye manifestations including cataracts and glaucoma, more labile hypertension and hypokalaemia. The risk for exacerbation of congestive heart failure is similar to non-steroid-treated patients[24]. Whether the psychological manifestations of corticosteroids are more prevalent in the elderly is controversial, with separate investigations suggesting an increased risk for developing mental status changes[24] and no difference compared to a younger population[6]. Nevertheless, when alterations in mental status do occur it becomes important to differentiate steroid-related effects from other causes, including ischaemic events. Adverse effects related to sulphasalazine and the newer 5-ASA agents appear to be no different from those younger patients[25]. Azathioprine also appears to be well-tolerated without an increased risk of bone marrow suppression[26]. Experience with cyclosporin in the elderly is limited. Although adverse events may generally be high with cyclosporin, particularly when used in conjunction with corticosteroids, limited data suggest that in the elderly the incidence of side-effects appears no greater than in the young population. As with all UC patients, anti-peristaltic agents should be used cautiously, if at all. The presence of interactions between all therapeutic agents employed for IBD and other drugs frequently prescribed for the elderly, notably cardiac medications, requires assessment. Lastly, there are practical issues that may arise regarding administration of rectal preparations to the elderly and home care support may be necessary.

Requirement for surgery

Notwithstanding the greater severity of the initial attack of UC in the elderly, the proportion of patients who require surgery either does not differ between older and younger (12% vs 8%) patients[20] or is higher in younger patients[18]. Although restorative proctocolectomy was initially recommended only for patients under 50 years of age, recent data suggest that the functional outcome after this operation in patients greater than 60 years of age is equivalent to patients less than 40 years of age[27,28].

Malignancy

Although the age-specific risk for the development of colorectal cancer in younger individuals is low, the presence of UC is recognized to increase the relative risk of colorectal cancer in a time-dependent manner. The converse seems to be present in elderly patients. In a study involving a retrospective cohort of 823 patients, Gyde *et al.*[29] reported a decrease in the relative risk of colorectal cancer when the onset of UC was over 40 years of age. Similarly, in a larger population-based cohort of 3117 patients, Ekbom *et al.*[30] found the relative risk of colorectal cancer adjusted for disease extent to be diminished by about one-half for each decade of age at which the diagnosis was made, and after age 60 the risk was only marginally increased. However, patients over age 40 do have a higher initial cumulative risk of colorectal cancer when compared to a younger age group[30]; the peak incidence occurs at the fifth decade and is independent of disease duration[29]. Thus, early endoscopic evaluation of the colon seems prudent in older UC patients. Although, in the healthy, elderly patient with long-standing quiescent UC, surveillance should still be considered, the presence of significant co-morbid disease may temper the enthusiasm for yearly colonoscopy.

Prognosis

In general, the clinical outcome of elderly patients with UC is comparable to younger patients. Indeed, in one study the relapse rate of 40% at 5 years in an older population of UC patients was one-half of that observed in the younger population[9]. Several recent studies[14,20,31,32] indicate that UC in the elderly is not associated with increased mortality and, when compared to age- and sex-matched controls, mortality is primarily related to co-morbid events. Therefore, UC in the elderly may be associated with an initially more severe attack and a longer length of hospital stay, but the remission rate is comparable to younger patients and the relapse rate may be less. Complications such as toxic megacolon may be more frequent with a greater requirement for surgery and an associated higher incidence of morbidity and mortality. However, the overall requirement for surgery is similar to a younger group and the presence of the disease itself is not reflected by a higher malignancy rate or a higher mortality rate. In selective patients restorative proctocolectomy undertaken in patients over 60 years of age will provide a functional outcome similar to patients less that 40 years of age.

CROHN'S DISEASE

Clinical characteristics

The spectrum of clinical symptoms, including diarrhoea, abdominal pain and weight loss and laboratory parameters is similar in CD of the elderly, when compared to younger patients[33-35]. Notwithstanding a comparable clinical presentation, the time to diagnosis of CD in the elderly may be quite variable compared to younger patients, as both longer and shorter time intervals to diagnosis have been reported. Whereas in one study[35] an average duration of 1.8 years to diagnosis was noted in the elderly compared to 2.7 years in young adults, other studies[36–38] have reported a period of more than 3 years to establish a diagnosis of CD in the older population. Differentiating CD from diverticular disease was the most common reason for the delay in diagnosis[37,38]. In the older population there also appears to be a difference in the distribution of CD. Several studies have found a greater proportion of elderly patients with CD have colonic involvement that on average was two-fold higher than younger patients. One analysis[6] compared the disease distribution from 12 studies comprising 450 elderly patients with the distribution of disease derived from the National Cooperative Crohn's Disease Study (NCCDS) and found colonic disease was more prevalent in the elderly (59% vs 15%), small intestinal disease was comparable (26% vs 30%) and combined disease was less frequent (15% vs 55%). The explanation for this dominant distribution of colonic CD in the elderly is not entirely clear, but is not a universal finding for all studies. Two recent retrospective reviews found that the majority of elderly patients presented with CD localized to the terminal ileum[39,40].

Medical management

Although the therapeutic armamentarium available for the management of elderly patients with CD is similar to younger patients, the requirement for systemic corticosteroid therapy may be less in older patients[38]. A proportionally larger group of elderly patients may receive metronidazole and ciprofloxacin[39] as this antibiotic combination seems particularly effective for CD involving the colon[41]. The rate and spectrum of complications related to drug therapy, notably corticosteroid treatment[24], are also similar to those observed in the management of patients with UC, as discussed above. The overall response to medical therapy appears to be comparable to younger patients[19]. Elderly patients with colonic involvement tend to respond better to medical management than patients with ileal involvement, and proportionally fewer patients require surgery[40,42]. Hospital admission appears to be less frequent for elderly patients with CD, but when required the length of stay may be up to three-fold greater than in younger patients[43,44].

Requirement for surgery

There is no universal consensus on the relative requirement for surgery in elderly CD patients. Reports on the indications for surgery based on the complications of the disease and the site of involvement are quite variable but, in general, suggest that the decision to operate in the elderly is no different from that in younger patients. Elderly patients with ileal disease may more frequently present initially with subacute intestinal obstruction from underlying stricture formation and require early surgery[40]. In a proportion of elderly patients with colonic CD the threshold for surgery may be lower due either to disease severity or the inability to differentiate benign strictures (CD or diverticular disease) from cancer. The initial operation of choice for colonic CD in elderly patients is panproctocolectomy, as segmental colonic resection seems to be associated with rapid recurrence and the frequent necessity for reoperation[40,44,45]. As with UC, the morbidity associated with operation may be marginally increased in the elderly, but co-morbid conditions are usually the major determinants of outcome. This notion is illustrated by data from a recent retrospective study[46], in which complication rates after surgery for CD in patients older than age 55 were compared to the outcome in a younger cohort. The anastomotic leak rate of 4.3% in older patients was similar to the rate of 5.3% in the younger group. There was one death in each group but the older patients had more cardiac (18.2% vs 0.8%) and respiratory (18.2% vs 2.4%) complications and a longer mean postoperative hospital stay. The necessity for emergency surgery may also be associated with a higher mortality in elderly patients. In one study[47] a 35% mortality rate was noted in 49 elderly patients with Crohn's colitis requiring emergency operation compared to a 7% mortality rate in a younger group. However, other studies[45,46] examining outcome after surgery in the elderly population have shown an overall mortality rate ranging from 1.3% to 9%; these values are comparable to surgical mortality rates reported for a younger group.

Recurrence

Although certain studies have demonstrated similar recurrence rates after surgery in elderly and younger groups[36,48], one large survey[49] found a five-fold lower symptomatic recurrence rate after surgery in patients greater than 50 years of age. This lower value of recurrence was particularly evident in patients operated upon for ileal disease. Interestingly, in one recent study the recurrence rate was also lower in elderly patients, but the duration to symptomatic recurrence of 3.7 years was shorter when compared to a duration of 5.8 years in a younger group[35]. As noted above, the recurrence rates after segmental colonic resection may be particularly rapid and high in the older population[40,45].

CONCLUSIONS

With the rising proportion of older individuals in the general population, and a high age-specific incidence of IBD in the elderly, physicians will more often be confronted with the challenges related to the diagnosis and management of UC and CD in the elderly. Although the clinical presentation is often similar to a younger population, important conditions that require differentiation from IBD include diverticulitis and its complications, ischaemic colitis and malignancy. The spectrum of drug therapy is comparable to that employed in younger individuals, but there is the potential for more drug-interaction complications because other medications are often required to treat co-morbid conditions. Psychosocial issues surrounding the home management of IBD in the elderly become an important consideration. Although the indications for surgery are similar to younger individuals, the threshold for operation may be lower, either to establish the diagnosis or because of disease-related complications. Upon hospital admission the length of stay may be prolonged, but with improved management strategies mortality is low and the overall prognosis is similar to, or perhaps even slightly better than, a younger population. Thus, from the available literature it is possible to gain some insight into the clinical features of IBD in the elderly. However, the paucity of prospective, multicentre evaluations of various therapeutic interventions and outcome measures in this growing subgroup of IBD patients suggests an important avenue for future study.

References

1. Kyle J. Crohn's disease in the northeastern and northern isles of Scotland: an epidemiological review. Gastroenterology 1992;103:392–9.
2. Bjornsson S. Inflammatory bowel disease in Iceland during a thirty-year period, 1950–1979. Scand J Gastroenterol 1989;24:47–9.
3. Hiatt RA, Kaufman L. Epidemiology of inflammatory bowel disease in a defined northern California population. West J Med 1988;149:541–6.
4. Stonnington CM, Phillips SF, Melton LJ, Zinsmeister AR. Chronic ulcerative colitis: incidence and prevalence in a community. Gut 1987;28:402–9.
5. Evans JG, Acheson ED. An epidemiological study of ulcerative colitis and regional enteritis in the Oxford area. Gut 1965;6:311–24.
6. Kadish SL, Brandt LJ. Inflammatory bowel disease in the elderly. In: Kirsner JB, Shorter RG, editors. Inflammatory Bowel Disease, 4th edn. Baltimore, MD: Williams & Wilkins, 1995:390–406.
7. Grimm IS, Friedman LS. Inflammatory bowel disease in the elderly. Gastroenterol Clin N Am 1990;19:361–89.
8. Ekbom A, Helmick C, Zack M, Adami H. Ulcerative proctitis in Central Sweden 1965–1983: a population-based epidemiological study. Dig Dis Sci 1991;36:97 102.
9. Sinclair TS, Brunt PW, Mowat NAG. Nonspecific proctocolitis in northeastern Scotland: a community study. Gastroenterology 1983;85:1–11.
10. Ekbom A, Helmick C, Zack M, Adami H. The epidemiology of inflammatory bowel disease: a large population-based study in Sweden. Gastroenterology 1991;100:350–8.
11. Zimmerman J, Gavish D, Rachmilewitz D. Early and late onset ulcerative colitis: distinct clinical features. J Clin Gastroenterol 1985;7:492–8.
12. Watts JM, Dombal FT, Goligher JC. Early course of ulcerative colitis. Gut 1966,7.16–31.
13. Greensteen AJ, Sachar DB, Gibas A et al. Outcome of toxic dilatation in ulcerative and Crohn's colitis. J Clin Gastroenterol 1985;7:137–43.
14. Ekbom A, Helmick CG, Zack M, Holmberg L, Adami HO. Survival and causes of death in patients with inflammatory bowel diseases: a population-based study. Gastroenterology 1992;103:954–60.
15. Carter AO, Borczyk AA, Carlson JA et al. A severe outbreak of Escherichia coli 0157:H7-associated hemorrhagic colitis in a nursing home. N Engl J Med 1987;317:1496–500.
16. Brandt, LJ, Boley SJ, Mitsudo S. Clinical characteristics and natural history of colitis in the elderly. Am J Gastroenterol 1982;77:382–6.
17. Brandt L, Boley S, Goldberg L, Mitsudo S, Berman A. Colitis in the elderly: a reappraisal. Am J Gastroenterol 1981;76:239–45.
18. Softley A, Myren J, Clamp SE, Bouchier IAD, Watkinson G, deDombal FT. Inflammatory bowel disease in the elderly patient. Scand J Gastroenterol 1988;23(Suppl. 144):27–30.
19. Watts JM, Dombal FT, Watkinson G, Goligher JC. Long-term prognosis of ulcerative colitis. Br Med J 1966;1:1447–53.
20. Jones HW, Hoare AM. Does ulcerative colitis behave differently in the elderly? Age Ageing 1988;17:410–14.
21. Gupta S, Saverymuttu SH, Keshavarzian A, Hodgson HJF. Is the pattern of inflammatory bowel disease different in the elderly. Age Ageing 1985;14:366–70.
22. Riley R. Crohn's disease and ulcerative colitis. Morbidity and mortality. Health Rep 1990;2:343–54.
23. Holt PR. Gastrointestinal drugs in the elderly. Am J Gastroenterol 1986;81:403–11.

24. Akerkar GA, Peppercorn MA, Hamel MB, Parker RA. Corticosteroid-associated complications in elderly Crohn's disease patients. Am J Gastroenterol 1997;92:461–4.
25. Lashner BA, Kirsner JB. Inflammatory bowel disease in older people. Clin Geriatr Med 1991;7:287–99.
26. Connell WR, Kamm MA, Ritchie JK, Lennard-Jones JE. Bone marrow toxicity caused by azathioprine in inflammatory bowel disease: 27 years of experience. Gut 1993;34:1981–5.
27. Takao Y, Gillard R, Nogueras JJ, Weiss EG, Wexner SD. Is age relevant to functional outcome after restorative proctocolectomy for ulcerative colitis? Prospective assessment of 122 cases. Ann Surg 1998;227:187–94.
28. Bauer JJ, Gorfine SR, Gelernt IM, Harris MT, Kreel I. Restorative proctocolectomy in patients older than fifty years. Dis Colon Rectum 1997;40:562–5.
29. Gyde SN, Prior P, Allan RN et al. Colorectal cancer in ulcerative colitis: a cohort study of primary referrals from three centres. Gut 1988;29:206–17.
30. Ekbom A, Helmick C, Zack M, Adami H. Ulcerative colitis and colorectal cancer. A population based study. N Engl J Med 1990;323:1228–33.
31. Hendriksen C, Kreiner S, Binder V. Long-term prognosis in ulcerative colitis – based on results from a regional patient group from the country of Copenhagen. Gut 1985;26:158–63.
32. Stonnington CM, Phillips SF, Zinsmeister AR, Melton LJ III. Prognosis of chronic ulcerative colitis in a community. Gut 1987;28:1261–6.
33. Rusch V, Simonowitz DA. Crohn's disease in the older patient. Surg Gynecol Obstet 1980;150:184–6.
34. Stalnikowicz R, Eliakim R, Diab R, Rachmilewitz D. Crohn's disease in the elderly. J Clin Gastroenterol 1989;11:411–15.
35. Wagtmans MJ, Verspaget HW, Lamers CB, von Hogezond RA. Crohn's disease in the elderly: a comparison with young adults. J Clin Gastroenterol 1998;27:129–33.
36. Foxworthy DM, Wilson JAP. Crohn's disease in the elderly. Prolonged delay in diagnosis. J Am Geriatr Soc 1985;33:492–5.
37. Serpell JW, Johnson CD. Complicated Crohn's disease in the over 70 age group. Aust NZ J Surg 1991;61:427–31.
38. Harper PC, McAuliffe TL, Beeken WL. Crohn's disease in the elderly. A statistical comparison with younger patients matched for sex and duration of disease. Arch Intern Med 1986;146:753–5.
39. Tai I, Greenberg GR. Inflammatory bowel disease in the elderly: a retrospective study of clinical manifestations. Can J Gastroenterol 1999;13(Suppl):83B.
40. Walmsley RS, Gillen CD, Allan RN. Prognosis and management of Crohn's disease in the over 55 age group. Postgrad Med J 1997;73:225–9.
41. Greenbloom SL, Steinhart AH, Greenberg GR. Combination ciprofloxacin and metronidazole for active Crohn's disease. Can J Gastroenterol 1998;12:53–6.
42. Fabricius PJ, Gyde SN, Shoulder P, Keighly MR, Alexander Williams J, Allan RN. Crohn's disease in the elderly. Gut 1985;26:461–5.
43. Carr N, Schofield PF. Inflammatory bowel disease in the older patient. Br J Surg 1982;69:223–5.
44. Tchirkow G, Lavery IC, Fazio VW. Crohn's disease in the elderly. Dis Colon Rectum 1983;26:177–81.
45. Wolfe BG. Factors determining recurrence following surgery for Crohn's disease. World J Surg 1998;22:364–9.
46. Norris B, Soloman MJ, Eyers AA, West RH, Glenn DC, Morgan BD. Abdominal surgery in the older Crohn's population. Aust NZ J Surg 1999;69:199–204.
47. Simpson CJ, Smith IS, Young S. Crohn's disease in the older patients. Gut 1986;27:A595.
48. Roberts PL, Schoetz J, Pricolo R, Veidenheimer MC. Clinical course of Crohn's disease in older patients. A retrospective study. Dis Colon Rectum 1990;33:458–62.
49. Softley A, Myren J, Clamp SE, Bouchier IA, Watkinson G, deDombal FT. Factors affecting recurrence after surgery for Crohn's disease. Scand J Gastroenterol 1988;23(Suppl. 144):31–4.

Section IV
Current therapy in inflammatory bowel disease

Moderators: **L. A. R. Boerr,** Buenos Aires
L. R. Sutherland, Calgary

11
Induction of remission in ulcerative colitis

S. B. HANAUER

ABSTRACT

Therapy for acute ulcerative colitis begins with an assessment of disease extent, severity and the response to prior treatments.

Mild–moderate activity can be treated with oral mesalamine in the setting of extensive colitis, or topical mesalamine or topical corticosteroids for distal disease. The dose–response is relevant for oral mesalamine, but is less important for topical therapy (in which case the frequency of topical administration and retention time correlate with efficacy).

Moderate–severe extensive colitis requires corticosteroid therapy whereas distal disease can still be treated with topical mesalamine or topical corticosteroids.

Severe–fulminant colitis requires hospitalization and parenteral corticosteroids. While there is no extensive evidence base for dose or product selection, there is sufficient clinical experience to arrive at sequential recommendations and contingencies. Significant improvement is anticipated within 3–5 days of initiating steroids at doses comparable to 40–60 mg of prednisolone or 200–400 mg of hydrocortisone. Patients who do not respond within 7 days are unlikely to improve. Failure to improve on parenteral steroids is indication for either colectomy or treatment with cyclosporin. Cyclosporin has been repeatedly demonstrated to provide prompt improvement in approximately 70–80% of patients within 3–5 days. Failure to respond with a reduction in bowel movements, cessation of bleeding and transfusion requirements and reduction in C-reactive protein (or erythrocyte sedimentation rate) within a week implies treatment failure and is an indication for colectomy. Total parenteral nutrition is adjunctive rather than primary therapy for patients with severe colitis who should be allowed to eat as long as they have an appetite. Narcotic analgesia is contraindicated, as are non-steroidal anti-inflammatory agents. The roles of topical mesalamine, infliximab and heparin in the setting of fulminant disease or toxic megacolon have not been established.

GENERAL PRINCIPLES

The initial recommendations for inductive therapy are based upon the extent and severity of colitis[1,2]. The extent is important due to the availability of effective topical (rectal) therapies when able to spread to the proximal margin of disease. Severity is relevant to estimate the intensity of anti-inflammatory therapy necessary to subdue inflammation and the risk of complications from the disease. Although no single definition of severity has gained uniform acceptance, the original classification by Truelove and Witts[3] offers simple and usable working definitions.

In the absence of a 'gold standard' measure of disease activity a working definition of *remission* used by the United States Food and Drug Administration is: 'the resolution of clinical symptoms attributed to ulcerative colitis *and* endoscopically documented mucosal healing (the regeneration of an intact mucosa *without* ulceration, granularity, or friability)'[4]. Although histological activity also can be quantified, scales have not been reproduced or validated that correlate well with endoscopic or clinical disease activity. In addition, an ultimate measure of disease activity may be the impact on a patient's *quality of life*[5]. Reproducible and validated quality of life indices have been developed for inflammatory bowel disease (IBD) that can be utilized in clinical trials[6].

Additional factors influencing the therapeutic approach are the chronicity of disease and response to prior therapies. Complications of the disease also need to be assessed because of their impact on therapy and prognosis before and after surgery.

Exogenous factors that influence the course of colitis or impact on efficacy of treatment include intercurrent infections recognized to initiate flare-ups of ulcerative colitis (UC)[7], including travellers' diarrhoea[8]. Patients with newly diagnosed UC or presenting with acute exacerbations should be evaluated for the possibility of a complicating enteric infection[9]. Dietary factors can also influence bowel habits in UC patients. Consumption of large quantities of non-absorbed carbohydrates such as lactose (in lactase-deficient patients), sorbitol or artificial fats such as Olestra® can induce symptoms of gas, bloating or diarrhoea. Conversely, patients with proctitis often present with constipation and will benefit from the addition of additional dietary fibre. A careful review of non-prescription vitamins, health foods, homeopathic agents or herbs may identify factors contributing to changes in bowel habits that are independent from the colitis. Complementary therapies are used in approximately one-half of patients with IBD[10].

Coexistent irritable bowel syndrome (IBS) is equally prevalent in UC patients as in the general population[9]. To differentiate IBS from active colitis patients presenting with abdominal cramping, diarrhoea or constipation in the absence of rectal bleeding should be evaluated for the presence of faecal leucocytes or undergo an endoscopic assessment.

Cigarette smoking has a major impact on the course of UC[11]. Ex-smokers have a worse course and are more likely to develop refractory disease, require immune modulation or colectomy[12]. Smoking also protects against sclerosing cholangitis[13] and pouchitis, but worsens osteoporosis in women[14]. Non-steroidal anti-inflammatory drugs (NSAID) are recognized to exacerbate UC[15,16] and contribute to refractory disease[9].

DISTAL ULCERATIVE COLITIS

The most common symptoms of distal UC are rectal bleeding and tenesmus. Diarrhoea is less often a problem than constipation, necessitating inquiry into the nature of *bowel movements* and *trips to the toilet*. Patients often describe a constant urge to evacuate blood and/or mucopus with less frequent passage of stool. The inability to distinguish flatus from stool can contribute to descriptions of constipation, bloating or a change in the odour of gas. Patients with distal colitis are rarely seriously ill, but may have chronic problems related to iron deficiency anaemia or complications of chronic steroid therapy. Topical aminosalicylates are the most effective initial approach for the treatment of distal UC[17,18]. Depending upon the proximal margin of disease, therapy can be initiated with mesalamine suppositories, enemas or foam. The initial dose is between 1000 and 4000 mg administered nightly or in divided doses for suppositories or foam. In contrast to the oral aminosalicylates there is not a topical dose–response between 1 and 4 g/daily[19,20]. Topical (rectal) mesalamine has been more effective, compared to oral aminosalicylate therapy at equal doses, for patients with distal colitis[17,21]. Combination treatment with both oral and topical mesalamine is superior to either single approach[21].

Alternatives to topical mesalamine are topical corticosteroids, again administered as suppository, enema or foam. Foam preparations are easier to retain and better tolerated, allowing maintenance of daily activities despite twice-daily administration. In general there is therapeutic equivalence between marketed steroid preparations although the 'non-systemic' formulations (budesonide, beclomethasone, prednisone–metasulphobenzoate) have the advantage of fewer side-effects and potential for adrenal suppression.

Oral aminosalicylates are less effective than topical therapies for distal UC[17], probably due to proximal colonic stasis in distal colitis and reduced delivery of 5-aminosalicylic acid (5-ASA) to the spastic, irritable rectum. Still, oral aminosalicylates have been used for decades for patients with mild–moderate symptoms of distal UC. In contrast to rectal mesalamine there is a dose–response for oral therapy[22]. Sulphasalazine, 2–6 g/day in divided doses, is the least expensive alternative, but is frequently compromised by dose-related side-effects. Non-sulpha containing formulations are preferable for patients with sulpha-allergy or for patients who develop sulpha-related intolerance or toxicity.

In the absence of a response to oral aminosalicylates, a topical mesalamine or steroid formulation should be added. Rectal instillation of combinations of mesalamine and steroids are most efficacious[23], but are not yet available in proprietary preparations.

It is rare that an oral steroid will be necessary to treat distal UC. All attempts should be made to optimize topical therapy with an oral aminosalicylate prior to initiating oral steroids. These measures include administration of intra-rectal mesalamine up to 4 g daily or utilizing combinations of topical therapy such a mesalamine and steroids together, in conjunction with oral mesalamine up to 4.8 g/day. Therapy is continued until the patient is asymptomatic, clinically manifest by the ability to pass flatus without the need to use the toilet. Depending upon the chronicity of symptoms a complete response may require 4–12 weeks.

Patients with left-sided colitis occasionally present with severe symptoms including toxic megacolon and/or extraintestinal manifestations. Severe left-sided UC requires treatment with systemic steroids as are indicated for extensive colitis.

EXTENSIVE ULCERATIVE COLITIS

UC extending proximal to the splenic flexure accounts for a minority of patients but a disproportionate proportion of hospitalizations and operations. Nevertheless, when patients with a history of pancolitis develop an exacerbation of quiescent disease they should be re-assessed to rule out regression to a distal colitis[24] and, as described above, can be treated more aggressively for left-sided disease. Newly diagnosed patients should undergo complete evaluations according to the severity of disease, and those with exacerbations should be assessed for complicating or aggravating factors.

Mild–moderate extensive colitis

Oral aminosalicylate therapy also is 'first-line' therapy for patients with mild–moderate, extensive colitis, but may be supplemented with topical mesalamine or steroids[2]. Again, the dose–response for oral aminosalicylates is more relevant than the specific preparation[25]. Response rates up to 80% can be anticipated with 4–6 g of sulphasalazine or 2–4.8 g of a mesalamine formulation, with approximately half of the patients achieving remission[2,26]. Therapy should be continued as long as the patient is improving to the point of clinical remission (i.e. normal bowel movements without blood or rectal urgency). If patients fail to improve completely, the dose should be 'optimized' up to 6 g/day of sulphasalazine or 4–5 g/day of a mesalamine formulation.

If the patient does not continually improve, or if there is any evidence of clinical deterioration, steroid therapy (equivalent to prednisone 40–60 mg/day) is added. Initiating therapy with 'low-dose' prednisone risks the failure to respond and typically results in prolongation of steroid exposure and eventually increasing doses. Rather, patients should be treated with effective doses from the onset to assure a complete response followed by more rapid tapering according to the time-course of improvement. The initial steroid dose is maintained until the patient is clinically well (as above), generally 2–4 weeks, and is then decreased by approximately 5 mg (prednisone) every week to 20 mg, and then by 2.5–5 mg every 1–2 weeks. Aminosalicylate therapy is continued as steroids are tapered.

Patients unable to taper prednisone despite optimal aminosalicylate therapy are candidates for azathioprine or 6-mercaptopurine[2]. Steroids are maintained at the lowest doses that prevent recurrence of symptoms for the 3–6 months required for purine antagonists to demonstrate therapeutic benefits[27,28]. If steroid therapy is prolonged, supplementation with calcium and vitamin D is indicated to prevent metabolic bone disease. If there is evidence of reduced bone density, then additional therapy with a biphosphonate, oestrogen replacement in postmenopausal women, or calcitonin may be indicated[29-31].

Moderate–severe extensive colitis

Patients with significant weight loss, fever, disabling extraintestinal manifestations, frequent nocturnal bowel movements, severe anaemia or a rapidly deteriorating course require hospitalization. Similarly, patients who do not improve within several weeks of introducing oral steroids for mild–moderate disease should be hospitalized.

Intravenous steroids are indicated for patients who are febrile in excess of 40°C, hypotensive, dehydrated, or with greater than 10–12 stools daily, persistent incontinence, severe rectal haemorrhage, protein depletion, peripheral oedema, or evidence of abdominal tenderness or distension[32-34]. Management of patients with severe colitis includes the prompt institution of general resuscitative measures to correct fluid and electrolyte imbalances and transfusions to maintain the haematocrit above 30%. Anticholinergics, antidiarrhoeals, and narcotic analgesics should be withheld to prevent inducing colonic dilation or masking peritoneal signs in debilitated patients or those on steroids[35].

Patients with severe colitis are treated with an intensive intravenous steroid regimen (e.g. prednisolone (40–60 mg/day), methylprednisolone (32–48 mg/day), or hydrocortisone (300–400 mg/day)) in divided doses or as a continuous infusion[35]. A continuous infusion of steroids provides reliability of blood levels, ease of administration (single intravenous bag or incorporation into total parenteral nutrition solution), and lower cost. There is no advantage to higher dose steroid therapy[36] which risks additional immunosuppression, opportunistic infections and osteonecrosis. A few clinicians continue to advocate infusions of intravenous adrenocorticotropic hormone (120 units daily) for patients who have not recently received corticosteroids[2,37]. A rectal steroid preparation can be added for patients with rectal urgency, to reduce tenesmus[38].

Oral aminosalicylates are discontinued due their minor anti-inflammatory effect compared to high-dose steroids and their potential to induce intolerant effects, as well as the rare instances when 5-ASA can worsen colitis[39,40]. There is no role for antibiotic therapy in the management of patients with moderate–severe UC[2].

There are no data supporting bowel rest for treatment of UC[2], although many patients are afraid to eat, fearing abdominal pain or rectal urgency, and many are unable to consume adequate diets. Therefore, parenteral nutrition is often useful as a caloric adjunct to assure sufficient caloric intake.

The intensive intravenous regimen is continued up to 7–10 days, as long as the patient is improving. Once clinical improvement has been established (normalization of vital signs, improved nutrition, stabilization of the haematocrit and white blood cells, the ability to tolerate a full diet with formation of bowel movements without blood or urgency) the patient can be changed on to an oral regimen. Full-dose therapy with an aminosalicylate is resumed and oral steroids replace the intravenous regimen.

If the patient does not improve within the first week of intensive intravenous steroid therapy the likelihood of improvement is small[41]. The failure rate for patients with severe colitis treated with intravenous steroids is nearly 40%[34] and correlates with the severity of diarrhoea, transfusion requirements and hypoalbuminaemia[42]. Therefore, if patients are not considerably improved within the first week of therapy they should be considered candidates for either surgery or the addition of cyclosporin[2,38].

Intravenous cyclosporin therapy has been an important advance in the therapy of severe UC as well as a controversial management issue[43–45]. There have been consistent benefits reported between centres using intravenous cyclosporin for severe UC with up to 80% of refractory patients responding within 7–10 days of therapy[46–48]. Most centres proceed with an initial dose of 4 mg/kg per 24 h as a continuous infusion, although some have reported equal results with 2 mg/kg dosing[49]. Prior to initiating cyclosporin the cholesterol level should be above 100 mg/dl to limit the risk of seizures. Recently, guidelines for monitoring cyclosporin therapy for UC have been published[50].

Whole blood levels of cyclosporin should be maintained between 200 and 400 ng/ml by high-performance liquid chromatography assay, although there is poor correlation between efficacy and side-effects within this range[45]. Dose reduction is necessary for elevations in blood urea nitrogen or creatinine. Persisting hypertension is treated with a calcium channel blocker, but care must be taken as these can also increase cyclosporin blood levels[50]. Minor side-effects such as headache, nausea or neuropathy are common and rarely require discontinuation of therapy[51].

Most patients begin to respond within 4–5 days[46]. Those who do not respond within 1 week are not likely to improve and should be referred to surgery[41]. Once in clinical remission (formed bowel movements without blood or urgency), the intravenous regimen is replaced with oral cyclosporin and prednisone. The daily dose of cyclosporin is doubled and administered in two divided doses[50]. Due to the high relapse rate after intravenous cyclosporin therapy[50–53], azathioprine or 6-mercaptopurine (6-MP) are added as maintenance therapy for virtually all patients responding to cyclosporin. Sulphamethoxazole–trimethoprim is added three times weekly as prophylaxis against *Pneumocystis* pneumonia. Thus, at discharge, a typical patient will be receiving prednisone 40 mg, cyclosporin b.i.d., mesalamine 2.4 g b.i.d., azathioprine 100 mg, and sulpha–trimethoprim q.o.d.

FULMINANT COLITIS AND TOXIC MEGACOLON

Fulminant colitis, with or without colonic dilation, is a medical emergency best managed by an experienced team of gastroenterology specialists and surgeons. Fulminant colitis represents transmural extension of inflammation to the serosa and is manifest by abdominal tenderness. Peritoneal irritation and perforation can occur in the absence of dilation. Toxic megacolon, caused by progression of inflammation through the bowel wall to the serosa, is associated with clinical signs of direct visceral tenderness, indistinguishable from a localized or free perforation. Toxic megacolon most commonly complicates extensive colitis, but has been documented in left-sided colitis or in settings of coexisting infections (e.g. cytomegalovirus or *Clostridium difficile*)[35]. Additional predisposing factors for toxic megacolon include medications such as anticholinergics, antidiarrhoeals, and opiates; electrolyte abnormalities, particularly hypokalaemia; and invasive diagnostic testing such as colonoscopy or barium enema.

Medical management of fulminant colitis or toxic megacolon is the same as described for severe colitis, with several modifications. Intensive monitoring by gastroenterological–surgical consultants is mandatory and support with fluid and electrolytes, transfusions and fresh-frozen plasma (in the presence of clotting abnormalities) and albumin are essential. Intravenous steroids are continued and, despite the absence of controlled evidence, broad-spectrum antibiotic coverage is added[32,35,38]. The rationale for antibiotics includes presumption of transmural extension of disease, risk of microperforation and systemic bacteraemia and, finally, as potential perioperative prophylaxis for patients with a high risk of emergent colectomy.

In contrast to those with moderate to severe disease, patients with fulminant colitis or toxic megacolon are made NPO (nothing by mouth) until clinically improved. In the presence of small bowel ileus a nasogastric tube should be inserted. Manoeuvres proposed to reduce distension by allowing redistribution and passage of colonic gas per rectum include rolling the patient from side to side, the insertion of a rectal tube, or assumption of the 'knee–elbow' position while prone[38,54].

The role for cyclosporin in the setting of fulminant colitis or toxic megacolon is controversial. There are no clinical trials in this setting, although in selected cases some have described rapid clinical improvement (as well as progressive deterioration)[38].

Signs of perforation or any deterioration are immediate indications for colectomy, as perforation greatly increases the morbidity and potential for mortality. Failure to improve within 24–72 h is another guidepost for abandonment of medical treatment as rapid surgical intervention minimizes the risk of complications and mortality[55]. A medically induced remission can be achieved in about 40–50% of patients with acceptable morbidity and rare mortality. However, the long-term 'viability' of the colon remains in question and many patients are destined for complications or resistant disease, including recurrent toxic megacolon[41,56,57].

REFRACTORY UC

The definition of refractory UC continues to evolve as therapeutic options and efficacy improve. In the setting of 'refractory disease' both endogenous and exogenous factors contributing to symptoms or inflammation should be examined[9,58]. In addition to adequate dosing, sufficient time must be allotted for a response to occur. The time-course depends upon the severity of disease, impact on quality of life, and tolerance to the therapeutic agent. In some settings (e.g. distal colitis) it may take several months for symptoms to completely resolve[59]. In the setting of more severe disease treated with intensive intravenous therapy response should be anticipated within 7–10 days[41].

Topical mesalamine has been the most efficacious therapy for distal UC. Patients refractory to oral aminosalicylates, oral steroids or topical steroids have a near-80% response to topical mesalamine as long as the formulation reaches the proximal extent of disease. Rarely, colitis is worsened by mesalamine. When this is suspected, a trial period off of all aminosalicylates is warranted. If patients do not respond to topical mesalamine alone, then the combination of rectal mesalamine with a steroid is often efficacious[23]. The intensive intravenous steroid regimen has also been effective for patients with distal disease refractory to oral steroid therapy[33]. Alternative approaches that may be useful in individual patients include administration of short-chain fatty acid, nicotine enemas, nicotine patches, or resumption of cigarette smoking[60].

Patients with extensive colitis failing inductive therapy with maximal doses of oral aminosalicylates and steroids should be treated with steroids alone, to determine whether 5-ASA paradoxically aggravates colitis. Azathioprine or 6-MP have been reported to be beneficial in steroid-resistant UC but require several months, making the option less acceptable than induction of remission with inpatient management and initiation of maintenance (steroid-sparing) therapy. Nicotine patches can be helpful in reducing symptoms, primarily in ex-smokers. A more reliable treatment is resumption of cigarette smoking, an approach that has yet to be given serious consideration compared to long-term steroids or immunomodulation. Finally, if outpatient therapy is not effective, hospitalization with the intensive intravenous steroid regimen is indicated, with or without cyclosporin.

References

1. Hanauer SB. Review Articles: Drug therapy: inflammatory bowel disease. N Engl J Med 1996;334:841–8.
2. Kornbluth A, Sachar DB. Ulcerative colitis practice guidelines in adults. American College of Gastroenterology, Practice Parameters Committee. Am J Gastroenterol 1997;92:204–11.
3. Truelove SC, Witts IJ. Cortisone in ulcerative colitis. Final report on a therapeutic trial. Br Med J 1995;2:1041–7.
4. Fredd S. Standards for approval of new drugs for IBD. Inflam Bowel Dis 1995;1:284–94.
5. Irvine EJ. Quality of life issues in patients with inflammatory bowel disease. Am J Gastroenterol 1997;92(12 Suppl.):18–24S.
6. Irvine EJ. Measuring quality of life: a review. Scand J Gastroenterol Suppl 1996;221:5–7.
7. Koutroubakis I et al. Environmental risk factors in inflammatory bowel disease. Hepatogastroenterology 1996;43:381–93.
8. Schumacher G, Sandsted B, Kollberg B. A prospective study of first attacks of inflammatory bowel disease and infectious colitis. Clinical findings and early diagnosis. Scand J Gastroenterol 1994;29:265–74.
9. Miner PB, Jr. Factors influencing the relapse of patients with inflammatory bowel disease. Am J Gastroenterol 1997;92(12 Suppl.):1–4S.
10. Hilsden RJ, Scott CM, Verhoef MJ. Complementary medicine use by patients with inflammatory bowel disease [see comments]. Am J Gastroenterol 1998;93:697–701.
11. Thomas GA, Rhodes J, Green JT. Inflammatory bowel disease and smoking–a review. Am J Gastroenterol 1998;93:144–9.
12. Fraga XF et al. Effects of smoking on the presentation and clinical course of inflammatory bowel disease. Eur J Gastroenterol Hepatol 1997;9:683–7.
13. Cohen RD, Hanauer SB. Protection from primary sclerosing cholangitis: smoke trails of just coattails? [editorial; comment]. Gastroenterology 1996;110:1658–62.

14. Silvennoinen JA, Lehtola JK, Niemela SE. Smoking is a risk factor for osteoporosis in women with inflammatory bowel disease. Scand J Gastroenterol 1996;31:367–71.
15. Bjarnason I *et al*. Side effects of nonsteroidal anti-inflammatory drugs on the small and large intestine in humans [see comments]. Gastroenterology 1993;104:1832–47.
16. Hamilton FA. Non-narcotic analgesics: renal and GI considerations. Clinician 1998;16:1–22.
17. Gionchetti P *et al*. Comparison of oral with rectal mesalamine in the treatment of ulcerative procitis. Dis Colon Rectum 1998;41:93–7.
18. Marshall JK, Irvine EJ. Rectal corticosteroids versus alternative treatments in ulcerative colitis: a meta-analysis. Gut 1997;40:775–81.
19. Campieri M *et al*. Optimum dosage of 5-aminosalicylic acid as rectal enemas in patients with active ulcerative colitis. Gut 1991;32:929–31.
20. Hanauer SB. Dose-ranging study of mesalamine (PENTASA) enemas in the treatment of acute ulcerative proctosigmoiditis: results of a multicentered placebo-controlled trial. The U.S. PENTASA Enema Study Group [In Process Citation]. Inflamm Bowel Dis 1998;4:79–83.
21. Safdi M *et al*. A double-blind comparison of oral versus rectal mesalamine versus combination therapy in the treatment of distal ulcerative colitis. Am J Gastroenterol 1997;92:1867–71.
22. Sutherland LR, Roth DE, Beck PL. Alternatives to sulfasalazine: a meta-analysis of 5-ASA in the treatment of ulcerative colitis. Inflam Bowel Dis 1997;3:65–78.
23. Mulder CJJ *et al*. A controlled randomized trial of beclomethasone dipropionate (3 mg) versus 5-aminosalicylic acid (1 g) versus the combination of both as retention enemas in active distal ulcerative colitis. Gastroenterology, 1994;106:A739.
24. Langholz E *et al*. Changes in extent of ulcerative colitis: a study on the course and prognostic factors. Scand J Gastroenterol 1996;31:260–6.
25. Sutherland L *et al*. Systematic review of the use of oral 5-aminosalicylic acid in the induction of remission in ulcerative colitis (Cochrane Review). The Cochrane Library. Vol. Issue 3 Oxford: Update Software; 1998.
26. Kornbluth AA *et al*. Meta-analysis of the effectiveness of current drug therapy of ulcerative colitis. J Clin Gastroenterol 1993;16:215–18.
27. George J *et al*. The long-term outcome of ulcerative colitis treated with 6-mercaptopurine. Am J Gastroenterol 1996;91:1711–14.
28. Sandborn WJ. Azathioprine: state of the art in inflammatory bowel disease. Scand J Gastroenterol Suppl 1998;225:92–9.
29. Andreassen H *et al*. Inflammatory bowel disease and osteoporosis. Scand J Gastroenterol 1997;32:1247–55.
30. Compston JE. Review article: osteoporosis, corticosteroids and inflammatory bowel disease. Aliment Pharmacol Ther 1995;9:237–50.
31. Ziegler R, Kasperk C. Glucocorticoid-induced osteoporosis: prevention and treatment. Steroids 1998;63:344–8.
32. Truelove SC *et al*. Further experience in the treatment of severe attacks of ulcerative colitis. Lancet 1978;2:1086–8.
33. Jarnerot G, Rolny P, Sandberg-Gertzen H. Intensive intravenous treatment of ulcerative colitis. Gastroenterology 1985;89:1005–13.
34. Kornbluth A *et al*. How effective is current medical therapy for severe ulcerative and Crohn's colitis? An analytic review of selected trials. J Clin Gastroenterol 1995;20:280–4.
35. Stein R, Hanauer SB. Life-threatening complications of IBD: how to handle fulminant colitis and toxic megacolon. J Crit Illness 1998;13:518–25.
36. Rosenberg W, Ireland A, Jewell DP. High-dose methylprednisolone in the treatment of active ulcerative colitis. J Clin Gastroenterol 1990;12:40–1.
37. Meyers S *et al*. Corticotropin versus hydrocortisone in the intravenous treatment of ulcerative colitis. A prospective, randomized, double blind clinical trial. Gastroenterology 1983;85:351–7.
38. Marion JF, Present DH. The modern medical management of acute, severe ulcerative colitis. Eur J Gastroenterol Hepatol 1997;9:831–5.
39. Chakraborty TK *et al*. Salicylate induced exacerbation of ulcerative colitis. Gut 1987;28:613–15.
40. Hanauer SB, Stathopoulos G. Risk–benefit assessment of drugs used in the treatment of inflammatory bowel disease. Drug Saf 1991;6:192–219.
41. Travis SP *et al*. Predicting outcome in severe ulcerative colitis. Gut 1996;38:905–10.
42. Chakravarty BJ. Predictors and the rate of medical treatment failure in ulcerative colitis. Am J Gastroenterol 1993;88:852–5.

43. Langford CA *et al.* Use of cytotoxic agents and cyclosporine in the treatment of autoimmune disease. Part 2: Inflammatory bowel disease, systemic vascultis, and therapeutic toxicity. Ann Intern Med 1998;129:49–58.
44. Atkinson KA *et al.* Intravenous cyclosporine for severe attacks of ulcerative colitis: a survey of Canadian gastroenterologists. Can J Gastroenterol 1997;11:583–7.
45. Sandborn W. A critical review of cyclosporine therapy in inflammatory bowel disease. Inflam Bowel Dis 1995;1:48–63.
46. Lichtiger S *et al.* Cyclosporine in severe ulcerative colitis refractory to steroid therapy [see comments]. N Engl J Med 1994;330:1841–5.
47. Van Gossum A *et al.* Short-and long-term efficacy of cyclosporin administration in patients with acute severe ulcerative colitis. Belgian IBD Group. Acta Gastroenterol Belg 1997;60:197–200.
48. Wenzl HH *et al.* Short-term efficacy and long-term outcome of cyclosporine treatment in patients with severe ulcerative colitis. Z Gastroenterol 1998;36:287–93.
49. Actis GC *et al.* Continuously infused cyclosporine at low dose is sufficient to avoid emergency colectomy in acute attacks of ulcerative colitis without the need for high-dose steroids. J Clin Gastroenterol 1993;17:10–13.
50. Kornbluth A *et al.* Cyclosporin for severe ulcerative colitis: a user's guide. Am J Gastroenterol 1997;92:1424–8.
51. Cohen RD, Stein R, Hanauer SB. Intravenous cyclosporin in ulcerative colitis: a five-year experience. Am J Gastroenterol 1999;94:1587–92.
52. Fernandez-Banares F *et al.* Azathioprine is useful in maintaining long-term remission induced by intravenous cyclosporine in steroid-refractory severe ulcerative colitis. Am J Gastroenterol 1996;91:2498–9.
53. Ramakrishna J *et al.* Combined use of cyclosporine and azathioprine or 6-mercaptopurine in pediatric inflammatory bowel disease. J Pediatr Gastroenterol Nutr 1996;22:296–302.
54. Panos MZ, Wood MJ, Asquith P. Toxic megacolon: the knee–elbow position relieves bowel distension [see comments]. Gut 1993;34:1726–7.
55. Seelig MH *et al.* Surgical therapy of severe colitis. Chirurg 1996;67:150–4.
56. Kornbluth A *et al.* How effective is current medical therapy for severe ulcerative and Crohn's colitis? An analytic review of selected trials. J Clin Gastroenterol 1995;20:280–4.
57. Sheth SG, LaMont JT. Toxic megacolon. Lancet 1998;351:509–13.
58. Griffin MG, Miner PB. Review article: Refractory distal colitis – explanations and options. Aliment Pharmacol Ther 1996;10:39–48.
59. Biddle WL, Miner PB. Jr. Long-term use of mesalamine enemas to induce remission in ulcerative colitis. Gastroenterology 1990;99:113–18.
60. Hanauer SB. No butts about it: put the fire out by lighting up [comment]. Inflamm Bowel Dis 1998;4:326 (discussion 327).

12
Remission maintenance in ulcerative colitis

J. SCHÖLMERICH

ABSTRACT

From a large patient cohort it is known that about 50% of all patients with ulcerative colitis who are in a continuous supervision programme are in remission each year. However, cumulatively 90% of patients have repetitive relapses over time. While in this cohort 25% of patients had been colectomized after 10 years, more than 90% were able to work at the same time.

These disease characteristics indicate that continuous supervision and remission maintenance contributes to such a generally positive outcome of this disease. Furthermore no increased carcinoma risk has been found in this large cohort from Copenhagen, which further supports the use of continuous remission maintenance treatment.

Remission maintenance is indicated in all patients having definitive ulcerative colitis with the goal of decreasing the number of relapses, and to normalize carcinoma risk.

A number of drugs has been used. Initially it was shown for sulphasalazine (SASP) that at a dose of 2 g per day it reduces relapses significantly compared to placebo. A dose of 4 g per day was even better, but the difference was not considered to be clinically relevant. The newer 5-aminosalicylic acid (5-ASA) releasing drugs have been tested for remission maintenance in a number of trials. They seem to be more or less equally effective, although a recent meta-analysis has shown that sulphasalazine seems to be slightly superior. However, in the trials used for this meta-analysis only patients already known to be tolerant for sulphasalazine had been included, thereby limiting the number of side-effects in the SASP group.

For patients who have frequent relapses in spite of such treatment, or can only be brought into remission using azathioprine, this drug has also been used for remission maintenance with a relatively good success rate. The same seems to be true for patients brought into remission using cyclosporin A, although this approach has not yet been formally tested.

Currently every patient with a definitive diagnosis of ulcerative colitis in remission should be treated with either sulphasalazine or the newer 5-ASA releasing drugs. The exact duration of such treatment is not yet known; indefinite treatment is normally recommended. Since this will normally not be accepted by the patient a withdrawal attempt can be made after 3–4 years of continuous maintenance treatment. In all patients who are difficult to treat and are having relapses in spite of 5-ASA, azathioprine should be considered. However, it should be kept in mind that surgery can cure the disease, although at a price.

INTRODUCTION

Since ulcerative colitis is a lifelong disorder, aside from treatment of the initial manifestation and relapses over the course of the years maintenance of remission is of major importance. While the first controlled trials showed that treatment of active disease and remission maintenance was possible using glucocorticosteroids (GCS) other modalities have been developed in the past 25 years. Relapse rate in ulcerative colitis is higher at younger ages and decreases with increasing duration of disease. In the majority of cases the disease never becomes completely quiescent. Large population-based studies demonstrate that in every given year about 50% of patients are completely in remission, but over the years 90% show relapses during a 25-year follow-up; 20% of patients have a relapse every year. On the other hand 90% of patients are able to work 10 years after disease onset. The colectomy rate in a large patient group reported was 25% in the first 10 years and there was no increased carcinoma risk in this group[1]. Ten-year survival is 96% of a normal population and is higher in proctitis (98%) than in pancolitis (93%)[2].

RATIONALE OF TREATMENT

Thus far it has never been shown that remission maintenance treatment improves the quality of life of patients. However, the data mentioned above indicate that continuous supervision and treatment are associated with a relatively good outcome overall when long-term analysis is performed[1]. Furthermore it has been shown that long-term treatment, in particular with sulphasalazine (SASP) or newer 5-aminosalicylic acid (5-ASA) releasing drugs decreases the risk of carcinoma development by 60%[3].

Meta-analyses of drug treatment have shown that treatment is effective in active disease (therapeutic advantage versus placebo 37–48%) and in remission maintenance (21% at 6 months and 46% at 12 months)[4,5]. Finally it has been shown that various drugs are effective in remission maintenance, e.g. GCS[6] and SASP[7] and more recently the new 5-ASA releasing drugs[8,9]. Thus, in spite of a relatively high placebo response[10] it is the consensus that maintenance treatment should be applied[11].

PREREQUISITES OF TREATMENT

As in active disease for treatment planning the extent of disease should be known, since treatment of left-sided or distal colitis is different from that of pancolitis. A number of small studies have found that rectal treatment is superior to oral treatment in remission maintenance[12], as has been shown for active disease[13,14]. A meta-analysis[5] has shown that the relative risk of not having a relapse is 16 times higher using 5-ASA enemas as compared to placebo.

STANDARD SITUATION

Distal colitis

A number of studies have demonstrated the ability of 5-ASA enemas to maintain remission in left-sided colitis[15,16] (Table 1). Application can be made every day, every second day or every third day, although efficacy will be slightly lower with the latter (Table 1).

For ulcerative proctitis suppositories have successfully been used; dose-finding studies indicated that two suppositories seem to be better than one per day[17] (Table 2). Combination of oral and rectal treatment has been found superior to oral treatment only[18] – this may seem to be merely an effect of higher local concentration. The advantage of this strategy is taking the enemas twice weekly and tablets every day.

Thus it can be concluded that rectal treatment is feasible and effective for remission maintenance of distal (left-sided) colitis. There are various possible schemes of application which can be tailored to the subjective needs of patients. It should be kept in mind that disease extension can change over time. It is reported that over 25 years proctosigmoiditis shows proximal expansion in about 53% of cases[19]; on the contrary extensive colitis or pancolitis showed a regression to more distal forms in about 70%. Thus if new symptoms occur, or remission maintenance no longer works, one should look for changes in extension before assuming drug failure.

Extensive colitis/pancolitis

There are numerous data showing that the oral application of SASP and 5-ASA is effective in maintenance of more extensive colitis (refs 7, 20, 21 and many others) (Table 3). Dose-finding studies showed that lower doses are effective[22] (Table 4). An intermittent treatment with 2.4 g every first week in a month

Table 1 Remission maintenance with 5-ASA enemas in distal UC[16]

	Placebo *(n = 44)*	*4 g 5-ASA every*		
		24 h *(n = 37)*	*48 h* *(n = 36)*	*72 h* *(n = 40)*
Remission				
6 weeks (%)	68	89	86	83
24 weeks (%)	48	81*	72*	65

*No difference for SE.

Table 2 5-ASA suppositories for maintenance in ulcerative proctitis[17]

	2 × 400 mg (n = 36)	*1 × 400 mg* (n = 40)	*Placebo* (n = 40)
Relapse (%)	10	30	47
Withdrawal due to adverse events (*n*)	3	2	2

Table 3 5-ASA orally for relapse prevention of UC[21]

	5-ASA (n = 103)	*Placebo* (n = 102)
Remission at 12 months (%)	64	38
Left-sided (%)	63	41
Extensive colitis (%)	67	31

Table 4 5-ASA (Asacol) for relapse prevention in UC[22]

	12 months		
	Placebo (n = 63)	*5-ASA, 0.8 g* (n = 68)	*5-ASA, 1.6 g* (n = 58)
Relapse (%)	60.3	41.2	34.5
SE (%)	39.1	32.2	41.4

shows very similar results when compared to 1.6 g daily[23] – 29% versus 34% relapses. More recently it has been shown that 5-ASA can be taken once a day instead of in divided doses[24] (Table 5).

There are several 5-ASA releasing drugs which have been compared in a number of studies. Mesalazine 0.8 g/day, is of identical efficacy as SASP, 2 g/day[25], and only the number of side-effects, in particular headache and abdominal discomfort, was much higher in the SASP group (Table 6). Studies comparing olsalazine with sulphasalazine showed no major differences[26,27] (Table 7). The theoretical advantage of a lower resorption leading to lower

Table 5 Divided doses of 5-ASA in IBD?[24]

	5-ASA/N-acetyl-5-ASA	
	3 × 400 mg	*1 × 1200 mg*
Faecal excretion (mg/24 h)	142/387	214/231
Mucosal concentration (AVC, ng.h/ml)	29/172	30/171
Serum AUC/peak and renal excretion not relevantly different!		

Table 6 Remission maintenance in UC[25]

	Mesalazine (0.8 g; n = 48)	SASP (2 g; n = 44)
Relapse rate (%)	38	39
Side-effects		
headache (%)	8	27
abdominal discomfort (%)	12	32

Table 7 Olsalazine versus SASP for relapse prevention in UC[27]

	6–18 Months	
	Olsalazine (1 g, n = 161)	SASP (2 g, n = 161)
Failure (%)	54.7	47.2
Relapse (%)	36.6	34.2
Withdrawal, AE (%)	7.5	5.0
Withdrawal, other (%)	10.6	8.1

plasma concentrations and lower urinary excretion[28] did not result in clinical differences. The comparison of balsalazide and mesalazine[29] also showed no clinically relevant differences, although such differences were claimed by the authors (Table 8). There are many more studies not showing any further relevant information. The data have been summarized in meta-analyses[8,9,30]. The most recent of these analyses compared sulphasalzine with all the other 5-ASA releasing drugs and found a slight advantage for SASP (Figure 1). The study showed no major difference regarding side-effects; this was probably due to the fact that only sulphasalazine-tolerant patients were included in the trials. In summary it is probably not relevant which of the available drugs is used. SASP tolerance should be known or be assessed. With olsalazine in particular diarrhoea has to be expected. The dose of 5-ASA should probably be in the range of 1.5–3 g. For sulphasalazine obviously 2 g is enough, and side-effects

Table 8 Balsalazide versus mesalazine for relapse prevention in UC[29]

	Balsalazide, 3 g	Mesalazine, 1.2 g
Asymptomatic		
nights (%)	90	77*
days (%)	58	50
Relapse		
3 months (%)	10	28
12 months (%)	42	42
AE (%)	61	65

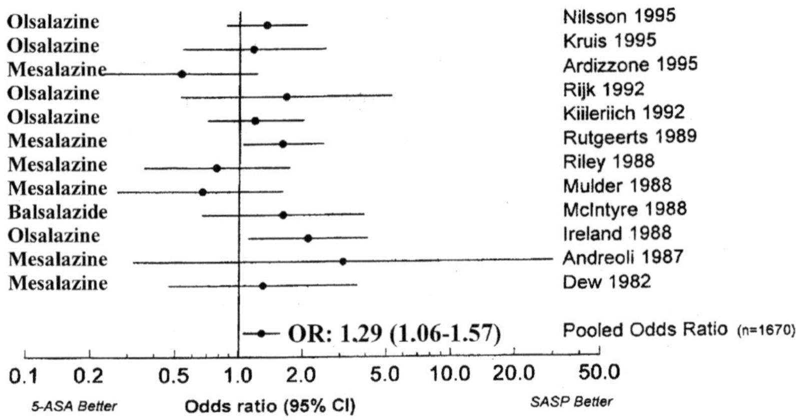

Figure 1   Sulphasalazine, mesalazine or olsalazine for remission maintenance in UC[9]

increase significantly with higher doses. For balsalazide and olsalazine 5-ASA amounts need to be calculated.

Whom to treat and when

A recent study[31] studied two groups of patients: those with remission for longer than 2 years at inclusion and those with shorter remission duration. It turned out that 5-ASA (1.2 g/day) did not significantly reduce the relapse rate versus placebo in the long-standing remission patients, but did so in those being in remission for shorter periods of time. Thus it may be that only patients having remission for less than 2 years should be treated. This is, however, controversial. Furthermore, there are interesting data on the time of relapses indicating that more patients have clinical activity in the winter months as compared to the summer[32] (Figure 2). Thus, we may use seasonally adapted treatment schedules in the future. Treatment should be individualized for each patient; some may want to continue treatment forever, some may want to stop it after 2 or 3 years. Other patients may prefer to take the drugs for 1 week a month, or at every weekend, or only in winter. It remains to be seen if such individualized treatment is equally effective, feasible and will increase compliance.

Alternatives

More recently a number of other substances have been studied for remission maintenance. For example an *Escherichia coli* preparation (mutaflor) has been found to be as effective as mesalazine[33] (Table 9); others have reproduced these results. Aside from such a 'probiotic' approach antibiotics have also been studied. In a controlled trial the addition of ciprofloxazin to standard treatment resulted in higher remission rates as compared to placebo in a controlled trial[34] (Table 10); it remains to be seen if this will be widely used. In contrast, the application of transdermal nicotine was not helpful[35]. Lipoxygenase inhibitors and PAF antagonists are not effective.

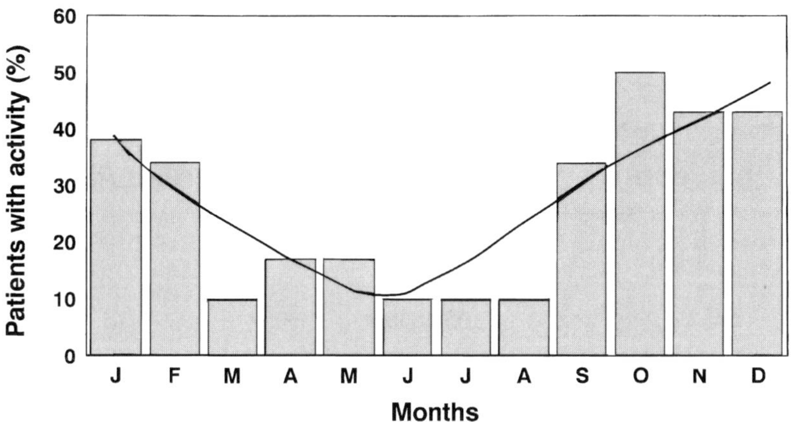

Figure 2 Influence of season on activity of UC[32]

Table 9 Mutaflor versus mesalazine for relapse prevention of UC[33]

	Mutaflor *$5×10^{10}$/day* *(n = 61)*	*Mesalazine* *1.5 g/day* *(n = 59)*
Relapse (6 months) (%)	11.5	11.9

Table 10 Ciprofloxacin for UC[34]

	Standard treatment	
	+ Placebo *(n = 36)*	*+ Ciprofloxacin* *(n = 29)*
Treatment failure (%)	44	17*
Surgery (%)	19	0*
Remission (6 months) (%)	56	83*

*Significant.

THE DIFFICULT PATIENT

For patients who are treatment refractory azathioprine has been advocated as second-line treatment. In a controlled study it was shown that, in those patients initially brought into remission with azathioprine, continued treatment reduced the relapse rate significantly[36] (Figure 3). Similar data have been reported by others indicating that azathioprine or 6-mercaptopurine treatment should be maintained over a period of years[37] (Figure 4). It is meanwhile clear that there is no significantly increased carcinoma risk due to azathioprine[38], although the risk of lymphoma may be increased[39]. Finally it has been found that

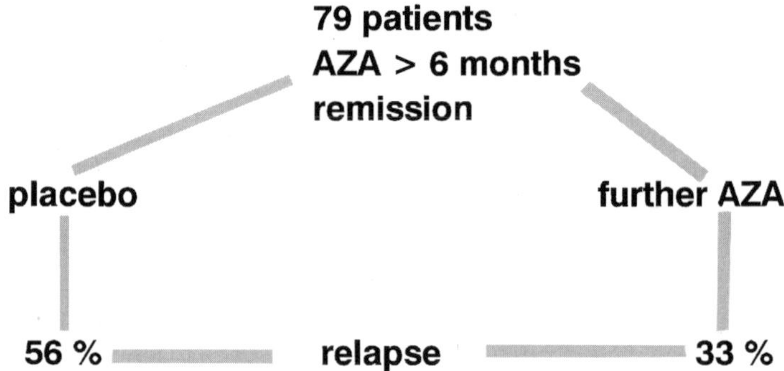

Figure 3 Azathioprine for maintenance of remission induced by azathioprine in UC[36].

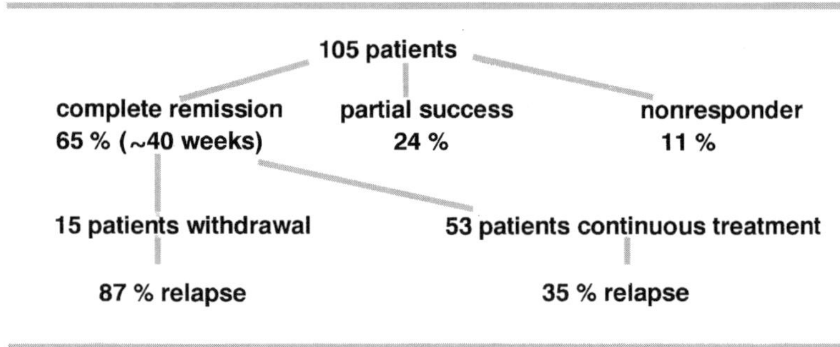

Figure 4 Long-term outcome of UC treated with 6-mercaptopurine[37]

azathioprine can be used in pregnancy but induces pregnancy problems if the father has been treated with this drug in the last 3 months before fertilization[40,41].

It has been shown meanwhile that severe and refractory ulcerative colitis can be treated successfully with intravenous cyclosporin[42]. Follow-up of those patients, however, indicated that oral cyclosporin treatment was not an optimal system, keeping only about 40–50% of patients in remission without colectomy. In addition the toxicity of cyclosporin has been found to be very high[43] (Table 11). Preliminary data suggest that application of 6-mercaptopurine or its mother substance azathioprine would be the treatment of choice to maintain cyclosporin-induced remission[44]. This, however, awaits proof from controlled trials which are under way.

SUMMARY

In summary, remission maintenance is effective. It decreases the number of relapses, probably decreases the carcinoma risk and improves the patient's quality of life. The most effective way of taking these drugs is not yet finally

Table 11 Toxicity of cyclosporin in IBD patients[43]

111 Patients (64 UC, 47 CD), m=8–9 months treatment	
Renal insufficiency	26 (23%)
Infections	22 (20%)
Seizures	3 (3%)
Anaphylaxis	1 (1%)
Death*	2 (2%)
Paraesthesias	57 (51%)
Hypertension	48 (43%)
Hypertrichosis	70 (27%)

*Septic shock: 1, haemorrhage: 1.

Table 12 Remission maintenance in UC – recommendations

Principles of optimal long-term treatment	Effective?	Therapeutic advantage ~50% (1 year)
	Tolerable?	Side-effects of mesalazine similar to placebo
1. **Effective**	Which drug?	SASP (if tolerated) or mesalazine – same effect, SASP cheaper
2. **Tolerable**		
3. **Simple**	Administration	Orally if possible (better acceptance, cheaper)
4. **Cheap**		
	How long?	>3 years
	Which patient?	All <2 years in remission
	Costs?	2000–5000 DM/avoided relapse

settled, and may need to be individualized. In selected patients, in particular those achieving remission only with immunosuppressants, the continuous application of 6-mercaptopurine or azathioprine is necessary and useful. Surgery should, however, not be forgotten.

The class of 5-ASA releasing drugs are the treatment of choice in the majority of patients. There seem to be no clinically relevant differences between these drugs; the choice of drug will be dominated by price differences and prices vary in given countries. Oral application probably has better acceptance, but rectal application as suppositories or enemas is more effective with distal disease. These drugs should be used for more than 3 years at least in all patients less than 2 years in remission (Table 12). Intermittent or otherwise individually tailored treatment seems advisable.

References

1. Langholz E, Munkholm P, Davidsen M, Binder V. Course of ulcerative colitis: analysis of changes in disease activity over years. Gastroenterology 1994;107:3–11.
2. Ekbom A, Helmick CG, Zack M, Holmberg L, Adami HO. Survival and causes of death in patients with inflammatory bowel disease: a population-based study. Gastroenterology 1992;103:954–60.
3. Pinczowski D, Ekbom A, Baron J, Yuen J, Adami HO. Risk factors for colorectal cancer in patients with ulcerative colitis: a case–control study. Gastroenterology 1994;107:117–20.

4. Kornbluth AA, Salomon P, Sacks HS, Mitty R, Janowitz HD. Meta-analysis of the effectiveness of current drug therapy of ulcerative colitis. J Clin Gastroenterol 1993;16:215–18.

5. Marshall JK, Irvine EJ. Rectal aminosalicylate therapy for distal ulcerative colitis: a metaanalysis. Aliment Pharmacol Ther 1995;9:293–300.

6. Powell-Tuck J, Bown RL, Chambers TJ, Lennard-Jones JE. A controlled trial of alternate day prednisolone as a maintenance treatment for ulcerative colitis in remission. Digestion 1981;22:263–70.

7. Dissanayke AS, Truelove SC. A controlled therapeutic trial of long-term maintenance treatment of UC with sulfasalazine. Gut 1973;14:923–8.

8. Sutherland LR, May GR, Shaffer EA. Sulfasalazine revisited: a meta-analysis of 5-aminosalicylic acid in the treatment of ulcerative colitis. Ann Intern Med 1993;118:540–9.

9. Sutherland L, Roth D, Beck P. Alternatives to sulfasalazine; a meta-analysis of 5-ASA in the treatment of ulcerative colitis. Inflam Bowel Dis 1997;3:665–78.

10. Meyers S, Janowitz HD. The 'natural history' of ulcerative colitis: an analysis of the placebo response. J Clin Gastroenterol 1989;33:33–7.

11. Schölmerich J. Therapie chronisch entzündlicher Darmerkrankungen. Klin Gegenwart 1996;16:1–44.

12. Andreoli A, Spinella S, Levenstein S, Prantera C. 5-ASA enemas versus sulfasalazine in maintaining remission in ulcerative colitis. Ital J Gastroenterol 1994;26:121–5.

13. Gionchetti P, Rizzello F, Venturi A et al. Comparison of oral with rectal mesalazine in the treatment of ulcerative proctitis. Dis Colon Rectum 1998;41:93–7.

14. Hamilton I, Pinder IF, Dickinson RJ, Ruddell WSJ, Dixon MF, Axon ATR. A comparison of prednisolone enemas with low-dose oral prednisolone in the treatment of acute distal ulcerative colitis. Dis Colon Rectum 1984;27:701–2.

15. Biddle WL, Greenberger JJ, Swan JT et al. 5-Aminosalicylic acid enemas: effective agent in maintaining remission in left-sided colitis. Gastroenterology 1988;94:1075–9.

16. Miner P, Daly R, Nester T and the Rowasa Study Group. The effect of varying dose intervals of mesalamine enemas for the prevention of relapse in distal ulcerative colitis. Gastroenterology 1994;106:A736.

17. D'Albasio G, Paoluzi P, Campieri M et al. Maintenance treatment of ulcerative proctitis with mesalazine suppositories: a double-blind placebo-controlled trial. The Italian IBD Study Group. Am J Gastroenterol 1998;93:799–803.

18. D'Albasio G, Pacini F, Camarri E et al. Combined therapy with 5-aminosalicylic acid tablets and enemas for maintaining remission in ulcerative colitis: a randomized double-blind study. Am J Gastroenterol 1997;92:1143–7.

19. Langholz E, Munkholm F, Davidsen M, Nielsen OH, Binder V. Changes in extent of ulcerative colitis: a study on the course and prognostic factors. Scand J Gastroenterol 1996;31:260–6.

20. Azad Khan AK, Howed DT, Pris J et al. Optimum dose of sulfasalazine for maintenance treatment in ulcerative colitis. Gut 1980;21:232–40.

21. Miner P, Hanauer S, Robinson M, Schwartz J, Arora S, U.C. Pentasa Maintenance Study Group. Safety and efficacy of controlled-release mesalamine for maintenance of remission in ulcerative colitis. Dig Dis Sci 1995;40:296–304.

22. Mesalamine Study Group. An oral preparation of mesalamine as long-term maintenance therapy for ulcerative colitis. A randomized, placebo-controlled trial. Ann Intern Med 1996;124:204–11.

23. Bardazzi G, D'Albasio G, Bonanomi AG et al. Intermittent versus continuous 5-aminosalicylic acid treatment for maintaining remission in ulcerative colitis. Ital J Gastroenterol 1994;26:334–37.

24. Hussain F, Ajjan R, Trudgill N, Riley S. Single and divided dose delayed-release mesalazine: are traditional dosing regimens in IBD outmoded? Gastroenterology 1996;110:A928.

25. Riley SA, Mani V, Goodman MJ, Herd ME, Dutt S, Turnberg LA. Comparison of delayed-release 5-aminosalicylic acid (mesalazine) and sulfasalazine as maintenance treatment of patients with ulcerative colitis. Gastroenterology 1988;94:1383–9.

26. Kruis W, Judmaier G, Kayasseh L et al. Double-blind dose-finding study of olsalazine versus sulfasalazine as maintenance therapy for ulcerative colitis. Eur J Gastroenterol Hepatol 1995;7:391–6.

27. Nilsson A, Danielsson A, Löfberg R et al. Olsalazine versus sulfasalazine for relapse prevention in ulcerative colitis: a multicenter study. Am J Gastroenterol 1995;90:381–7.

28. Becker K, Ewe K, Ueberschaer B. Absorption of 5-ASA from a mesalazine and an olsalazine preparation in ulcerative colitis in remission. Gut 1995;37(Suppl. 2):A31.
29. Green JR, Lobo AJ, Holdsworth CD *et al*. Balsalazide is more effective and better tolerated than mesalamine in the treatment of acute ulcerative colitis. Gastroenterology 1998;114:15–22.
30. De Franchis R, Vecchi M, Carpinelli L, Meucci G, Torgano G. Comparison of the efficacy and safety of sulfasalazine and mesalazines in the maintenance treatment of ulcerative colitis: a meta-analysis. Eur J Gastroenterol Hepatol 1993;5:505–10.
31. Ardizonne S, Petrillo M, Imbesi B, Cerutti R, Bollani S, Bianchi-Porro G. Is maintenance therapy always necessary for patients with ulcerative colitis in remission? Aliment Pharmacol Ther 1999;13:373–9.
32. Myszor M, Calam I. Seasonality of ulcerative colitis. Lancet 1984;2:522–3.
33. Kruis W, Schütz E, Fric P, Fixa B, Judmaier G, Stolte M. Double-blind comparison of an oral *Escherichia coli* preparation and mesalazine in maintaining remission of ulcerative colitis. Aliment Pharmacol Ther 1997;11:853–8.
34. Turunen UM, Färkkilä MA, Hakala K *et al*. Long-term treatment of ulcerative colitis with ciprofloxacin: a prospective, double-blind, placebo-controlled study. Gastroenterology 1998;115:1072–8.
35. Thomas GAO, Rhodes J, Mani V *et al*. Transdermal nicotine as maintenance therapy for ulcerative colitis. N Engl J Med 1995;332:988–92.
36. Hawthorne AB, Logan RFA, Hawkey CJ *et al*. Randomized controlled trial of azathioprine withdrawal in ulcerative colitis. Br Med J 1992;305:20–2.
37. George J, Present DH, Pou R *et al*. The long-term outcome of ulcerative colitis treated with 6-mercaptopurine. Am J Gastroenterol 1996;91:1711–14.
38. Connell WR, Kamm M, Dickson M, Balkwill A, Richie J, Lennard-Jones J. Long-term neoplasia risk after azathioprine treatment in inflammatory bowel disease. Lancet 1994;343:1249–52.
39. Farrell RJ, Kileen P, Mahmud N *et al*. Increased risk of non-Hodgkin's lymphoma with immunomodulatory therapy in inflammatory bowel disease. Gastroenterology 1997;112:A969.
40. Alstead EM, Ritchi JK, Lennard-Jones JE, Farthing MJ, Clark ML. Safety of azathioprine in pregnancy in inflammatory bowel disease. Gastroenterology 1990;99:443–6.
41. Rajapakse RO, Korelitz BI, Zlatanic J, Baiocco PJ, Gleim GM. Outcome of pregnancies when fathers are treated with 6-mercaptopurine for inflammatory bowel disease. Gastroenterology 1998;114:A1066.
42. Lichtiger S, Present DH, Kornbluth A *et al*. Cyclosporin in severe ulcerative colitis refractory to steroid therapy. N Engl J Med 1994;330:1841–5.
43. Sternthal JG, Kornbluth A, Lichtiger S, Present D. Toxicity associated with the use of cyclosporin in patients with inflammatory bowel disease (IBD). Gastroenterology 1996;110:A1019.
44. Actis GC, Rocca G, Pinna-Pintor M, Rizzetto M. Azathioprine (AZA) to maintain the response of acute ulcerative colitis (CU) to cyclosporin. Gastroenterology 1998;114:A917.

13
Induction therapy for Crohn's disease

A. H. STEINHART

ABSTRACT

The choice of therapies available for the induction of remission in Crohn's disease is becoming increasingly complex. For many years sulphasalazine and conventional corticosteroids were the mainstays of induction therapy. Although these therapies continue to be used, advances in the understanding of the pathogenesis of inflammatory diseases of the gastrointestinal tract and mechanisms of drug action have led to the development and clinical use of novel therapies. Identification of 5-aminosalicylic acid (mesalazine) as the principally active portion of the sulphasalazine molecule led to the development of mesalazine formulated in various controlled-release preparations targeted to release in the areas of the bowel most commonly affected by Crohn's disease. The potent anti-inflammatory effects of corticosteroids spurred the development of safer, topically active corticosteroids such as budesonide. The immunosuppressive agents azathioprine and 6-mercaptopurine, once thought to be principally useful for maintenance therapy because of slow onset of action, probably have a role in induction therapy when used in combination with corticosteroids. Methotrexate has also been shown to be of value in the patient with chronically active corticosteroid-resistant Crohn's disease. Antibiotics, particularly metronidazole and ciprofloxacin, are used not only to treat septic complications of Crohn's disease but have also been found to be effective in treating active intestinal inflammatory disease. The advent of biological agents, which are targeted against specific aspects of the mucosal immune response, is likely to change the approach to induction therapy. The chimeric monoclonal anti-tumour necrosis factor antibody (Infliximab) has been shown to induce remission in up to 48% of patients at 4 weeks following a single infusion and to improve drainage in patients with fistulas. Other agents, such as IL-10 and antisense ICAM-1 oligonucleotide, continue to undergo clinical trial evaluation. With the development of an ever more varied armamentarium of therapeutic agents, all of which have some degree of efficacy with variable safety profiles and financial costs, the challenge will be to determine the optimal induction therapy for the individual patient.

INTRODUCTION

The primary goals of medical therapy for Crohn's disease are to induce and maintain remission. Additional goals include the avoidance of long-term complications or sequelae of the disease or its therapy and the maintenance of what the individual patient would consider to be a good quality of life. The induction of remission involves the treatment of patients presenting with symptoms and signs of active intestinal inflammation or occasionally with extraintestinal findings associated with inflammatory bowel disease. The goal of induction therapy is, in general, to adequately minimize or, if possible, to eliminate these signs and symptoms with the minimum treatment-related morbidity. The definition of adequate symptom reduction is highly dependent upon the patient's and physician's interpretation but, for the purposes of most clinical trials, has generally been defined as a Crohn's Disease Activity Index (CDAI) score of less than 150. Unfortunately, the induction of remission as defined by the CDAI is not always the endpoint desired by the patient, who may still be suffering from significant symptoms despite a CDAI score that indicates 'clinical remission'. In addition, apparent clinical remission is often not associated with endoscopic or histological remission and it is this discordance which may be responsible for the fact that many patients who are in 'clinical remission' by standard measures still do not feel entirely well and in good health. These limitations need to be considered when evaluating the results of controlled clinical trials and attempting to extrapolate those results to the care of the individual patient.

There are several therapies currently available and used for the induction of remission of Crohn's disease. Remission rates vary between 36% and 92% depending on the patient groups treated, the medications and doses that are prescribed, the duration of therapy and the definition of remission or treatment success.

The ideal induction therapy should probably be one that is highly effective, associated with few adverse effects, cost-effective, equally effective and safe with repeated use, able to reduce the risk of long-term complications and positively affect the natural history of Crohn's disease. At the present time there is no therapeutic agent that fulfils all of these criteria.

SULPHASALAZINE AND MESALAZINE (5-AMINOSALICYLIC ACID)

Prior to 1980, sulphasalazine was a mainstay of Crohn's disease therapy. The first study to carefully examine the effectiveness of sulphasalazine in a controlled manner was the National Co-operative Crohn's Disease Study (NCCDS)[1]. This randomized multicentre study showed sulphasalazine to be superior to placebo when given at a dose of 1 g per 15 kg body weight per day (to a maximum of 5 g per day). However, despite the fact that the proportion of patients in remission (CDAI <150) at the end of 17 weeks of therapy was greater in the sulphasalazine group than in the placebo group (43% versus 30%) this difference was not statistically significant by conventional definitions.

The problem with sulphasalazine, beyond that of the modest degree of efficacy for the induction of remission, is the associated adverse event profile. Gastrointestinal intolerance, in particular, is a problem with the higher doses required to induce remission, and may be dose-limiting for many patients. It is clear that the adverse event profile of sulphasalazine resides primarily in the sulphapyridine part of the molecule and that the 5-aminosalicylic acid (mesalazine) part of the molecule contains much of the anti-inflammatory activity. A number of controlled-release preparations of mesalazine have been manufactured and several of these preparations have undergone clinical trials as induction therapy in Crohn's disease, with variable results.

The largest study of mesalazine, in the form of Pentasa, is a placebo-controlled dose finding study carried out in the United States[2,3]. In that study 310 patients with Crohn's disease of the terminal ileum alone or terminal ileum and colon were randomly assigned to receive placebo, 1, 2 or 4 g of Pentasa daily. After 8 weeks of treatment the patients receiving 4 g per were found to have fared better than those receiving placebo (43% in remission versus 18% in the placebo group). There were no statistically or clinically significant differences between the placebo, 1 g/day or 2 g/day arms with respect to CDAI scores or proportion of patients in remission at the end of treatment. However, a second similar study of 232 patients was not able to demonstrate the superiority of Pentasa over placebo[4]. In a smaller study, Tremaine et al.[5] randomized 38 patients with Crohn's disease of the colon with or without terminal ileum involvement to receive mesalazine, in the form of the Eudragit S coated Asacol 800 mg q.i.d., or placebo for 16 weeks. Forty-five per cent of the Asacol group were found to have achieved clinical remission as compared with 22% of the placebo-treated patients.

More recently, mesalazine (Pentasa) was compared to controlled ileal release budesonide (Entocort CIR) in patients with active Crohn's disease of the terminal ileum with or without involvement of the right side of the colon[6]. Patients were randomized to receive either mesalazine 2 g twice daily or budesonide (Entocort CIR) 9 mg once daily for 16 weeks. Sixty-nine per cent of the budesonide-treated patients were in remission after 8 weeks as compared with only 45% of the mesalazine-treated group. The proportion of patients still in remission after 12 and 16 weeks showed a slight decrease in both arms but budesonide continued to be statistically superior to mesalazine (62% versus 36% remission rates). In addition 27 of the 61 patients randomized to receive mesalazine were withdrawn from the study because of worsening Crohn's disease as compared to only 10 of 63 budesonide-treated patients. Although the results seem to clearly demonstrate the superiority of budesonide over mesalazine it should be noted that the remission rate in the budesonide-treated group was higher than that reported in any of the previous trials of budesonide[7-9]. Similarly, the remission rate observed in the Pentasa-treated group was somewhat lower than that observed in the Singleton et al. study[2]. The absence of a placebo arm makes any conclusion regarding the absolute effectiveness of Pentasa problematic.

The evidence presently available regarding the effectiveness of mesalazine for the treatment of active Crohn's disease is not consistent from one study to the next. However, the studies do appear to indicate only a modest effect with respect to induction of remission. The conflicting study results may be due to the patient selection criteria used by the individual studies and the inherent heterogeneity of the Crohn's disease patient population. It may not be that mesalazine is ineffective, but that physicians and investigators have not adequately defined subgroups of patients who are most likely to benefit from therapy. If mesalazine, which is thought to be primarily a topically active compound with little effect or penetration into the deeper layers of the gut wall, is to have any appreciable clinical benefit it will probably be in patients with early or superficial disease. The inclusion in clinical trials of patients with extensive transmural inflammation and deep ulcers, fissures or fistulas has probably obscured a larger benefit that might have been observed if only patients with more superficial disease or less-advanced disease had been studied.

CORTICOSTEROIDS

Corticosteroids have been the mainstay of Crohn's disease therapy for many years. The NCCDS clearly showed superiority of prednisone, 0.5–0.75 mg/kg per day, over placebo in the induction of remission but at the cost of a significant adverse event profile[1]. Prednisone also appeared to have a therapeutic advantage over sulphasalazine and azathioprine throughout the 17-week study period. Higher doses of corticosteroids may further improve response rates. In an open prospective study, Modigliani *et al.*[10] found a 92% remission rate after 7 weeks of prednisolone 1 mg/kg per day.

A potential drawback associated with the use of corticosteroid therapy is the fact that it has not been demonstrated to be effective and safe for the maintenance of remission for the majority of patients who achieve remission on 2–4 months of acute therapy[1,11,12]. Although this problem is not unique to corticosteroids the potential risks of long-term therapy have made many physicians and patients reluctant to initiate treatment of acute symptoms with corticosteroids. It has also been the impression of some clinicians, although never clearly demonstrated, that corticosteroids somehow change the clinical behaviour of Crohn's disease. It has been shown, however, that a large proportion of Crohn's disease patients become steroid-resistant or steroid-dependent within 1 year of starting corticosteroid therapy[13]. Management of these patients' disease poses a particularly difficult problem for their physicians.

More recently the development of topically active corticosteroids which undergo rapid first-pass metabolism in the liver has permitted therapy that has the potential to achieve the efficacy of conventional corticosteroids with a much more acceptable short- and long-term adverse event profile. Budesonide 9 mg/day, in a controlled-release preparation (Entocort CIR), has been shown to be more effective than both placebo and mesalazine and similarly effective to conventional corticosteroids in patients with Crohn's disease of the terminal ileum[6–9]. Most striking was the safety of the budesonide preparation and the low incidence of usual corticosteroid side-effects. Corticosteroid-associated side-effects were no more common in budesonide-treated patients as compared to placebo-treated patients, and significantly less common as compared to patients treated with conventional corticosteroids[7–9]. A different type of pH-dependent release formulation of budesonide has been found to have efficacy and safety similar to that of Entocort CIR[14–16]. Although it is not known if the use of budesonide to induce remission will affect the incidence of steroid resistance and dependence, and permit safe and effective long-term use of corticosteroids, it can be safely and effectively used to induce remission in patients with mildly to moderately active Crohn's disease.

IMMUNOSUPPRESSIVE AGENTS

The purine analogues, azathioprine and 6-mercaptopurine (6-MP), are becoming more widely used and accepted in the long-term management of Crohn's disease. However, their ability to quickly reduce symptoms of active Crohn's disease is not that great and may, therefore, limit their use as single-drug therapy for the induction of remission[1,17]. It appears that the mean time to response following the use of daily oral azathioprine or 6-MP is approximately 3–4 months. It has been suggested that the use of an intravenous loading dose of azathioprine followed by daily oral administration may shorten the time to response, so as to make its use more suitable for that clinical setting[18]. However, the use of an oral daily dose of a purine analogue, in combination with a corticosteroid, may provide substantial benefits as compared with a corticosteroid alone[19–21]. In a study of paediatric CD patients, Markowitz and colleagues showed that patients who were started on corticosteroids for the treatment of acute symptoms required less prednisone and achieved better long-term remission rates when 6-MP (1.5 mg/kg per day) was started concomitantly and maintained following weaning off prednisone[22].

An area of increasing interest in the use of purine analogue therapy is the use of patient genotyping, enzyme-level measurement and purine metabolite measurement. The use of these techniques is likely to allow better selection of patients and to permit optimization of drug dosing so as to facilitate more rapid and complete therapeutic responses.

Methotrexate is an often-overlooked, but frequently useful, choice for the treatment of patients with chronically active corticosteroid-resistant Crohn's disease. The available evidence supports the use of weekly intramuscular injections of 25 mg to induce remission and allow tapering of prednisone[23]. The drug is generally well tolerated with the occasional occurrence of nausea or asymptomatic liver enzyme elevations. Patients who respond to acute therapy over a 16-week period often do well on maintenance therapy of 15 mg weekly but, at present time, there are not sufficient data available to draw conclusions regarding longer-term efficacy and safety in the Crohn's disease population.

Oral low-dose cyclosporin has been previously shown to be ineffective for the treatment of patients with inactive or mildly active Crohn's disease[24]. However, intravenous cyclosporin followed by the microemulsion oral preparation may be useful in selected situations. Brynskov and colleagues[25] studied a group of patients with chronically active Crohn's disease of the colon and found that the subgroup receiving steroids improved when treated with high-dose oral cyclosporin. In patients with severe refractory Crohn's colitis intravenous cyclosporin is an option that can be considered prior to surgery.

However, as is the case with ulcerative colitis, the optimal maintenance therapy following induction of remission is not well established. It appears that long-term oral cyclosporin may not be effective maintenance therapy and that it is often associated with significant adverse events such as renal toxicity, hypertension and tremor[24]. Other strategies, such as institution of a purine analogue, should be tried for the long-term maintenance therapy of patients successfully treated with cyclosporin.

ANTIBIOTICS

Antibiotics are commonly used to treat the septic complications of Crohn's disease and to reduce drainage from external fistulas. However, their use for the treatment of symptoms due to intestinal mucosal inflammation and ulceration is not universally accepted. This may, in part, be due to the unimpressive results obtained in the controlled trials of antibiotics. The Swedish Co-operative study compared the use of sulphasalazine and metronidazole in an 8-month crossover design and found the drugs to be roughly equivalent with respect to clinical parameters of disease activity[26]. Metronidazole, given at a dose of 0.4 g b.i.d., did have a beneficial effect on inflammatory activity as measured by the serum orosomucoid level. More recently Sutherland and co-workers compared two doses of metronidazole to placebo and found that, although metronidazole produced statistically significant reductions in the mean CDAI scores, the number of patients who achieved clinical remission while receiving metronidazole was no greater than those receiving placebo[27]. However, careful examination of the data shows that metronidazole produced a much more noticeable clinical benefit in patients with colonic disease, who experienced a reduction in their mean CDAI score of 145 points (as compared with a mean reduction of 60 points in patients with both small and large intestinal involvement). This latter observation has certainly coincided with our unit's experience with antibiotic use in the treatment of Crohn's disease. We typically use a combination of ciprofloxacin 500 mg twice daily and metronidazole at a dose of 250 mg two or three times daily depending on the patient's body weight. Antibiotics are often utilized as first-line therapy, particularly in patients with colonic disease. Our initial open-label experience demonstrated a 76% response rate to the combination, and this was associated with very good tolerability and few discontinuations due to side-effects[28]. Others have also demonstrated efficacy of either single or combination antibiotic therapy comparable to that of mesalazine and close to that of systemic corticosteroids[29,30].

BIOLOGICAL AGENTS

The next 10 years will see a number of new therapeutic agents released for use in Crohn's disease. Many of these so-called 'biologicals' have been developed with the benefit of new insights regarding the altered mucosal immune response that is thought to play a central role in the pathogenesis of Crohn's disease, and they are specifically targeted to block or enhance certain aspects of that immune response. These drugs have the potential to improve the therapy of Crohn's disease by specifically targeting critical or important directors or mediators of the immune response, thereby resulting in increased efficacy and safety.

A chimaeric mouse–human antibody against tumour necrosis factor-α (infliximab) has recently been released in the United States for the treatment of patients with active intestinal Crohn's disease and those with draining fistulas. In each of these two clinical settings pivotal studies have demonstrated the effectiveness of one or multiple infusions of infliximab at a dose of 5 mg/kg body weight per infusion[31,32]. In the first study the drug produced a measurable clinical response in 81% of patients and clinical remission in 48% at 4 weeks following a single 5 mg/kg dose[28,32]. There was a definite fall-off of response and remission rates with the higher doses of 10 and 20 mg/kg. A follow-up study suggested that repeated infusions given every 8 weeks can effectively maintain the improvement obtained from a single infusion[33]. What makes these results even more impressive is the fact that the majority of the patients included in the study were already receiving corticosteroid and/or immunosuppressive therapy and not adequately responding.

In a study of patients with draining fistulas, treatment with three infusions of infliximab 5 mg/kg given at 0, 2 and 6 weeks resulted in closure of the fistulas for at least 1 month in 55% of patients and a reduction in the number of draining fistulas in another 13%[31]. However, approximately 50% of patients relapsed after a further 12 weeks of follow-up. The short-term safety of infliximab appears to be quite good, but there have been reports of malignancies in patients treated with this drug, thus raising some concerns about the effect of anti-TNF-α on the ability of the immune system to effectively monitor and eliminate malignant clones of cells.

Other biological agents undergoing clinical trial evaluation include interleukin-10, interleukin-11, ICAM-1 anti-sense oligonucleotide, soluble anti-TNF-α receptor-Fc fusion protein and monoclonal human anti-TNF-α antibody (CDP 571). It is likely that one or more of these, and other biological agents not listed above, will receive regulatory approval over the next 5–10 years.

CONCLUSIONS

The burgeoning number of options available for the treatment of symptoms of active Crohn's disease will make therapeutic choices even more complicated than they are today. However, these new options should ultimately improve patient outcomes and result in both short and long-term improvements in symptom control and reduction in disease complications. Further advances are likely to be made in the area of combination drug therapy as we come to understand more about the pathogenesis of Crohn's disease. The use of multiple drugs, although commonly employed by clinicians, has generally been neglected by investigators and pharmaceutical companies. It should, however, be considered another way of improving the treatment of Crohn's disease using the currently available medical therapies and should be a focus of future investigation.

References

1. Summers RW, Switz DM, Sessions JT *et al*. National Cooperative Crohn's Disease Study: results of drug treatment. Gastroenterology 1979;77:847–69.
2. Singleton JW, Hanauer SB, Gitnick GL *et al*. Mesalamine capsules for the treatment of active Crohn's disease: results of a 16-week trial. Pentasa Crohn's Disease Study Group. Gastroenterology 1993;104:1293–301.
3. Singleton JW, Hanauer S, Robinson M. Quality-of-life results of double-blind, placebo-controlled trial of mesalamine in patients with Crohn's disease. Dig Dis Sci 1995;40:931–5.
4. Singleton J. Second trial of mesalamine therapy in the treatment of active Crohn's disease. Gastroenterology 1994;107:632–3.
5. Tremaine WJ, Schroeder KW, Harrison JM, Zinsmeister AR. A randomized, double-blind, placebo-controlled trial of the oral mesalamine (5-ASA) preparation, Asacol, in the treatment of symptomatic Crohn's colitis and ileocolitis. J Clin Gastroenterol 1994;19:278–82.
6. Thomsen OO, Cortot A, Jewell D *et al*. A comparison of budesonide and mesalamine for active Crohn's disease. International Budesonide–Mesalamine Study Group. N Engl J Med 1998;339:370–4.
7. Campieri M, Ferguson A, Doe W, Persson T, Nilsson LG. Oral budesonide is as effective as oral prednisolone in active Crohn's disease. The Global Budesonide Study Group. Gut 1997;41:209–14.
8. Greenberg GR, Feagan BG, Martin F *et al*. Oral budesonide for active Crohn's disease. Canadian Inflammatory Bowel Disease Study Group. N Engl J Med 1994;331:836–41.
9. Rutgeerts P, Lofberg R, Malchow H *et al*. A comparison of budesonide with prednisolone for active Crohn's disease. N Engl J Med 1994;331:842–5.
10. Modigliani R, Mary JY, Simon JF *et al*. Clinical, biological, and endoscopic picture of attacks of Crohn's disease. Evolution on prednisolone. Groupe d'Etude Therapeutique des Affections Inflammatories Digestives. Gastroenterology 1990;98:811–18.
11. Malchow H, Ewe K, Brandes JW *et al*. European Cooperative Crohn's Disease Study (ECCDS): results of drug treatment. Gastroenterology 1984;86:249–66.
12. Smith RC, Rhodes J, Heatley RV *et al*. Low dose steroids and clinical relapse in Crohn's disease: a controlled trial. Gut 1978;19:606–10.
13. Munkholm P, Langholz E, Davidsen M, Binder V. Frequency of glucocorticoid resistance and dependency in Crohn's disease. Gut 1994;35:360–2.
14. Bar-Meir S, Chowers Y, Lavy A *et al*. Budesonide versus prednisone in the treatment of active Crohn's disease. The Israeli Budesonide Study Group. Gastroenterology 1998;115:835–40.
15. Caesar I, Gross V, Roth M *et al*. Treatment of active and postactive ileal and colonic Crohn's disease with oral pH-modified-release budesonide. German Budesonide Study Group. Hepatogastroenterology 1997;44:445–51.
16. Gross V, Andus T, Caesar I *et al*. Oral pH-modified release budesonide versus 6-methylprednisolone in active Crohn's disease. German/Austrian Budesonide Study Group. Eur J Gastroenterol Hepatol 1996;8:905–9.
17. Present DH, Korelitz BI, Wisch N, Glass JL, Sachar DB, Pasternack BS. Treatment of Crohn's disease with 6-mercaptopurine. A long-term, randomized, double-blind study. N Engl J Med 1980;302:981–7.
18. Sandborn WJ, Van OE, Zins BJ, Tremaine WJ, Mays DC, Lipsky JJ. An intravenous loading dose of azathioprine decreases the time to response in patients with Crohn's disease. Gastroenterology 1995;109:1808–17.
19. Candy S, Wright J, Gerber M, Adams G, Gerig M, Goodman R. A controlled double blind study of azathioprine in the management of Crohn's disease. Gut 1995;37:674–8.
20. Ewe K, Press AG, Singe CC *et al*. Azathioprine combined with prednisolone or monotherapy with prednisolone in active Crohn's disease. Gastroenterology 1993;105:367–72.
21. Lemann M, Bonhomme P, Bitoun A, Messing B, Modigliani R, Rambaud JC. Treatment of Crohn's disease with azathioprine or 6-mercaptopurine. Retrospective study of 126 cases. Gastroenterol Clin Biol 1990;14:548–54.

22. Markowitz J, Rancher KG, Kohn N, Daum F. The multicenter pediatric Crohn's disease 6-mercaptopurine trial. Final results. Gastroenterology 1999;116:A771.
23. Feagan BG, Rochon J, Fedorak RN *et al*. Methotrexate for the treatment of Crohn's disease. The North American Crohn's Study Group Investigators. N Engl J Med 1995;332:292–7.
24. Feagan BG, McDonald JW, Rochon J *et al*. Low-dose cyclosporine for the treatment of Crohn's disease. The Canadian Crohn's Relapse Prevention Trial Investigators. N Engl J Med 1994;330:1846–51.
25. Brynskov J, Freund L, Norby Rasmussen S *et al*. Final report on a placebo-controlled, double-blind, randomized, multicentre trial of cyclosporin treatment in active chronic Crohn's disease. Scand J Gastroenterol 1991;26:689–95.
26. Ursing B, Alm T, Barany F *et al*. A comparative study of metronidazole and sulfasalazine for active Crohn's disease: the cooperative Crohn's disease study in Sweden. II. Result. Gastroenterology 1982;83:550–62.
27. Sutherland L, Singleton J, Sessions J *et al*. Double blind, placebo controlled trial of metronidazole in Crohn's disease. Gut 1991;32:1071–5.
28. Greenbloom SL, Steinhart AH, Greenberg GR. Combination ciprofloxacin and metronidazole for active Crohn's disease. Can J Gastroenterol 1998;12:53–6.
29. Colombel JF, Lemann M, Cassagnou M *et al*. A controlled trial comparing ciprofloxacin with mesalazine for the treatment of active Crohn's disease. Groupe d'Etudes Therapeutiques des Affections Inflammatoires Digestives (GETAID). Am J Gastroenterol 1999;94:674–8.
30. Prantera C, Zannoni F, Scribano ML *et al*. An antibiotic regimen for the treatment of active Crohn's disease: a randomized, controlled clinical trial of metronidazole plus ciprofloxacin. Am J Gastroenterol 1996;91:328–32.
31. Present DH, Rutgeerts P, Targan S *et al*. Infliximab for the treatment of fistulas in patients with Crohn's disease. N Engl J Med 1999;340:1398–405.
32. Targan SR, Hanauer SB, van Deventer SJ *et al*. A short-term study of chimeric monoclonal antibody cA2 to tumor necrosis factor alpha for Crohn's disease. Crohn's Disease cA2 Study Group. N Engl J Med 1997;337:1029–35.
33. Rutgeerts P, D'Haens G, van Deventer SJ *et al*. Retreatment with anti-TNF-α chimeric antibody (cA2) effectively maintains cA2-induced remission in Crohn's disease. Gastroenterology 1997;112:A1078.

14
Maintenance of remission in Crohn's disease

P. RUTGEERTS

Flares of Crohn's disease can be controlled in 50–70% of the patients within 8–12 weeks of start of therapy. Relapses upon discontinuation of therapy, however, are frequent and most patients will receive maintenance therapy.

MAINTENANCE IN MEDICALLY ACHIEVED REMISSION

The NCCDS[1] and the ECCDS[2] failed to demonstrate efficacy for sulphasalazine to maintain remission of Crohn's disease.

Meta-analyses of 5-ASA trials[3,4] showed efficacy with a reduction of the relapse rate of about 50% predominantly in patients with ileal and ileocolonic disease. A provocative Getaid trial[5] suggested that Pentasa 2 g/day for 2 years is effective only when initiated within 3 months after achieving remission, and that 5-ASA maintenance is not beneficial if the patients were already in remission for longer than 3 months. This has not yet been confirmed. It is not clear whether higher doses of 5-ASA up to 4 g may be more effective to maintain remission or to facilitate GCS withdrawal[6].

Standard GCS were not useful for maintenance of remission of Crohn's disease but there was hope that the newer topically acting GCS might be effective without severe side-effects. Although two large trials[7,8] showed that 6 mg of budesonide (Entocort) prolongs the activity-free interval in comparison with placebo, the drug was not efficacious to maintain remission of Crohn's disease over 1 year. Pulse therapy with 9 mg of budesonide o.m. when the disease flares seems preferable over maintenance therapy with lower doses because of the rapid onset of its action.

The immunosuppressors azathioprine and 6-mercaptopurine are currently the only medications that predictably maintain medically induced remission[9,10] There are no clear answers, however, as to how long this therapy needs to be continued. A group of French investigators[11] compared relapse rates in 157 patients in remission who continued azathioprine or 6-mercaptopurine for more than 6 months after steroid withdrawal with 42 patients who stopped therapy for reasons other than relapse. Relapse rates at 1 and 5 years were 11% and 32% in the immunosuppressive group versus 38% and 75% in the group that had discontinued immunosuppressives. The authors also observed that the benefit of continuing immunosuppressive therapy tended to disappear after 4 years. This finding, however, may be biased by the relatively low number of patients and potential lack of power, as suggested by the authors themselves.

There is great hope that immunomodulation will change the long-term management of Crohn's disease. The results of TNF antibodies in active Crohn's disease were excellent but long-term data are also promising. In a follow-up trial[12] after induction of remission with cA2, it was demonstrated that retreatment with cA2 infusions in patients responding to the treatment maintained the treatment benefit over a period of 1 year, whereas in patients treated with repeated placebo infusions the initial treatment benefit was gradually lost. Repeated treatment with cA2 was generally well tolerated. One patient who was already on immunosuppression for a very long time, developed a lymphoma in the course of placebo retreatments.

Conflicting data have been reported on the efficacy of ω-3 fatty acids to maintain remission. In an Italian placebo-controlled trial[13] therapy with 4.5 g of fish oil containing 40% eicosapentanoic acid and 20% docosahexanoic acid resulted in relapse rate of 28% compared with 69% in the placebo group ($p<0.001$). In a German trial[14] 5 g/day of ω-3 fatty acids was not beneficial for maintenance of remission.

PROPHYLACTIC STRATEGIES AFTER CURATIVE SURGERY FOR CROHN'S DISEASE

Recurrence of Crohn's disease is the main complication of ileal resection and partial colectomy and ileocolonic anastomosis for complicated Crohn's ileitis. Before defining risk factors for recurrence of Crohn's disease and discussing prophylaxis one must give clear definitions. We use the definitions proposed by the late E. Lee in his excellent review paper[15].

Crohn's recurrence: the appearance of objective signs – defined radiologically, endoscopically or pathologically – of Crohn's disease in the bowel of a patient who has previously had a resection of all microscopically diseased tissue.
Crohn's relapse: the appearance of the clinical features of Crohn's disease after a symptom-free interval in patients with known disease; provided that other non-related causes of these symptoms have been excluded.

The term 'recurrence' can be used only after radical or curative resection. A *radical resection* involves the excision of a sufficient length of normal bowel from either side of the diseased gut together with lymph nodes draining the region to remove all the disease. Nowadays the segment of normal bowel removed is rather limited (5–15 cm) in order to avoid short bowel syndrome upon repeated surgery. This type of resection can still be called '*curative resection*'. *Local or segmental resections* are designed to remove segments of Crohn's disease which are causing the symptoms, such as fistulas and obstructions. No attempt is made to carry out a curative resection and areas of inflammation may be left behind. *Bypass operations* divert the faecal stream from the diseased segment to improve the inflammation in the dysfunctioned gut.

NATURAL HISTORY OF RECURRENCE OF CROHN'S DISEASE IN THE NEOTERMINAL ILEUM

Systematic endoscopic studies[16] of the neoterminal ileum at different times after ileal resection have shown that within 1 year after resection almost 80% of the patients present with new lesions in the neoterminal ileum. In most of these patients aphthous ulcers are the only lesions visualized. Patients examined at a longer interval after resection have more severe lesions. A higher percentage already presents with severe oral, longitudinal, serpiginous ulcers, while nodularity and strictures develop. The proportion of patients, however, presenting with recurrent lesions seems to stay more or less the same over the years.

The aphthous ulcer is an early lesion. Biopsies taken around these lesions show blunting of the villi, mixed inflammatory infiltrate, with frequent predominance of eosinophils. It seems that the natural evolution of Crohn's lesions mimics the course of the disease at onset. If this is the case postoperative recurrence is the best model available for the study of the pathogenesis of Crohn's disease. This means that it is critical to study the earliest changes, and this might reveal whether mucosal damage occurs first, or whether submucosal inflammatory changes lead to mucosal ulcerations. Sankey *et al.*[17] recently identified a sequence of superficial changes occurring before the development of the aphthous ulcer. They describe disruption of the capillary basement membrane with haemorrhage and trails of fibrinogen in the surrounding lamina propria emptying into the bowel lumen. They found this 'summit' lesion before local inflammatory changes occurred. The authors suggest that vascular lesions lead to mucosal ulcerations. The question remains, however, whether these early changes are specific[18] for Crohn's disease.

TRIGGER OF EARLY RECURRENT LESIONS IN THE NEOTERMINAL ILEUM

Crohn's disease is probably a diffuse disease of the entire digestive tract. Even in intestinal areas that seem macroscopically unaffected at barium meal X-ray follow-through small lesions can be identified at very careful examination, and focal inflammatory infiltrate can be found at serial biopsies. Perioperative endoscopy[19] of the whole small bowel proximal to the section line shows that lesions are found at that time scattered over the intestine. Frequently these lesions are not recognized by preoperative evaluation or surgical inspection of the serosal surface. Although focal isolated lesions can be found throughout the small bowel, recurrence after surgery is always located in a well defined segment of the neoterminal ileum. The same group of investigators who performed the perioperative endoscopy of the whole small bowel studied the relationship between the lesions found at preoperative enteroscopy and postoperative recurrence pattern. They found no relationship between the presence of small bowel lesions at perioperative endoscopy and recurrence patterns after resection[20]. Other authors[21] performed intraoperative endoscopy and found no lesions in the segment where recurrence developed after surgery. In another study[22] intraoperative biopsies in the segment proximal to the section line (the neoterminal ileum) showed no inflammatory changes in 19 of 22 patients, whereas 6 months after surgery clear-cut Crohn's recurrence was present in 21/22 patients, showing that neoterminal ileal lesions recurring after ileal resection are indeed 'new lesions'. More and more it seems that the recurrence pattern is characteristic for the disease of each individual patient. In a very interesting study D'Haens et al.[23] demonstrated that the length of recurrent ileitis after ileocolonic resection correlates closely with the presurgical extent of the disease. This is another manifestation of disease patterns that are currently better understood[24].

So not only the clinical pattern of Crohn's disease[25] remains unchanged after surgery but also the morphological distribution of the lesions[23].

Smedh and co-authors[26] link the recurrence of ileal inflammation to an increase in mucosal phospholipase A2 activity.

The trigger for development of recurrent lesions is probably a luminal factor[27]. When the ileocolonic anastomosis is protected by a proximal ileostomy and no faecal stream passes through the anastomosis Crohn's lesions do not recur. However, as soon as the bowel continuity is restored recurrent ulcers develop in the neoterminal ileum and the evolution of the disease resumes its natural course.

The importance of the faecal stream was also emphasized by the study of Cameron et al.[28]. These authors found that recurrent ileal disease after ileocolonic resection with side-to-end anastomosis involves the ileum adjacent to the colon but spares the ileum in the blind pouch.

PREVENTION OF RECURRENCE OF CROHN'S DISEASE IN THE NEOTERMINAL ILEUM

Altering luminal contents of the bowel – metronidazole

Since there exists a close relationship between the severity of early recurrent Crohn's disease in the neoterminal ileum after ileal resection and clinical reactivation of the disease, prevention of early recurrence must be a major goal in the therapeutic approach to patients submitted to ileal resection. As the faecal stream seems to be the trigger for recurrence, studies of elimination of certain foods resulting in changes of intestinal contents might be of benefit. There is, however, no basis to exclude foods, and long-term trials with elemental diet are very difficult to perform. Antibiotics alter the bacterial intraluminal content of the bowel and might be useful for recurrence prevention. In a double-blind placebo-controlled trial[29] using metronidazole 20 mg/kg body weight during 3 months active treatment resulted in significantly less severe recurrent endoscopic lesions than placebo. Treatment was started within 1 week of ileal resection with partial colectomy and ileocolonic anastomosis. The overall endoscopic recurrence rates at 3 months were lower in the metronidazole group (12/23; 52%) than in the placebo group (21/28; 75%) but the difference was not significant. However, severe lesions were found significantly more frequently in the placebo group (12/28; 43%) than in the metronidazole group (3/23; 13%; $p=0.02$). A drawback in this study was the high incidence of side-effects in the metronidazole group. Symptomatic recurrence rates were significantly different at 1 year but the difference had disappeared by year 3.

Anti-inflammatory treatment with sulphasalazine or 5-ASA

In a multicentre prevention trial for clinical recurrence Ewe *et al.*[30] found that sulphasalazine (3 g/day) was significantly more effective in the first 2 years of therapy to maintain clinical remission of the disease after resection than placebo, and surprisingly the recurrence rate was significantly higher in the group of patients treated with radical resection than in patients with more limited Crohn's resection. Both strategies were additive: non-radical operation and sulphasalazine had the best prognosis.

In a multicentre randomized trial for prevention of postoperative recurrence reported on by Caprilli and coauthors[31], 110 patients were randomized to Asacol 2.4 g/day or no treatment 2 weeks after a first ileal resection and ileocolonic anastomosis. Recurrence was defined on the basis of endoscopic criteria and classified as mild or severe. The cumulative proportion of recurrence at 6, 12 and 24 months was significantly lower in the 5-ASA group than in the untreated group ($p=0.0023$). At 24 months the cumulative proportion of recurrence was 0.52 ± 0.12 and 0.85 ± 0.07. At the same time the cumulative proportion (CP) of symptomatic recurrence was 0.18 ± 0.09 and 0.41 ± 0.09 ($p=0.0062$). The CP of the severe recurrence was also significantly lower in the 5-ASA group (0.17 ± 0.09 vs 0.38 ± 0.09; $p=0.21$). Although the total duration of this study will be 5 years this preliminary analysis shows that administration of oral 5-ASA prevents endoscopic and symptomatic recurrence of Crohn's ileitis at 2 years. The authors estimated that Asacol therapy prevented 39% of all recurrences and 55% of the severe recurrences.

An important weakness of this study is that there was no placebo involved. Patients took Asacol or no medication at all. This could have led to observer bias.

Another Italian placebo-controlled prevention trial[32] with Pentasa in a dose of 3 g/day started within 1 month of ileal resection and ileocolonic anastomosis showed that endoscopic lesions were significantly less severe in the Pentasa-treated patients ($p=0.008$). The overall rate of severe endoscopic and radiological recurrences amounted to 24% in the Pentasa group versus 56% in the placebo group ($p<0.004$); difference 32% (95% CI 22–52). Florent *et al.*[33] performed a placebo-controlled trial of Claversal 1.5 g b.i.d. during 12 weeks for prevention of endoscopic recurrence after ileal resection with ileocolonic anastomosis started within 15 days of surgery; 126 patients were included in the study. An endoscopic relapse was observed in 50% of the patients treated with Claversal and in 63% of the patients treated with placebo. Although there was a trend in favour of 5-ASA the difference is not significant ($p=0.16$). There was no further clinical or endoscopic follow-up reported.

In another prevention study of Eudragit-L coated 5-ASA 1.5 g/day Fiasse *et al.*[34] started therapy only at 3 months after resection. Only preliminary results were published in abstract form. There was no significant difference as far as clinical relapse rates or severity of radiological lesions at 1 year in 37 patients (19 placebo, 18 5-ASA) who completed the trial. A major drawback of this study is that the medication was started only 3 months after surgery, whereas it has been shown by endoscopic studies that in the majority of the patients lesions recur as early as the first 3 months.

A multicentre North American study[35] compared mesalamine 3 g/day with placebo for prophylaxis of postoperative Crohn's disease recurrence.

The symptomatic recurrence rate in the treatment group was 31% (27 of 87) compared with 41% (31 of 76) in the control group at 3 years ($p=0.031$). The relative risk of developing recurrent disease was 0.628 (90% CI 0.40–0.97) for the treatment group patients on intention-to-treat analysis. The endoscopic and radiological risk was also decreased significantly with a relative risk of 0.654 (90% CI 0.47–0.91). There were a number of drawbacks in that study: there was switching of 5-ASA formulation, lumping of patients with different disease location and patients were included only 8 weeks postsurgically.

A recently large multicentre German study[36] showed that mesalazine (4 g/day) for 18 months after surgery for Crohn's disease tended to decrease postoperative relapse rates, but the study failed to show a significant overall effect. Subgroup analysis showed a significant effect on patients with isolated small bowel disease, while no benefit was seen in patients with Crohn's disease including the colon.

A meta-analysis by Camma *et al.*[37] calculated a pooled risk difference of –13.1% (95% CI –21.8–4.5%) for symptomatic recurrence after surgery on prophylaxis with mesalamine.

BUDESONIDE FOR RECURRENCE PREVENTION IN POSTOPERATIVE CROHN'S DISEASE[38]

Comparing budesonide 6 mg/day o.m. with placebo, the frequency of endoscopic recurrence did not differ between the groups (intent-to-treat analysis) at 3 months (45% vs 46%) or at 12 months (63% vs 63%). The recurrence rates were, however, different with respect to the indication for surgery. There was no difference between the treatments in patients who had undergone surgery for fibrostenosis whereas endoscopic recurrence rates were lower in the BUD group, both at 3 months (21% vs 47%; $p=0.12$) and at 12 months (32% vs 65%; $p=0.048$) in patients who had undergone surgery for disease activity.

IMMUNOSUPPRESSION FOR CROHN'S DISEASE RECURRENCE PROPHYLAXIS

Since intestinal inflammation in Crohn's disease is probably the consequence of increased mucosal immune activation immunosuppression is a logical therapy to prevent recurrent Crohn's disease. Preliminary data[39] on recurrence prevention using 6-mercaptopurine published by Adler and Korelitz suggest there is a role for 6-MP in prevention. A multicentre placebo-controlled trial comparing 6-MP and Pentasa has been completed recently[40]; 50 mg of 6-MP consistently decreased endoscopic and clinical recurrence rates. The full data will be published soon.

CONCLUSIONS

Recurrence of Crohn's lesions after ileal resection is the best model presently available to study the natural evolution and pathogenetic factors in Crohn's disease. Although prevention studies are scarce at present, preliminary results suggest that medical therapy can influence the course of the disease after surgery by decreasing the rate of early recurrent mucosal lesions. The aim must be to totally prevent new lesions. More well-designed studies are much needed.

References

1. Summers RW, Switz DM, Sessions JT Jr *et al*. National Cooperative Crohn's Disease Study: results of drug treatment. Gastroenterology 1979;77:847–69.
2. Malchow H, Ewe K, Brandes JW *et al*. European Co-operative Crohn's Disease Study (ECCDS): results of drug treatment. Gastroenterology 1984;86:249–66.
3. Messori A, Brignola C, Trallori G *et al*. Effectiveness of 5-aminosalicylic acid for maintaining remission in patients with Crohn's disease: a meta-analysis. Am J Gastroenterol 1994;89:692–8.
4. Steinhart AH, Hemphill D, Greenberg GR. Sulfasalazine and mesalazine for the maintenance therapy of Crohn's disease: a meta-analysis. Am J Gastroenterol 1994;89:2116–24
5. Hanauer SB, Krawitt EL, Robinson M, Rick GG, Safdi MA and the Pentasa Crohn's Disease Compassionate Use Study Group. Long term management of Crohn's disease with mesalamine capsules (Pentasa). Am J Gastroenterol 1993;88:1343–50.
6. Modigliani R, Colombel JF, Dupas JL *et al*., for GETAID. Mesalamine in Crohn's disease with steroid-induced remission: effect on steroid withdrawal and remission maintenance. Gastroenterology 1996;110:688–93.
7. Greenberg GR, Feagan BG, Martin F *et al*. and the Canadian IBD group. Oral budesonide as maintenance treatment for Crohn's disease: a placebo-controlled, dose-ranging study. Gastroenterology 1996;110:45 51.
8. Löfberg R, Rutgeerts P, Malchow H *et al*. Budesonide prolongs time to relapse in ileal and ileocaecal Crohn's disease: a placebo-controlled one-year study. Gut 1996;39:82–6.
9. Pearson DC, May GR, Fick GH, Sutherland LR. Azathioprine and 6-mercaptopurine in Crohn's disease: a meta-analysis. Ann Intern Med 1995;122:132–42.
10. O'Donoghue DP, Dawson AM, Powell-Tuck J, Bown RL, Lennard-Jones JE. Double-blind withdrawal trial of azathioprine as maintenance treatment for Crohn's disease. Lancet 1978;2:955–7.
11. Bouhnik Y, Lémann M, Mary JY *et al*. Long-term follow-up of patients with Crohn's disease treated with azathioprine or 6-mercaptopurine. Lancet 1996;347:215–19.
12. Rutgeerts P, D'Haens G, van Deventer SJH *et al*. Retreatment with anti-TNFα chimeric antibody (cA2) effectively maintains cA2-induced remission in Crohn's disease. Gastroenterology 1997;112:A1078.
13. Belluzi A, Brignola C, Campieri M, Pera A, Boschi S, Miglioli M. Effect of an enteric-coated fish-oil preparation in relapses in Crohn's disease. N Engl Med 1996;334:1557–60.
14. Lorenz-Meyer H, Bauer P, Nicolay C *et al*. and study group members of the German Crohn's Disease Study Group. Omega-3 fatty acids and low carbohydrate diet for maintenance of remission in Crohn's disease. Scand J Gastroenterol 1996;31:778 85.
15. Lee ECG, Papainannou N. Recurrence following surgery for Crohn's disease. Clin Gastroenterol 1980;9:419–38.
16. Rutgeerts P, Geboes K, Vantrappen G. Natural history of recurrent Crohn's disease at the ileocolonic anastomosis after curative surgery. Gut 1984;25:665–72.
17. Sankey EA, Dhillon AP, Anthony A *et al*. Early mucosal changes in Crohn's disease. Gut 1993;34:375–81.

18. Rutgeerts P, Geboes K. Inflammatory bowel disease – Crohn's disease and pre-aphthoid lesions. Lancet 1993;341:1443–4.
19. Lescut D, Vanco D, Bonnière P et al. Perioperative endoscopy of the whole small bowel in Crohn's disease. Gut 1993;34:647–9.
20. Lescut D, Vanco D, Colombel JF et al. Influence des lésions endoscopiques d'amont sur les lésions endoscopiques anastomatiques au cours de la maladie de Crohn. Gastroenterol Clin Biol 1990;14:A20.
21. Olaison G, Smedh K, Sjödahl R. Natural course of Crohn's disease after ileocolic resection: endoscopically visualized ileal ulcers preceding symptoms. Gut 1992;33:331–5.
22. Rutgeerts P, Geboes K, Vantrappen G et al. Predictability of the postoperative course of Crohn's disease. Gastroenterology 1990;99:450–63.
23. D'Haens GR, Gasparaitis AE, Hanauer SB. The length of recurrent ileitis after ileocolonic resection correlates with presurgical extent of Crohn's disease. Gastroenterology 1993;104:A692.
24. Sachar DB, Andrews HA, Farmer RG et al. Proposed classification of patient subgroups in Crohn's disease. Gastroenterol Int 1992;5:141–54.
25. Pallone F, Boivirant M, Antonietta M, Cosintino R, Pranthera C, Torsoli A. Analysis of clinical course of postoperative recurrence in Crohn's disease of distal ileum. Dig Dis Sci 1992;37:215–19.
26. Smedh K, Olaison G, Sjödahl R. Initiation of anastomotic recurrence of Crohn's disease after ileocolic resection. Onset proximal to the junction and preceded by increased phospholipase A_2 activity. Scand J Gastroenterol 1992;27:691–4.
27. Rutgeerts P, Geboes K, Peeters M et al. Effect of faecal stream diversion on recurrence of Crohn's disease in the neoterminal ileum. Lancet 1991;338:771–4.
28. Cameron JL, Hamilton SR, Coleman J et al. Patterns of ileal recurrence in Crohn's disease. A prospective randomized study. Ann Surg 1992;215:546–52.
29. Rutgeerts P, Hiele M, Geboes K et al. Controlled trial of metronidazole treatment for prevention of Crohn's recurrence after ileal resection. Gastroenterology 1995;108:1617–21.
30. Ewe K, Herfarth C, Malchow H et al. Postoperative recurrence of Crohn's disease in relation to radicality of operation and sulfasalazine prophylaxis: a multicenter trial. Digestion 1989;42:224–32.
31. Caprilli R, Andreoli A, Capurso L et al. Oral 5-aminosalicylic acid (Asacol) for prevention of Crohn's disease postoperative recurrences. Aliment Pharmacol Ther 1994;8:35–43.
32. Brignola C, Cottone M, Pera A et al. Mesalamine in the prevention of endoscopic recurrence after intestinal resection for Crohn's disease. Gastroenterology 1995;108:345–9.
33. Florent Ch, Cortot A, Quandale P et al. Placebo-controlled trial of Claversal[R](C) in the prevention of early endoscopic relapse after 'curative' resection for Crohn's disease. Gastroenterology 1992;102:A623.
34. Fiasse R, Fontaine F, Vanheuverzwyn R. Prevention of Crohn's disease recurrences after intestinal resection with Eudragit-L-coated 5-aminosalicylic acid. Preliminary results of a one-year double-blind placebo controlled study. Gastroenterology 1991;100:A208.
35. McLeod RS, Wolff BG, Steinhart AH et al. Prophylactic mesalamine treatment decreases postoperative recurrence of Crohn's disease. Gastroenterology 1995;109:404–13.
36. Lochs H, Mayer M, Fleig WE, Mortensen PB, Bauer P and the ECCDS VI Study Group. Prophylaxis of postoperative relapse in Crohn's disease with mesalazine (Pentasa®) in comparison with placebo. Gastroenterology 1997;112:A1027.
37. Camma C, Giunta M, Rosselli M, Cottone M. Mesalamine in the maintenance treatment of Crohn's disease: a metaanalysis adjusted for confounding variables. Gastroenterology 1997;113:1465–73.
38. Hellers G, Löfberg R, Rutgeerts P et al. Oral budesonide for prevention of recurrence following ileocolonic resection of Crohn's disease. A one year placebo-controlled study. Gastroenterology 1996;110:A923.
39. Adler DJ, Korelitz BI. The long-term efficacy of 6-mercaptopurine in the treatment of inflammatory bowel disease. In: MacDermott RP, editor. Inflammatory Bowel Disease: Current Status and Future Approach. New York: Elsevier; 1991:731–35.
40. Korelitz B, Hanauer S, Rutgeerts P, Present D, Peppercorn M. Postoperative prophylaxis with 6-MP, 5-ASA or placebo in Crohn's disease: a 2 year multicenter trial. Gastroenterology 1998;114:G4141.

Section V
Bone disease in inflammatory bowel disease

Moderator: **R. F. Bursey,** St John's

15
Risk factors and prevalence of bone disease in inflammatory bowel disease

C. N. BERNSTEIN

ABSTRACT

The prevalence rates of decreased bone mineral density (BMD) in patients with inflammatory bowel disease (IBD) range from 40% to 50%. Osteoporosis, as defined by a BMD Z score of -2.5, has been reported in a range of 2–30%. There are a paucity of data reporting the fracture incidence rate among patients with IBD. Fractures are a hard endpoint and the main morbidity associated with osteopenia of any cause. Osteoporosis which places subjects at risk for fractures has been a term applied to histomorphometric diagnoses, radiological diagnoses, and most recently to BMD diagnoses. We have recently reported that there is an increased rate of fractures at the hip, ribs and forearm among patients with IBD compared with an age, gender and geographically matched cohort drawn from the general population. We found a tendency towards increased fractures at the spine, but this was not statistically significant.

The following is a discussion of risk factors for the development of osteoporosis and fractures in patients with IBD. Measurable risk factors, such as BMD or serum and urine markers of bone resorption and formation, will be discussed in the context of patients with IBD. Similarly, modifiable risk factors will also be discussed.

INTRODUCTION

We have recently reported that there is an increased rate of fractures, at the hip, ribs and forearm among patients with inflammatory bowel disease (IBD) compared with an age, gender and geographically matched cohort drawn from the general population[1]. We found a tendency towards increased fractures at the spine but this was not statistically significant. Fractures are a hard endpoint and the main morbidity associated with osteopenia of any cause. Osteoporosis which places subjects at risk for fractures has been a term applied to histomorphometric diagnoses, radiological diagnoses, and most recently to bone densitometry diagnoses. The most complete histomorphometric data available in the IBD population reported on iliac crest biopsies from 19 patients[2]; this revealed that IBD patients had diminished trabecular bone, decreased adjusted appositional rates, decreased maximal cavity depth and length and increased mineralization lag time. The study found no difference in osteoid area or seam width. It was concluded that IBD-associated osteoporosis is characterized by decreased bone formation at a cellular and tissue level consistent with a negative remodelling balance. Other recent bone biopsy and bone turnover studies suggested that reduced bone formation was a key factor in the osteopenia seen in IBD[3].

By bone mineral densitometry (BMD) osteoporosis is diagnosed when the T score[4] is less than –2.5. Recently the flaws with our current 'gold standards' of diagnosing osteoporosis have been discussed[5]. One important issue is that the BMD definition ignores the importance of architectural abnormalities. Furthermore, the role of biphosphonates in reducing fracture risk among patients with postmenopausal osteoporosis is out of proportion to their effects on BMD[5]. This underscores the rationale for using fracture as the endpoint of studies investigating these issues rather than BMD. This is even more critical when addressing bone risks and IBD, since most data available do not reflect IBD specifically.

Because there is significant morbidity associated with hip fractures in particular, which we have shown to be increased in IBD, it is important to review risk factors including diminished bone mass. We will also review the prevalence of osteopenia in IBD and the implications of these data.

RISK FACTORS

In terms of preventing fractures there are two types of risk factors to be addressed. The first to be addressed will be measurable markers that serve as warnings of a heightened fracture risk. Then a discussion of modifiable risk factors that affect bone mass will follow.

Measurable risk factors

Bone mineral densitometry

BMD is the single best predictor of hip fractures in postmenopausal women, particularly when a measurement is taken at the femoral neck[6–8]. It is not known whether this holds also for a population of patients with IBD who would typically be much younger than the postmenopausal population. In the past, decreased BMD has often been viewed as a diagnosis unto itself as opposed to being a risk factor (for fracture). Not all patients with markedly decreased BMD will sustain a fracture, much like not all smokers will sustain vascular disease. Decreased BMD was relegated to risk factor status for bone fragility in 1991[9].

One difficulty in extrapolating the risk conferred by BMD measures for fracture from the postmenopausal osteoporosis literature is the evidence that among some groups using corticosteroids fractures may occur at higher BMD than that which would be predictive for postmenopausal osteoporosis[10]. The normal population with T scores of –2 to 0 may not have an increased fracture risk, but this risk has been studied in elderly mostly postmenopausal populations, who have other confounding risk factors such as the risk of falling. Thus, the high prevalence of T scores between –1 and –2.5 among patients with IBD who are non-corticosteroid users[11–15] may not necessarily confer an increased risk of fracture. It is possible that a patient with IBD who is a non-corticosteroid user with normal sex hormone profile and normal body mass may have no increased risk of fracture even if the BMD T score falls below –1. Thus, even if it is true that non-corticosteroid-using IBD patients may have decreased BMD, they may not necessarily have an increased fracture risk and the BMD may prove to be of minimal importance.

BMD gives us an apparent areal measure of bone density rather than volumetric BMD, which has been suggested to be a truer measure of bone mineral content and to have a truer association with fracture risk[16,17]. This is because volumetric BMD is less dependent on body and bone sizes. Finally, BMD measures do not equate exactly with intrinsic bone fragility. There may be local defects or biomechanically critical areas of weakness that are not reflected in BMD measures integrated over larger areas[18].

Markers of bone formation and resorption

Several studies have evaluated the relationship between serum 25-OH vitamin D levels and osteopenia. In Crohn's disease, ileal resection and increased malnutrition in general would be suspected to lead to lower levels of 25-OH vitamin D than normal controls or even patients with ulcerative colitis. One group found these levels to be below the lower limit of normal in 65% of 82 patients with Crohn's disease[19] and another found low levels in 44% of 115 patients with Crohn's disease[20]. This latter study found no relationship between 25-OH vitamin D level and BMD, underscoring the difficulty in knowing how to interpret these levels. Another study found low 25-OH vitamin D levels only in 8% of 66 IBD patients[15]. Furthermore, in a Finnish study IBD patients had normal levels of 25-OH vitamin D and the levels also did not correlate with BMD[21]. Others have also found no clear relationship between measured serum hormone levels (vitamin D metabolites, or parathyroid hormone, PTH) and BMD among IBD patients[22,23]. In a small study it was shown that in three subjects who had bone biopsies showing osteomalacia ($n=2$) or osteoporosis ($n=1$) with normal serum 25-OH vitamin D levels there was no improvement on bone biopsy after treatment with vitamin D. However, the three subjects who had osteomalacia on bone biopsy and low levels of 25-OH vitamin D did respond to vitamin D with improvement on bone biopsy[19].

Bone formation markers such as serum osteocalcin, pro-collagen-carboxy terminal propeptide (PICP), and bone-specific alkaline phosphatase are normal in Crohn's disease[13,24]. Non-carboxylated osteocalcin is the marker most highly associated with hip fracture in postmenopausal osteoporosis[25] and for corticosteroid-induced osteoporosis serum osteocalcin and PICP levels were decreased[26]. Two studies did find low osteocalcin levels in some patients[3,22]; however, only one study found a correlation between osteocalcin levels and BMD[3]. These findings underscore the difficulty in extrapolating one form of osteoporosis to others.

Bone resorption marker such as urinary deoxypyridoline (DPD) was found to be increased in 63% of patients with Crohn's disease[13]. Elsewhere urinary DPD was increased in IBD patients[27], while another marker of bone resorption, carboxy terminal telopeptide of type 1 collagen (ICTP) was reportedly increased[24].

Modifiable risk factors

Corticosteroids

Studies on states of corticosteroid excess or insufficiency with replacement have shown that corticosteroids cause diminution in BMD, which is reversible upon correcting the corticosteroid imbalance[28–30]. There are recently reported data that patients with active IBD treated with corticosteroids will have increased BMD after the corticosteroids are discontinued[31]. This, however, does not resolve the issue as to whether the corticosteroids or the active inflammatory disease is the culprit for the diminished BMD.

It has been estimated that up to 30–50% of patients using prolonged corticosteroids may experience vertebral compression fractures[32]. There are data that suggest that corticosteroid-induced osteopenia may be highest in growing children[33,34]. This is important obviously for young children with IBD. However, it may also be true that since children and young adults can continue to have a positive bone remodelling balance, these effects are more readily reversible in this group upon withdrawing the corticosteroids.

Corticosteroids primarily reduce trabecular bone but also diminish cortical bone[35–39]. The hip is composed of about 75% cortical bone[40]. Estimates of cortical bone at the transcervical measurement are at 57% while Ward's triangle is thought to comprise predominantly trabecular bone[41]. Thus, factors that affect trabecular bone will obviously also affect the hip. One study showed similar reductions in BMD in the proximal femur as in the lumbar spine among 32 corticosteroid-using patients with chronic inflammatory diseases (none of whom had IBD)[42]. However, only one of these subjects had BMD Z scores of less than –2.5. Studies have shown an increased rate of vertebral fractures in corticosteroid users[38,39]. Our data showed a trend of increased vertebral fractures[1]. We simply did not know the degree to which our IBD population was using corticosteroids, and it is possible that we might have different results if we analysed the corticosteroid-using patients separately. Even if we assume that a substantial number of IBD patients had used corticosteroids, studies have shown that many IBD patients may have diminished bone mass in the absence of ever having used corticosteroids[43]. Even bone mass data from corticosteroid users with a variety of chronic conditions (i.e. asthma, polymyalgia rheumatica, rheumatoid arthritis) may not be directly extrapolated to IBD since among these conditions there are wide ranges as to the effects of corticosteroids[44,45].

There has been confusion among clinicians as to when it is most appropriate to intervene regarding bone status in patients using corticosteroids. It has been suggested by some that there is more rapid loss of bone in the first 6 months than in patients on long-term corticosteroids[42,46]. A recent study showed no change in BMD after 1 year in patients enrolled in the study who had already used corticosteroid for greater than 12 months[47]. Some have suggested that low doses can have differential effects on bone mass depending on the underlying disease state[45,46,48]. A significant correlation was found between amount of steroids used and spinal trabecular bone loss in males[49], and larger amounts reduce bone mass more notably than do smaller cumulative amounts[15]. Other data also suggest that cumulative corticosteroid doses correlate with bone loss[50]. This does not refute the possibility that the highest amount of bone loss is in the first 6 months of therapy. It is also suggested that the bone loss will remain for as long as high doses of corticosteroids are used[50]. Thus, constant corticosteroid dosing may perpetuate the diminution in BMD.

One important study showed that not all corticosteroid-using patients will have impaired calcium homeostasis[51]. One group of patients ($n=29$) had vertebral compression fractures and they also had a significantly decreased intestinal calcium absorption and BMD. A second group ($n=31$) had no vertebral compression fractures and they also had normal calcium absorption and BMD. Thus, it would be ideal to have some marker of predicting which corticosteroid users might encounter bone homeostasis problems.

Corticosteroids inhibit bone formation by inhibiting osteoblasts[36,52]. They also increase bone resorption directly by stimulating osteoclasts and indirectly by inhibiting intestinal absorption of calcium, which in turn increases PTH activity[53,54].

Other drugs

Purine analogues are increasingly used in the long-term management of patients with IBD. Two studies have suggested azathioprine does not pose any risk to bones[55,56]. Methotrexate has been associated with some deleterious effects on bone in postmenopausal women with primary biliary cirrhosis[57]. This is obviously a situation that does not equate with many patients with IBD, because of the confounding effects of the postmenopausal state and cirrhosis which is known also to be associated with decreased bone mass. In a study of children with juvenile rheumatoid arthritis, methotrexate had no deleterious effects on bone mass[58].

Sex hormones

The lack of oestrogen is thought to be a main contributor to postmenopausal osteoporosis[59]. After 1 year treatment with oestrogen, BMD was increased in the spine, mid radius and femoral trochanter, although no changes were seen at the femoral neck[60]. More importantly, a reduced rate of vertebral fractures was seen. In a study of premenopausal women, oestrogen status and incidence of menstrual irregularities were the major determinants of bone loss[61]. In IBD a non-randomized study of postmenopausal women using oestrogens did show an increase in distal radius and spine bone mass[62]. In a group of amenor-rhoeic women using long-term corticosteroids, oestrogen and progesterone therapy increased spine BMD compared to those women not taking this therapy[63]. Glucocorticoids can reduce both oestrogens and androgens through adrenal atrophy, inhibition of pituitary gonadotropin secretion and by direct gonadal effects[64,65]. Oestrogen's effects on calcium balance are towards a net gain through increased intestinal absorption and decreased urinary excretion[66]. Oestrogens also inhibit bone resorption[67]. Males with IBD may be hypoandrogenized, possibly related to corticosteroid therapy or systemic inflam-mation[68], and testosterone therapy may improve bone mass.

Trauma risk

It might be that young patients with IBD, despite a low BMD, are less susceptible to falls than the elderly; therefore low BMD in IBD patients may correlate less well with fracture incidence. Alternatively, young males with IBD who may be more hypoandrogenized compared to young males in the general population[68] may have a greater fracture risk at lesser of a decrease in BMD. Thus, the correlation between BMD and fracture risk in this population needs to be studied. Furthermore, there is evidence that, among some groups using corticosteroids, fractures may occur at higher BMD than that which would be predictive for postmenopausal osteoporosis[10]. Thus, although younger patients may have lower short-term fracture risk they have higher lifetime fracture risks, by virtue of the extended period at which they are at risk[18].

Exercise, body weight, body size

Lack of exercise and low body weight may also place patients at fracture risk[59,69,70]. There are mechanical effects on bone secondary to direct effects of loading (weight bearing, impact) or indirectly through muscle tension. Length of the femoral neck predicts risk for hip fracture independent of BMD[71]. Thus, assessments of bone macrostructure through morphometry will be an important advance in risk stratification. Body mass index proved to be a significant predictor of decreased BMD in a multivariate analysis among patients with Crohn's disease[72,73]. In a case–control study of Crohn's disease patients, body weight (as well as age and gender) was a significant predictor of decreased BMD[74]. Volumetric adjustments are necessary to truly understand the meaning of BMD and fracture risk. DEXA areal BMD may underestimate true volumetric bone density if bone size variability secondary to stunted size exists (for instance, secondary to stunted growth, or malnutrition)[16]. Thus, assessing fracture risk based on areal DEXA measurements, which do not account for bone or body size, may be inaccurate.

Patients with IBD can exercise without necessarily adversely affecting their disease state[75]. Exercise can increase muscle strength, balance, mobility and overall physical function and thereby reduce the risk of falling[70]. Conversely, prolonged bedrest can increase urinary calcium losses[76]. Physical exercise was shown to have a positive influence on bone mass in young women in their third decade[77]. Thus, being sedentary is harmful to bones and being physically active is beneficial.

Smoking

Smoking is a known risk factor for fracture risk. This has been shown in males[78], in females[79] and even specifically in IBD[80]. It is known that patients with Crohn's disease are more likely be smokers[81], although patients with ulcerative colitis are more likely to be ex-smokers[82]. Tobacco use may decrease circulating oestrogens, and thus have indirect effects on decreasing bone mass, or may have direct effects on increasing bone resorption. In a twin study for every 10 pack-year smoking history, the BMD of the twin who smoked more heavily was 2% lower at the spine ($p=0.01$) and 1.4% lower at the femoral shaft ($p=0.04$). This effect was not confounded by lifestyle measures[79]. These investigators suggested that smoking one pack a day throughout adulthood until menopause could contribute a 5–10% decrease in BMD[79]. Female IBD patients who smoke have significantly decreased BMD at the spine, femoral neck, trochanter and Ward's triangle, although these changes were not seen among male smokers[80]. Perhaps the increased metabolism of oestrogen among smokers enhances the effect of smoking on bones[83,84].

Diet

The bone remodelling balance favours continued bone gain up until age 30 years and one group found that the calcium:protein ratio of the diet was the most important determinant of the amount of gain[85]. For patients with IBD this may be a very critical fact since the ages of highest incidence of IBD are the second and third decades[86], which are important years in determining final adult bone mass. Most calcium intake data are in studies of postmenopausal women. Calcium intake inversely correlated with bone mass in postmenopausal women. A 400 mg increment in dietary calcium correlated with a 1.3% increase in femoral neck BMD[59]. This effect in this study was less than that seen for the effects of oestrogen. Groups have shown that the use of 1200 mg/day of calcium (with 800 IU of vitamin D)[87] or 1750 mg/day of calcium[88] could suppress age-related bone loss in postmenopausal women. However, 1000 mg of calcium/day plus 0.6 µg of $1,25(OH)_2$ vitamin D for 1 year saved bone loss at the spine but not at the femoral neck or distal radius[89]. It has also been shown that 1200 mg/day of calcium with 800 IU vitamin D over 18 months could decrease hip fractures by 43% and other non-vertebral fractures by 32%[90], and even 500 mg/day of calcium with 700 IU of vitamin D over 3 years could reduce fracture rates[91]. These fracture reduction data are the most compelling evidence for the benefit of calcium (and vitamin D) in postmenopausal states. Calcium intake also positively correlated with BMD among healthy adolescent girls[92].

Dietary restrictions may limit the calcium intake of patients with IBD, which may further exacerbate fracture risk. Studies have shown that patients with IBD ingest approximately 800–900 mg/day of calcium[93,94]. Even in geographic areas where a matched control population ingested a mean of 1334 mg/day, IBD patients ingested only a mean of 1093 mg/day and 53% of IBD patients ingested less than 1000 mg/day[21]. Particularly for patients who may lack in sex hormones, or who are receiving corticosteroids, this may simply be far below recommended requirements.

The average daily vitamin D intake in one US study of IBD patients was a mere 128 IU[93]. Similar dietary vitamin D intakes were reported in an Austrian study of patients with Crohn's disease, and this intake was not different from controls[95]. In a study in Finland IBD patients had the same vitamin D intake as controls and there was no correlation between the vitamin D intake and BMD[96].

There is suggestive but inconclusive evidence that lower intakes of zinc, copper, magnesium, manganese and vitamin K correlate with lower BMD among Crohn's disease patients[94].

Genetics

Heredity has been deemed for some time as contributing to risk for osteoporosis[97]. The second most significant determinant of bone loss in a study of premenopausal women was a family history of osteoporosis[61,98]. Recently genotypes have been explored. Polymorphisms in the vitamin D receptor gene, oestrogen receptor gene and most recently in the alleles of the collagen type Ial gene have been assessed[99–101]. Ultimately genetic variants that may predict osteoporosis in ageing or postmenopausal populations will also have to be assessed in IBD populations. Genetic predisposition may explain why some patients using corticosteroids or with long-standing IBD do not have osteoporosis.

Other

Disease location and disease duration do not correlate with BMD among patients with IBD[27,73,74]. However, disease diagnosis (Crohn's disease versus ulcerative colitis) did correlate with BMD in some studies[22,73]. Disease activity may also contribute to lowering BMD. Studies have shown that patients with IBD can have lowered BMD at first presentation, possibly implicating the disease process[44]. This may reflect the altered systemic cytokine milieu during active disease, since several proinflammatory cytokines have a detrimental effect on bone mass[102]. Bone loss in middle-aged males has also been shown to be correlated with alcohol consumption, although this is not likely to be a major contributor in patients with IBD[78].

PREVALENCE

The prevalence of osteopenia among patients with inflammatory bowel disease (IBD) ranges from 40% to 50% and frank osteoporosis is seen in a range of as low as 2% and as high as 30%[11–15] (Table 1). These estimates are based on BMD data, where osteoporosis is defined as a bone mass T score < -2.5[4]. Some investigators found a similar reduction in BMD at the spine and hip whereas others found increased loss of BMD at the hip vs the spine[27,73,74,103]. Most studies typically used BMD measurements in IBD patients compared with the normal data from the DEXA company's software database. In case–control studies recently reported, but not fully published, there was no difference

Table 1. Studies published in full form that describe prevalence of osteoporosis in IBD

Reference	Crohn's/UC	Measure	Osteoporosis definition %	Major risk factors for decreased BMD	Sites
Compston 1987[108]	56/17	SPA qCT	Z<–2 31%	Lifetime steroid dose BMI weight	spine or radius
Pigot 1992[109]	27/12	DEXA	Z<–2 28%	Daily steroid dose (spine) Body weight (hip) Calcium intake (hip)	spine or hip
Ghosh 1994§[3]	15/15	DEXA	Z<–2 3%	Disease dx (Crohn's vs UC)	spine + forearm
Bernstein 1994[22]	26/23	DEXA	Z<–2 18%(spine) 24%(hip)	Steroid use (vs nonuser)	spine or hip
Abitbol 1995[3]	34/32	DEXA	Z<–2 16%*	Lifetime steroid dose Age	spine or hip
Silvennoinen 1995[15]	78/67	DEXA	Z<–2 5% (spine) 5% (hip)	Lifetime steroid dose	spine + hip
Roux 1995[23]	14/9	DEXA	Z<–2 26%	Steroid use for hip only	spine or hip
Bjarnason 1997[27]	44/35	DEXA	T<–2.5 18% (spine) 29% (hip)	More likely to have received larger steroid dose (no statistical correlation to lifetime steroid dose)	spine + hip

Table 1. Continued

Reference	Crohn's/UC	Measure	Osteoporosis definition %	Major risk factors for decreased BMD	Sites
Jahnsen 1997[73]	60/60	DEXA	Z<−2.5 2%(spine) 4%(hip)	Disease dx (Crohn's vs UC) Male sex BMI Steroid use in Crohn's only	spine + hip
Robinson 1998[13]	117/0	DEXA	Z<−2 12%		spine or hip
Fries 1998[14]	22/11	DEXA	T<−2.5 9%	Lifetime steroid dose	spine
Andreassen 1999[74]	113/0	DEXA	Z<−2.5 3%	Age, gender, weight	hip
Dinca 1999[110]	54/49	DEXA	T<−2.5 6%	Lifetime steroid dose	

§This study included only those patients with new diagnoses of IBD.
*The denominator for this calculation includes 18 patients who had prior colectomy.
Hip or spine implies that the determination of % of patients with osteroporosis (Z or T score <−2 to −2.5) was reported for either or both sites but not individually.
Where studies included UC patients post-colectomy these numbers were excluded from the study denominators.

between BMD and age- and gender-matched controls[104,105]. This was corroborated in another case–control study among males but not for females[74]. A consistent theme among the studies included in Table 1 is that corticosteroids correlate with BMD. Corticosteroid use may simply be a proxy measure for disease activity, so these associations do not prove that the drugs are causing the lowered BMD. Furthermore, it should be highlighted that these data are for BMD measures of osteoporosis but cannot be translated into specific morbidity, since data on fracture incidence are not represented in Table 1.

Some longitudinal data of BMD in patients with IBD reveal evidence of ongoing decreased BMD while other reports suggest stable BMD over time. One study using quantitative computerized tomography found a mean decrease in bone mass of 3% over 1 year[72]. This group later reported no mean change in bone mass over 4 years in the IBD cohort compared to normal populations[49], although patients with low BMD using corticosteroids represented a subgroup that had continued diminution in BMD. Another study using DEXA found a decrease of BMD of 3.1% among Crohn's disease patients and 6.4% among ulcerative colitis patients over a mean period of 19 months[23]. On the other hand, by DEXA two studies found no change over 1 year[44,93] and by single-photon absorptiometry one study found no change among men and a decrease of –0.74%/year among women when followed for an average of 7.9 years[103]. This latter study included postmenopausal women, which somewhat confounds the results regarding bone loss in relation to IBD. One study reported the 2-year follow-up of 80 patients with Crohn's disease by DEXA[31]. It was found that only patients with active disease requiring corticosteroids during the follow-up had a diminution in BMD.

Should we be surprised that the fracture rates are not higher in IBD? Most studies that have reported osteopenia by bone density measures have used company software normal data as a control. Two case–control studies matched for age and sex reported lower BMD among IBD patients than controls[15,73], but, two recent case–control studies found no difference among IBD patients[104,105]. The peak incidence of IBD is in the second and third decades[86,106], thus IBD patients are often young people who still have the potential to increase their bone mass, since a positive bone remodelling balance occurs until age 30–35 years. If disease activity diminishes, and corticosteroids are withdrawn, with no further interventions it remains possible that bone mass may stabilize or even increase. In contrast in postmenopausal or age-related osteoporosis, ongoing bone mass decrements are inevitable in the absence of interventions.

In a Consensus conference and report the Osteoporosis Society of Canada issued the following statement: 'the use of bone densitometry can be justified only when the results will help the physician and the patient make a management decision'[107]. There is no proven therapy for osteoporosis specifically in patients with IBD. I would argue therefore that any patient ultimately being found to have low BMD should certainly have sufficient risk to warrant starting unproven therapy (even if some therapies such as biphosphonates have been used for other corticosteroid-treated conditions; or are simple such as calcium and vitamin D which have been tested mostly in the postmenopausal setting). Thus, rather than pursuing screening DEXA tests on all patients, physicians following patients with IBD should be selective. Patients with Crohn's disease who smoke, are physically inactive, are underweight or malnourished, have active disease and have used chronic or recurrent courses of corticosteroids, have a positive history of an osteoporosis-associated fracture in a first-degree relative and have irregular menses should be screened. If DEXA T scores are less than -2.5 treatment should be initiated. If scores are -1 to -2 perhaps risk factor intervention and subsequent DEXA testing should be undertaken. For all other patients each physician will have to develop the criteria he/she wants to follow in terms of deciding who to screen with a DEXA test.

References

1. Bernstein CN, Hopper Y, Leslie W, Blanchard JF. The incidence of spine and hip fractures among patients with IBD: a population-based cohort study. Gastroenterology 1999;116:A667.
2. Croucher PI, Vedi S, Motley RJ, Garrahan NJ, Stanton MR, Compston JE. Reduced bone formation in patients with osteoporosis associated with inflammatory bowel disease. Osteoporos Int 1993;3:236–41.
3. Abitbol V, Roux C, Chaussade S *et al*. Metabolic bone assessment in patients with inflammatory bowel disease. Gastroenterology 1995;108:417–22.
4. Kanis JA, Melton LJ III, Christiansen C *et al*. The diagnosis of osteoporosis. J Bone Min Res 1994;9:1137–41.
5. Heaney RP. Bone mass, bone fragility, and the decision to treat. J Am Med Assoc 1998;280:2119–20.
6. Hui SL, Slemenda CW, Johnston CC. Age and bone mass as predictors of fracture in a prospective study. J Clin Invest 1988;81:1804–9.
7. Ross PD, Genant HK, Davis JW, Miller PD, Wasnich RD. Predicting vertebral fracture incidence from prevalent fractures and bone density among non-black osteoporotic women. Osteoporosis Int 1993;3:120–6.
8. Cummings SR, Black DM, Nevitt MC *et al*. Bone density at various sites for prediction of hip fractures. The Study of Osteoporotic Fractures Research Group. Lancet 1993;341:72–5.
9. Consensus development conference: Prophylaxis and treatment of osteoporosis. Am J Med 1991;90:107–11.
10. Leungo M, Picado C, Del Rio L, Guanabens N, Montserrat JM, Setoain J. Vertebral fractures in steroid dependent asthma and involutional osteoporosis: a comparative study. Thorax 1991;46:807–10.
11. Bernstein CN. Calcium and bone issues in inflammatory bowel disease. Gastroenterol Int 1997;10:71–7.
12. Compston JE. Review article: Osteoporosis, corticosteroids and inflammatory bowel disease. Aliment Pharmacol Ther 1995;9:237–50.
13. Robinson RJ, Iqbal SJ, Abrams K, Al-Azzawi F, Mayberry JF. Increased bone resorption in patients with Crohn's disease. Aliment Pharmacol Ther 1998;12:699–705.
14. Fries W, Dinca M, Luisetto G, Peccolo F, Bottega F, Martin A. Calcaneal ultrasound bone densitometry in inflammatory bowel disease – a comparison with double energy x-ray absorptiometry. Am J Gastroenterol 1998;93:2339–44.
15. Silvennoinen JA, Karttunene TJ, Niemela SE, Manelius JJ, Lehtola JK. A controlled study of bone mineral density in patients with inflammatory bowel disease. Gut 1995;37:71–6.
16. Bertelloni S, Baroncelli GI, Ferdeghini M, Perri G, Saggese G. Normal volumetric bone mineral density and bone turnover in young men with histories of constitutional delay of puberty. J Clin Endocrinol Metab 1998;83:4280–3.
17. Seeman E. Editorial: Growth in bone mass and size – are racial and gender differences in bone mineral density more apparent than real? J Clin Endocrinol Metab 1998;83:1414–19.
18. Melton LJ III, Kan SH, Wahner HW, Riggs BL. Lifetime fracture risk: an approach to hip fracture risk assessment based on bone mineral density and age. J Clin Epidemiol 1988;41:985–94.
19. Driscoll RH Jr, Meredith SC, Sitrin M, Rosenberg IH. Vitamin D deficiency and bone disease in patients with Crohn's disease. Gastroenterology 1982;83:1252–8.
20. Andreassen H, Rix M, Brot C, Eskildsen P. Regulators of calcium homeostasis and bone mineral density in patients with Crohn's disease. Scand J Gastroenterol 1998;33:1087–93.

21. Silvennoinen J, Lamberg-Allardt C, Karkkainen M, Niemela S, Lehtola J. Dietary calcium intake and its relation to bone mineral density in patients with inflammatory bowel disease. J Intern Med 1996;240:285–92.

22. Bernstein CN, Seeger LL, Sayre JW, Anton PA, Artinian L, Shanahan F. Decreased bone density in inflammatory bowel disease is related to corticosteroid use and not disease diagnosis. J Bone Miner Res 1995;10:250–6.

23. Roux C, Abitbol V, Chaussade S et al. Bone loss in patients with inflammatory bowel disease: a prospective study. Osteoporosis Int 1995;5:156–60.

24. Silvennoinen J, Risteli L, Karttunen T, Risteli J. Increased degradation of type I collagen in patients with inflammatory bowel disease. Gut 1996;38:223–8.

25. Delimas PD. Biochemical markers of bone turnover. I: Theoretical considerations and clinical use in osteoporosis. Am J Med 1993;95 (Suppl 5A):11–15S.

26. Ristelli L, Ristelli J. Biochemical markers of bone metabolism. Ann Med 1993;25:385–93.

27. Bjarnason I, Macpherson A, Mackintosh C, Buxton-Thomas M, Forgacs I, Moniz C. Reduced bone density in patients with inflammatory bowel disease. Gut 1997;40:228–33.

28. Zelissen PMJ, Croughs RJM, van Rijk PP, Raymakers JA. Effect of glucocorticoid replacement therapy on bone mineral density in patients with Addison's disease. Ann Intern Med 1994;120:207–10.

29. Bressot C, Meunier PJ, Chapuy MC et al. Histomorphometric profile, pathophysiology and reversibility of corticosteroid-induced osteoporosis. Metab Bone Dis 1979;1:303–9.

30. Pocock NA, Eisman JA, Dunstan CR et al. Recovery from steroid-induced osteoporosis. Ann Intern Med 1987;107:319–23.

31. Andreassen H, Hylander E, Rix M, Eskildsen P. Rate of bone loss in patients with Crohn's disease: a longitudinal study of 80 patients. Bone 1998;23 (5 Suppl.):S587.

32. Adinoff AD, Hollister JR. Steroid-induced fractures and bone loss in patients with asthma. N Engl J Med 1983;309:265–8.

33. Darling DB, Loridan L, Senior B. The roentgenographic manifestations of Cushing's syndrome in infancy. Radiology 1970;96:503–8.

34. Lukert BP, Raisz LG. Glucocorticoid-induced osteoporosis: pathogenesis and management. Ann Intern Med 1990;112:352–64.

35. Meunier PJ. Is steroid-induced osteoporosis preventable? N Engl J Med 1993;328:1781–2.

36. Reid IR. Pathogenesis and treatment of steroid induced osteoporosis. Clin Endocrinol (Oxf) 1989;30:83–103.

37. Rickers H, Deding AA, Christiansen C, Rodbro P. Mineral loss in cortical and trabecular bone during high-dose prednisone treatment. Calcif Tissue Int 1984;36:269–73.

38. Baylink DJ. Glucocorticoid induced osteoporosis. N Engl J Med 1983;309:306–8.

39. Avioli LV. Effects of chronic corticosteroid therapy on mineral metabolism and calcium absorption. Adv Exp Med Biol 1984;171:81–9.

40. Seeman E, Wahner HW, Offord KP, Kumar R, Johnson WJ, Riggs BL. Differential effects of endocrine dysfunction on the axial and appendicular skeleton. J Clin Invest 1982;69:1302–6.

41. Bohr H, Schaadt O. Bone mineral content of the femoral neck and shaft: relation between cortical and trabecular bone. Calcif Tissue Int 1985;37:340–4.

42. Sambrook P, Birmingham J, Kempler S et al. Corticosteroid effects on proximal femur bone loss. J Bone Miner Res 1990;5:1211–16.

43. Ghosh S, Cowen S, Hannan WJ, Ferguson A. Low bone mineral density in Crohn's disease, but not in ulcerative colitis, at diagnosis. Gastroenterology 1994;107:1031–9.

44. Genarri C, Civitelli R. Glucocorticoid induced osteoporosis. Clin Rheum Dis 1986;12:637–55.

45. Reid DM, Kennedy NSJ, Smith MA, Tothill P, Nuki G. Total body calcium in rheumatoid arthritis; effects of disease activity and corticosteroid treatment. Br Med J 1982;285:330–2.

46. Lo Cascio V, Bonuccci E, Ballanti P et al. Glucocorticoid osteoporosis: a longitudinal study. In: Christiansen C, Johansen JS, Riis BJ, (editors). Osteoporosis 1987. Copenhagen: Osteo Press ApS; 1987:1044–6.

47. Goemare S, Correa-Rotter R, Saag K et al., for the Alendronate Study Group, Gent UZ. Alendronate increases spine BMD irrespective of glucocorticoid dose or duration. Bone 1998; 23 (5 Suppl.): S182.

48. Leboff MS, Wade JP, Mackowiak S, El hajj FG, Zangari M, Liang M. Low dose prednisone does not affect calcium homeostasis or bone density in post menopausal women with rheumatoid arthritis. J Rheumatol 1991;18:339–44.

49. Motley RJ, Clements D, Evans WD *et al.* A four-year longitudinal study of bone loss in patients with inflammatory bowel disease. Bone Miner 1993;23:95–104.
50. Ruegsegger P, Medici TC, Anliker M. Corticosteroid-induced bone loss: a longitudinal study of alternate day therapy in patients with bronchial asthma using quantitative computed tomography. Eur J Clin Pharmacol 1983;25:615–20.
51. Morris HA, Need AG, O'Loughlin PD, Horowitz M, Bridges A, Nordin BEC. Malabsorption of calcium in corticosteroid-induced osteoporosis. Calcif Tissue Int 1990;46:305–8.
52. Chavassieux P, Pastoureau P, Chapuy MC, Delmas PD, Meunier PJ. Glucocorticoid-induced inhibition of osteoblastic bone formation in ewes: a biochemical and histomorphometric study. Osteoporosis Int 1993;3:97–102.
53. Klein RG, Arnaud SB, Gallagher JC *et al.* Intestinal calcium absorption in exogenous hypercortisolism. Role of 25-hydroxy vitamin D and corticosteroid dose. J Clin Invest 1977;60:253–69.
54. Gennari C. Differential effect of glucocorticoids on calcium absorption and bone mass. Br J Rheumatol 1993;32(Suppl.2):11–14.
55. Bryer HP, Isserow JA, Armstrong EC *et al.* Azathioprine alone is bone sparing and does not alter cyclosporin A induced osteopenia in the rat. J Bone Miner Res 1995;10:132–8.
56. Flores CH, Ahren B, Bengtsson M, Bartosik J, Obrant K. Bone mineral density in patients with Crohn's disease during long term treatment with azathioprine. J Int Med 1998;243:123–6.
57. Blum M, Wallenstein S, Clark J, Luckey M. Effect of methotrexate treatment on bone in postmenopausal women with primary biliary cirrhosis. J Bone Miner Res 1996;11(Suppl.1):S436.
58. Bianchi ML, Bardare M, Cimaz R, Galblati E, Corona F, Chorubini R. Does methotrexate have an effect on bone mass? J Bone Miner Res 1996;11(Suppl. 1):S225.
59. Orwoll ES, Bauer DC, Vogt TM, Fox KM for the Study of Osteoporotic Fractures Research Group. Axial bone mass in older women. Ann Intern Med 1996;124:187–96.
60. Lufkin EG, Wahner HW, O'Fallon WM *et al.* Treatment of postmenopausal osteoporosis with transdermal estrogen. Ann Intern Med 1992;117:1–9.
61. Armamento-Villareal R, Villareal DT, Avioli LV, Civitelli R. Estrogen status and heredity are major determinants of premenopausal bone mass. J Clin Invest 1992;90:2464–71.
62. Clements D, Compston JE, Evans WD, Rhodes J. Hormone replacement therapy prevents bone loss in patients with inflammatory bowel disease. Gut 1993;34:1543–46.
63. Lukert BP, Johnson BE, Robinson RG. Estrogen and progesterone replacement therapy reduces glucocorticoid-induced bone loss. J Bone Miner Res 1992;7:1063–9.
64. Crilly RG, Cawood M, Marshall DH, Nordin BE. Hormonal status in normal, osteoporotic, and corticosteroid-treated postmenopausal women. J R Soc Med 1978;71:733–6.
65. MacAdams MR, White RH, Chipps BE. Reduction of serum testosterone levels during chronic glucocorticoid therapy. Ann Intern Med 1986;104:648–51.
66. Heaney RP, Recker RR, Stegman MR, Moy AJ. Calcium absorption in women: Relationships to calcium intake, estrogen status and age. J Bone Miner Res 1989;4:469–75.
67. Meunier PJ, Bressot C. Endocrine influences on bone cells and remodeling evaluated by clinical histomorphometry. In: Parsons JA, (editor). Osteoporosis. New York: Grune & Stratton; 1988:257–65.
68. Reid IR, Wattie DJ, Evans MC, Stapleton JP. Testosterone therapy in glucocorticoid-treated men. Arch Intern Med 1996;156:1173–7.
69. Bauer DC, Browner WS, Cauley JA *et al.* for The Study of Osteoporotic Fractures Research Group. Factors associated with appendicular bone mass in older women. Ann Intern Med 1993;118:657–65.
70. Gregg EW, Cauley JA, Seeley DG, Ensrud KE, Bauer DC for The Study of Osteoporotic Fractures Research Group. Physical activity and osteoporotic fracture risk in older women. Ann Intern Med 1998;129:81–8.
71. Faulkner KG, Gluer CC, Palermo L, Black D, Genant HK, Cummings SR. Geometric measurements from dual x-ray absorptiometry scans predict hip fracture. J Bone Miner Res 1992;4(Suppl.):S326.
72. Motley RJ, Crawley EO, Evans C, Rhodes J, Compston JE. Increased rate of spinal trabecular bone loss in patients with inflammatory bowel disease. Gut 1988;29:1332–6.
73. Jahnsen J, Falch JA, Aadland E *et al.* Bone mineral density is reduced in patients with Crohn's disease but not in patients with ulcerative colitis: a population based study. Gut 1997;40:313–19.

74. Andreassen H, Hylander E, Rix M. Gender, age, and body weight are the major predictive factors for bone mineral density in Crohn's disease: a case–control cross-sectional study of 113 patients. Am J Gastroenterol 1999;94:824–8.

75. Loudon CP, Corroll V, Butcher J, Rawsthorne P, Bernstein CN. The effects of physical exercise on patients with Crohn's disease. Am J Gastroenterol 1999;94:697–703.

76. Hulley SB, Vogel JM, Donaldson CL, Bayers JH, Friedman RJ, Rosen SN. The effect of supplemental oral phosphate on the bone mineral changes during prolonged bed rest. J Clin Invest 1971;50:2506–18.

77. Recker RR, Davies M, Hinders SM, Heaney RP, Stegman MR, Kimmel DB. Bone gain in young adult women. J Am Med Assoc 1992;268:2403–8.

78. Slemenda CW, Christian JC, Reed T, Reister TK, Williams CJ, Johnston CC Jr. Long-term bone loss in men: effects of genetic and environmental factors. Ann Intern Med 1992;117:286–91.

79. Hopper JL, Seeman E. The bone density of female twins discordant for tobacco use. N Engl J Med 1994;330:387–92.

80. Silvennoinen JA, Lehtola JK, Niemela SE. Smoking is a risk factor for osteoporosis in women with inflammatory bowel disease. Scand J Gastroenterol 1996;31:367–71.

81. Tobin MV, Logan RFA, Langamn MJS, McConnel RB, Gilmore IT. Cigarette smoking and inflammatory bowel disease. Gastroenterology 1987;93:316–21.

82. Motley RJ, Rhodes J, Ford GA et al. Time relationship between cessation of smoking and onset of ulcerative colitis. Digestion 1987;37:125–7.

83. Jensen J, Christiansen C, Rodbro P. Cigarette smoking, serum estrogens, and bone loss during hormone-replacement therapy early after menopause. N Engl J Med 1985;313:973–5.

84. Cassidenti DL, Vijod AG, Vijod MA, Stanczyk FZ, Lobo RA. Short term effects of smoking on the pharmacokinetic profiles of micronized estradiol in postmenopausal women. Am J Obstet Gynecol 1990;163:1953–60.

85. Recker RR, Davies M, Hinders SM, Heaney RP, Stegman MR, Kimmel DB. Bone gain in young adult women. J Am Med Assoc 1992;268:2403–8.

86. Bernstein CN, Blanchard JF, Rawsthorne P, Wajda A. The epidemiology of Crohn's disease and ulcerative colitis in a central Canadian province: a population-based study. Am J Epidemiol 1999;149:916–24.

87. Dawson-Hughes B, Dallal GE, Krall EA, Sadowski L, Sayhoun N, Tannenbaum S. A controlled trial of the effect of calcium supplementation on bone density in post menopausal women. N Engl J Med 1990;323:878–83.

88. Reid IR, Ames RW, Evans MC, Gamble GD, Sharpe SJ. Effect of calcium supplementation on bone loss in postmenopausal women. N Engl J Med 1993;328:460–4.

89. Sambrook P, Birmingham J, Kelly P et al. Prevention of corticosteroid osteoporosis: a comparison of calcium, calcitriol, and calcitonin. N Engl J Med 1993;328:1747–52.

90. Chapuy MC, Arlot ME, Duboeuf F et al. Vitamin D3 and calcium to prevent hip fractures in elderly women. N Engl J Med 1992;327:1637–42.

91. Dawson-Hughes B, Harris SS, Krall EA, Dallal GE. Effect of calcium and vitamin D supplementation on bone density in men and women 65 years of age or older. N Engl J Med 1997;337:670–6.

92. Matkovic V, Fontana D, Tominac C, Goel P, Chesnut CH III. Factors that influence peak bone mass formation: a study of calcium balance and the inheritance of bone mass in adolescent females. Am J Clin Nutr 1990;52:878–88.

93. Bernstein CN, Seeger LL, Anton PA et al. A randomized placebo-controlled study of calcium supplementation for decreased bone density in corticosteroid-using patients with inflammatory bowel disease: a pilot study. Aliment Pharmacol Ther 1996;10:777–86.

94. Reed CA, Nichols DL, Bonnick SL, DiMarco NM. Bone mineral density and dietary intake in patients with Crohn's disease. J Clin Densit 1998;1:33–40.

95. Vogelsang H, Resch H, Klamert M, Ferenci P. Dietary vitamin D intake in patients with Crohn's disease. Wien Klin Wochenschr 1995;107:578–81.

96. Silvennoinen J. Relationship between vitamin D, parathyroid hormone and bone mineral density in inflammatory bowel disease. J Intern Med 1996;239:131–7.

97. Krall EA, Dawson Hughes B. Heritable and lifestyle determinants of bone mineral density. J Bone Miner Res 1993;8:1–9.

98. Pocock NJ, Eisman JA, Hopper JL, Yeates MG, Sambrook PN, Eberi S. Genetic determinants of bone mass in adults. J Clin Invest 1987;80:706–10.
99. Morrison NA, Qi JC, Tokita A *et al.* Prediction of bone density from vitamin D receptor alleles. Nature 1994;367:284–7.
100. Smith EP, Boyd J, Frank GR *et al.* Estrogen resistance caused by a mutation in the estrogen-receptor gene in a man. N Engl J Med 1994;331:1056–61.
101. Uitterlinden AG, Burger H, Huang Q *et al.* Relation of alleles of the collagen type$1\alpha1$ gene to bone density and the risk of osteoporotic fractures in postmenopausal women. N Engl J Med 1998;338:1016–21.
102. Manolagas SC, Jilka RL. Bone marrow, cytokines, and bone remodeling. Emerging insights into the pathophysiology of osteoporosis. N Engl J Med 1995;332:305–11.
103. Clements D, Motley RJ, Evans WD *et al.* Longitudinal study of cortical bone loss in patients with inflammatory bowel disease. Scand J Gastroenterol 1992;27:1055–60.
104. Schoon EJ, Blok BM, Geerling BJ, Russel MG, Stockbrugger RW, Brummer RJ. Is bone mineral density in patients with inflammatory bowel disease low at diagnosis? A case–control study. Bone 1998;23(5 Suppl.):S287.
105. Haugeberg G, Stallemo A, Stokkeland M, Vetvik K. BMD in patients with Crohn's disease better than expected: a cross sectional study in a Norwegian community. Bone 1998;23 (5 suppl):S504 (abstract).
106. Russel MGVM, Stockbrugger RW. Epidemiology of inflammatory bowel disease: an update. Scand J Gastroenterol 1996;31:417–27.
107. Sturtridge W, Lentle B, Hanley DA. The use of bone density measurement in the diagnosis and management of osteoporosis. Can Med Assoc J 1996;155:924–9.
108. Compston JE, Judd D, Crawley EO *et al.* Osteoporosis in patients with inflammatory bowel disease. Gut 1987; 28:410–15.
109. Pigot F, Roux C, Chaussade S *et al.* Low bone mineral density in patients with inflammatory bowel disease. Dig Dis Sci 1992;37:1396–403.
110. Dinca M, Fries W, Luisetto G *et al.* Evolution of osteopenia in inflammatory bowel disease. Am J Gastroenterol 1999;94:1292–7.

16
Management of low bone mass in patients with inflammatory bowel disease

A. TENENHOUSE

ABSTRACT

Prevention of osteoporosis requires first that those at increased risk be identified. Risk factors for osteoporosis include age, gonadal hormone deficiency, chronic illness such as inflammatory bowel disease (IBD) and rheumatoid arthritis, drugs such as glucocorticoids, low body mass index, and smoking. Since patients with IBD generally have two or more risk factors they must be considered at increased risk to develop osteoporosis. They therefore should, as part of the initial medical work-up, have bone mineral density (BMD) measured. If the BMD is decreased they should be treated.

The strategies for prevention and treatment are the same and are based on the assumption, supported by considerable evidence, that decreasing BMD is due primarily to a relative increase in bone resorption. The ultimate objective of therapy is to prevent fracture. This objective is best accomplished by eliminating risk factors and using drugs to inhibit bone resorption. Elimination of risk factors includes optimizing nutritional status, especially calcium and vitamin D intake, ensuring normal gonadal function, encouraging weight-bearing physical activity, eliminating smoking and excess alcohol consumption, and where possible eliminating or diminishing total consumption of drugs such as glucocorticoids and agents such as psychoactive drugs and antihypertensives, which tend to increase the risk of falling. All patients should have a baseline BMD measurement of lumbar spine and hip and these measurements should be repeated as risk changes, e.g. introduction of glucocorticoid therapy, weight loss or other evidence of failing nutrition, and fracture. If BMD is decreased antiresorptive drugs should be introduced. Those approved for use in Canada include oestrogen, bisphosphonates, calcitonin, and selective oestrogen receptor modulators (SERMs). In postmenopausal women the treatment of choice, according to most published guidelines is hormone replacement therapy (HRT), with one of the bisphosphonates as a second choice. In premenopausal women and men the antiresorptive agent of choice is a bisphosphonate. Response to therapy should be monitored with bone density measurements. Evidence of treatment failure includes decreasing BMD, and occurrence of a 'fragility' fracture. If this occurs combination therapy, e.g. HRT+bisphosphonate, may be considered.

Bisphosphonates are very poorly and unpredictably absorbed from the normal gastrointestinal tract. The rate of absorption of these drugs from the intestine of IBD patients is unknown. It may therefore be desirable or necessary to use intravenous bisphosphonate therapy in IBD patients.

The efficacy and safety of drugs which increase BMD (fluoride) and/or normal bone formation (intermittent parathyroid hormone) have yet to be demonstrated.

PREAMBLE

Loss of bone tissue with resultant increase in fracture risk is a relatively frequent consequence of chronic inflammatory illness and the drugs used to treat them. This is particularly true of gastrointestinal diseases which are often associated with decreased absorption of nutrients essential to the growth and maintenance of bone and treated with prolonged courses of drugs such as glucocorticoids which can cause a rapid decrease in bone mass. The estimated prevalence of low bone mass, osteopenia and osteoporosis, in patients with IBD is 30–60%[1–3]. This review will briefly describe those characteristics of bone relevant to an understanding of the processes involved in the development of low bone mass and present one approach to its prevention and treatment. It will also attempt to answer the most frequently asked questions about the management of osteoporosis. Who to treat? How to treat? How long to treat?

INTRODUCTION

Bone growth

The accumulation of bone mass occurs very rapidly from birth to reach a maximum, the peak bone mass (PBM), some time during the second or third decade of life. The actual PBM and the age at which it is reached vary somewhat between skeletal sites. It is a characteristic of the individual and is determined largely by genetic factors; however, achievement of the genetically determined PBM in any individual is greatly influenced by 'environmental' factors such as nutrition, general health, gonadal function, use of drugs such as glucocorticoids, and sedentary life style[4–8]. In both men and women, once PBM is achieved, bone mass remains constant for some variable time, after which a slow loss of bone begins. The age at which this bone loss begins is different at each skeletal site; e.g. the lumbar spine maintains bone mass at peak until age 40–45 years, whereas the femoral neck begins losing bone mass almost immediately after PBM is reached[9] (Tenenhouse et al., unpublished). This age-dependent bone loss continues for life, although the rate of loss is not constant. In women the rate of loss accelerates significantly at the time of the menopause and this rapid rate is maintained for a prolonged period of time, possibly for life. In men the rate of age-dependent bone loss appears to continue unchanged for life.

Table 1 General risk factors for osteopenia and osteoporosis

Age	Low BMI
Sex	Nutrition
Race	Calcium
Family history	Vitamin D
	Lifestyle
	Sedentary
	Smoking
	Excess alcohol

The rate of age-dependent bone loss is independent of PBM, i.e. a person who has achieved a high PBM loses bone at the same rate as one who achieved a lower PBM. It follows that the higher the PBM, the lower the risk of developing osteoporosis; also, since fracture risk is in large part determined by bone mass, this means that, all else being equal, the greater the PBM, the smaller the lifetime risk for fracture. The prevention of osteoporosis and fracture should therefore begin in the very young with efforts to maximize PBM.

In normal bone the rates of resorption and formation are tightly coupled. Prior to achievement of PBM, the rate of formation is greater than that of resorption, resulting in a net increase in bone mass. For a variable time after PBM is reached the rates of formation and resorption are equal so there is no net change in bone mass. However, as noted above, with advancing age resorption rate becomes relatively greater than that of formation and there is a net loss of bone mass. This latter situation continues for life. When the difference between the rates of resorption and formation is large enough and persists for a long enough period of time, osteoporosis results.

Osteopenia and osteoporosis

Osteoporosis is defined as a 'disease characterized by low bone mass and microarchitectural deterioration which leads to enhanced bone fragility and increased fracture risk'[10]. The mechanisms that cause osteoporosis are not known; however, it is clear that the bone loss is due to a relative increase in the rate of osteoclast-mediated bone resorption. The rate of bone loss is variable and unpredictable and is determined by both genetic and environmental factors, some of which are listed in Tables 1 and 2. On the left side of Table 1 are listed the non-modifiable risk factors such as advanced age, sex, race, and family history, and on the right are listed those risk factors which can be modified and in most individuals completely eliminated. These include nutritional deficiencies, gonadal insufficiency, and high-risk lifestyle choices such as smoking. Table 2 lists those risk factors that are more related to the IBD and are often very difficult to manage. Particularly devastating is the prolonged use of corticosteroids[1,11,12] which can cause significant bone loss in weeks to months

Table 2 Disease-specific risk factors for osteopenia and osteoporosis

---

Severity of disease
  Duration
  Bowel segment involved
  Bowel resection
  Recent/sustained weight loss
Therapy
  Glucocorticoids
General nutrition

An expert committee of the World Health Organization (WHO) suggested that in postmenopausal women osteopenia and osteoporosis may be defined in terms of bone mineral density (BMD) as measured by dual-energy X-ray absorptiometry (DEXA)[13]. They suggested that osteopenia exists when there is a decrease in BMD equal to or greater than 1 standard deviation (SD) below PBM. Osteoporosis exists when the BMD decrease is equal to or greater than 2.5 SD below PBM and severe osteoporosis is defined as osteoporosis with a fragility fracture. The deviation of BMD from PBM expressed in terms of SDs is known as the 'T' score; i.e. by WHO criteria a T score$\leq$–1.0 is osteopenia whereas a T score$\leq$–2.5 is osteoporosis. These WHO criteria have been widely adopted and are now often applied to premenopausal women as well as men. Low BMD is the single most important risk factor for fracture[14]; fracture risk increases 1.5–2.5-fold for each SD decrease in BMD[15–17].

Osteoclast-mediated bone resorption may be inhibited by a variety of agents including estrogen, bisphosphonates, calcitonin, and selective oestrogen receptor modulators (SERMs) such as raloxifene. These drugs, particularly oestrogen and bisphosphonates, are the ones most widely used in the prevention and treatment of osteopenia and osteoporosis. Safe and efficient methods for stimulation of bone formation, which is desirable particularly in people who have already lost a significant proportion of their total bone mass, are not yet available. To date the only drugs that act to stimulate bone formation, and have been shown in clinical trials to increase BMD, are fluoride[18] and parathyroid hormone (PTH)[19–21]. There is some evidence that the bone formed in response to fluoride administration is abnormal and that this drug may actually increase fracture risk[22]. Other studies report a decreased fracture risk in response to fluoride therapy[23,24]. Because of this uncertainty fluoride is rarely a drug of choice in the treatment of osteoporosis. Parathyroid hormone is still in the developmental stage, although early results are encouraging[19–21].

MANAGEMENT OF LOW BONE MASS

Assessment of risk

A careful assessment of each individual patient's risk to fracture is essential to determine who should be treated and how aggressive that treatment should be. The risk factors fall into two broad categories: those that increase risk of

Table 3 Routine laboratory work-up for individuals at risk for osteopenia and osteoporosis

Serum
  Calcium (total, ionized)
  Inorganic phosphate
  Alkaline phosphatase
  Parathyroid hormone
  Creatinine
Urine
  Calcium
  Creatinine
  Phosphate

falling and those that result in increased bone fragility. Although this review is restricted to a consideration of factors which cause increased bone fragility, a complete fracture prevention programme must include removal, to the extent possible, of those factors that increase the risk of falling.

The most important determinant of fracture risk which can be conveniently and accurately assessed is bone mass as measured by DEXA[14]. However, it has also been shown that, at any given BMD, other factors such as advanced age, smoking, and use of drugs such as glucocorticoids, can dramatically increase the risk of hip fracture. Cummings et al.[25] found that, independent of BMD, the addition of five or more other risk factors increases hip fracture risk approximately 10-fold.

The initial assessment of IBD patients should include a complete medical history to screen for risk factors and a BMD measurement of the hip and lumbar spine. The activity of the disease, current use and cumulated dose of corticosteroids, BMI≤19 and/or recent weight loss, bowel resection, and nutritional deficiencies are among the most important risk factors seen in these patients[26–28]. If the BMD of either the lumbar spine or hip is decreased ($T<-1.0$), aggressive therapy should be considered.

Biochemical tests are of limited use in establishing a diagnosis of osteoporosis or for assessing fracture risk; however, they are useful for eliminating some secondary causes of osteoporosis and assessing calcium and vitamin D nutrition. Table 3 lists the tests that should be done in all patients. The results of these few relatively inexpensive biochemical tests, along with the routine biochemical and haematological tests done in the general work-up of IBD patients, will help eliminate other causes of osteoporosis and will provide estimates of the rate of urinary excretion of calcium, and the state of vitamin D nutrition.

On occasion it might be useful to determine serum vitamin D metabolite concentrations, particularly 25-hydroxyvitamin D, to confirm the presence of vitamin D deficiency and to measure the blood and/or urine concentrations of various markers of bone resorption (N-telopeptides, deoxypyridinolines) and bone formation (osteocalcin, bone-specific alkaline phosphatase). Using markers of bone resorption it has been possible to detect response to therapy after a very few weeks to months[29–31]. With DEXA response to therapy may not be detectable before 1–2 years[29–32]. Measurement of bone resorption markers may be useful in patients with IBD since intestinal absorption of oral bisphosphonates is unpredictable, particularly in these patients.

Drug therapy

The strategy for prevention and treatment of osteopenia, osteoporosis, and fracture in patients with IBD is the same as that used in any other at-risk population. Identify and eliminate modifiable risk factors to the extent possible and if, after doing this, the patient remains at increased risk, use antiresorptive drugs. This approach is schematically outlined in Figure 1.

Before beginning treatment it is important to ensure that the low BMD is not due to osteomalacia. Bone densitometry cannot distinguish between low bone mass due to osteoporosis and osteomalacia. X-rays are often not helpful and bone biopsy, which is the definitive diagnostic procedure, is often not available or practical. The prevalence of vitamin D insufficiency is surprisingly high among Canadian men and women, particularly the elderly[33]. It is most common in northern latitudes and is seasonal in that it is most severe in the winter[34–38]. Vitamin D deficiency may be inferred from the results of the simple biochemical screen shown in Table 3. Serum calcium and inorganic phosphate concentrations are often at the lower end of the normal range while serum PTH concentration is moderately elevated or at the upper end of the normal range. Urinary calcium excretion is very low. Administration of calcium and vitamin D will increase serum calcium and phosphate concentrations, decrease serum PTH, and increase urinary calcium excretion. The dose of vitamin D needed varies, and may be as much as 50 000 IU (1.25 mg) per week. If this dose fails to achieve the desired response, activated metabolites such as 1α-cholecalciferol or 1,25-dihydroxycholecalciferol may be used. When using pharmacological doses of vitamin D or the activated metabolites, it is essential that serum and urine calcium concentrations be monitored at least every 3 months until a stable endpoint is reached. If hypercalciuria or hypercalcaemia occurs the dose must be reduced.

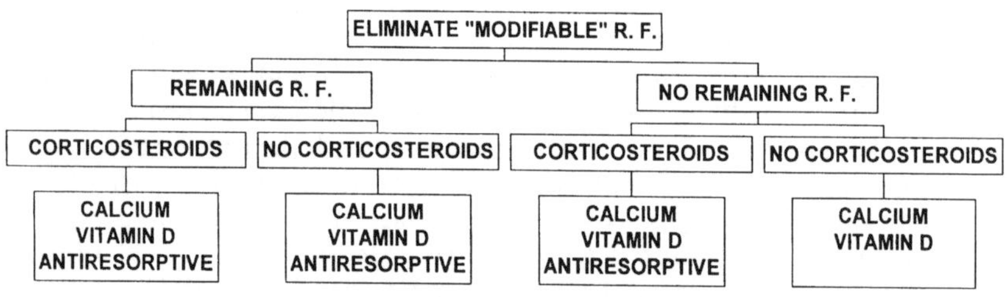

Figure 1 A general scheme for prevention and treatment of osteopenia and osteoporosis (R.F. refers to 'risk factors')

If the risk for osteoporosis and fracture remains high after elimination of modifiable risk factors and restoration of adequate calcium and vitamin D nutrition then the use of antiresorptive drugs must be considered. Because of the frequency with which they cause bone loss, corticosteroids are separated from other risk factors in the 'management scheme' (Figure 1). It is recommended that whenever corticosteroids are used, antiresorptive drugs be administered.

There have been very few studies of the efficacy of antiresorptive agents to prevent bone loss and/or fracture in IBD patients specifically, although IBD patients have been included in a number of studies of the efficacy of these agents for the prevention of corticosteroid-induced bone loss. In all these trials the vast majority of participants had inflammatory joint rather than bowel disease; however, in none of these studies did patients with IBD behave differently on average from patients with any other inflammatory disease. Antiresorptive agents, particularly the bisphosphonates, have also been shown to effectively inhibit osteoclast-mediated bone resorption whatever the cause. There is therefore no reason to believe that IBD patients will not respond to antiresorptive drugs.

A number of bisphosphonates have been found to prevent bone loss and fractures in patients receiving corticosteroids. Cyclical etidronate proved effective in preventing bone loss from the lumbar spine and also reduced the rate of vertebral fractures in patients who had recently started corticosteroid therapy[39]. It has also been shown that the beneficial effects of cyclical etidronate on spine BMD persist for at least 1 year after the drug is discontinued[40]. Saag et al.[41] found that alendronate treatment of patients who were taking corticosteroids for a variable period of time resulted in an increase BMD of the lumbar spine and femoral neck, but they did not find a significant reduction in vertebral fracture rate. In 1992 Gallacher et al.[42] reported that treatment with intravenous pamidronate of patients with corticosteroid-dependent lung disease (infusion of 30 mg every 3 months for 1 year) resulted in a significant increase of the BMD of the lumbar spine but not the femoral neck. Boutsen et al.[43] gave a loading dose of 90 mg intravenous pamidronate along with 800 mg calcium simultaneously with the initiation of corticosteroid therapy. Subsequently each patient received an intravenous infusion of 30 mg pamidronate every 3 months for 1 year. The control group received calcium only. Boutsen et al. found a significant increase in BMD of the lumbar spine and femoral neck in patients in the treatment group, whereas those in the control group had a significant reduction of BMD at these skeletal sites.

Etidronate and alendronate are oral preparations while pamidronate is available for intravenous administration. All oral bisphosphonates are very poorly and unpredictably absorbed from the normal gastrointestinal tract; nothing is known of their absorption from the intestine of IBD patients. Because their absorption is further reduced by many foods and minerals it is recommended that these drugs be taken with water only, at least 2 h after the last food and at least 30–60 min before the next. The interaction of these drugs with most other medication is not known. Because IBD patients often do not tolerate oral drugs, and because absorption is so unpredictable, it may be an advantage to treat these patients with an intravenous preparation such as pamidronate. Intravenous therapy may have additional advantages. Compliance is no longer a problem and bone markers, which respond to oral bisphosphonates only after months of therapy, have been found to respond to intravenous pamidronate in days[44]. In the experience of the author patients often prefer the once every 3 months intravenous administration of drug to daily pills.

Duration of drug therapy

Sufficient calcium and vitamin D supplementation to maintain adequate nutrition should be continued, with adjustments as necessary, for life. Antiresorptive drug therapy should continue as long as increased risk for osteoporosis and fracture remain. If therapy is discontinued, the patient should be monitored with BMD measurements every 1 or 2 years until it is demonstrated that bone mass is stable. Therapy should be restarted with any increase in risk. In general, an antiresorptive drug should be continued for as long as corticosteroid therapy or should be started whenever a new course of corticosteroid therapy begins.

SUMMARY

The risk for osteoporosis and fracture is substantially increased in patients with IBD, particularly in those taking corticosteroids. A recent study found that in the UK only 14% of patients receiving corticosteroids have received any preventive treatment for osteoporosis[45]. There is no reason to believe that physicians in North America are doing any better. There are now safe and effective drugs for the prevention and treatment of osteopenia and osteoporosis. Prevention of these potentially devastating outcomes must become an integral part of the treatment plan for all patients with IBD.

References

1. Compston JE. Osteoporosis, corticosteroids and inflammatory bowel disease. Aliment Pharmacol Ther 1995;9:237–50.
2. Roux C, Abitbol V, Chaussade S *et al*. Bone loss in patients with inflammatory bowel disease: a prospective study. Osteoporosis Int 1995;5:156–60.
3. Andreassen H, Rungby J, Dahlerup JF, Mosekilde L. Inflammatory bowel disease and osteoporosis. Scand J Gastroenterol 1997;32:1247–55.
4. Slemenda CW, Miller JZ, Hui SL, Reister TK, Johnston CC. Role of physical activity in the development of skeletal mass in children. J Bone Miner Res 1991;6:1227–33.
5. Recker RR, Davies KM, Hinders M, Heaney RP, Stegman MR, Kimmel DB. Bone gain in young adult women. J Am Med Assoc 1992;268:2403–8.
6. Krall EA, Dawson-Hughes B. Heritable and life-style determinants of bone mineral density. J Bone Miner Res 1993;8:1–9.
7. Bonjour JP, Carrie AL, Ferrari S *et al*. Calcium-enriched foods and bone mass growth in prepubertal girls: a randomized, double-blind, placebo-controlled trial. J Clin Invest 1997;99:1287–94.
8. Weaver CM, Peacock M, Johnston CC. Commentary. Adolescent nutrition in the prevention of postmenopausal osteoporosis. J Clin Endocrinol Metab 1999;84:1839–43.
9. Slemenda CL, Peacock M, Hui S, Johnston CC. Sex steroids, bone mass, and bone loss. A prospective study of pre-, peri-, and postmenopausal women. J Clin Invest 1996;97:14–21.
10. Consensus development conference. Diagnosis, prophylaxis, and treatment of osteoporosis. Am J Med 1993;94:646–50.

11. Sambrook P, Birmingham J, Kempler S, *et al.* Corticosteroid effects on proximal femur bone loss. J Bone Miner Res 1990;5:1211–16.
12. Sambrook P, Birmingham J, Kelly P *et al.* Prevention of corticosteroid osteoporosis. A comparison of calcium, calcitriol, and calcitonin [see comments]. N Engl J Med 1993;328:1747–52.
13. WHO. Assessment of fracture risk and its application to screening for postmenopausal osteoporosis. Technical report series 843. Geneva: WHO;1994.
14. Miller PD, Zapalowski C, Kulak CAM, Bilezikian JP. Commentary. Bone densitometry: the best way to detect osteoporosis and to monitor therapy. J Clin Endocrinol Metab 1999;84:1867–71.
15. Hui SL, Slemenda CW, Johnston CC, Jr. Age and bone mass as predictors of fracture in a prospective study. J Clin Invest 1988;81:1804–9.
16. Cummings SR, Black DM, Nevitt MC *et al.* Bone density at various sites for prediction of hip fractures. The Study of Osteoporotic Fractures Research Group [see comments]. Lancet 1993;341:72–5.
17. Kroger H, Huopio J, Honkanen R *et al.* Prediction of fracture risk using axial bone mineral density in a perimenopausal population: a prospective study. J Bone Miner Res 1995;10:302–6.
18. Kleerekoper M. The role of fluoride in the prevention of osteoporosis. Endocrinol Metab Clin N Am 1998;27:441–52.
19. Finkelstein JS, Klibanski A, Schaefer EH, Hornstein MD, Schiff I, Neer RM. Parathyroid hormone for the prevention of bone loss induced by estrogen deficiency. N Engl J Med 1994;331:1618–23.
20. Sone T, Fukunaga M, Ono S, Nishiyama T. A small dose of human parathyroid hormone (1–34) increased bone mass in the lumbar vertebrae in patients with senile osteoporosis. Miner Electrolyte Metab 1995;21:232–5.
21. Hodsman AB, Fraher LJ, Watson PH *et al.* A randomized controlled trial to compare the efficacy of cyclical parathyroid hormone versus cyclical parathyroid hormone and sequential calcitonin to improve bone mass in postmenopausal women with osteoporosis. J Clin Endocrinol Metab 1997;82:620–8.
22. Riggs BL, Hodgson SF, O'Fallon WM *et al.* Effect of fluoride treatment on the fracture rate in postmenopausal women with osteoporosis [see comments]. N Engl J Med 1990;322:802–9.
23. Pak CY, Sakhaee K, Zerwekh JE, Parcel C, Peterson R, Johnson K. Safe and effective treatment of osteoporosis with intermittent slow release sodium fluoride: augmentation of vertebral bone mass and inhibition of fractures. J Clin Endocrinol Metab 1989;68:150–9.
24. Pak CY, Sakhaee K, Piziak V *et al.* Slow-release sodium fluoride in the management of postmenopausal osteoporosis. A randomized controlled trial [see comments]. Ann Intern Med 1994;120:625–32.
25. Cummings SR, Nevitt MC, Browner WS *et al.* Risk factors for hip fracture in white women. Study of Osteoporotic Fractures Research Group. N Engl J Med 1995;332:767–73.
26. Robinson RJ, al-Azzawi F, Iqbal SJ *et al.* Osteoporosis and determinants of bone density in patients. Dig Dis Sci 1998;43:2500–6.
27. Valentine JF, Sninsky CA. Prevention and treatment of osteoporosis in patients with inflammatory bowel disease. Am J Gastroenterol 1999;94:878–83.
28. Reed CA, Nichols DL, Bonnick SL, DiMarco NM. Bone mineral density and dietary intake in patients with Crohn's disease. J Clin Densit 1998;1:33–40.
29. Ravn P, Hosking D, Thompson D *et al.* Monitoring of alendronate treatment and prediction of effect on bone mass by biochemical markers in the early postmenopausal intervention cohort study. J Clin Endocrinol Metab 1999;84:2363–8.
30. Ravn P, Clemmesen B, Christiansen C, Group AOPS. Biochemical markers can predict the response in bone mass during Alendronate treatment in early postmenopausal women. Bone 1999;24:237–44.
31. Hannon R, Blumsohn A, Naylor K, Eastell R. Response of biochemical markers of bone turnover to hormone replacement therapy: impact of biological variability. J Bone Miner Res 1998;13:1124–33.
32. Delmas PD, Bjarnason NH, Mitlak BH *et al.* Effects of raloxifene on bone mineral density, serum cholesterol concentrations, and uterine endometrium in postmenopausal women. N Engl J Med 1997;337:1641–7.
33. Yendt ER. Vitamin D and osteoporosis. Osteoporosis Society of Canada Bulletin 1994;2.

34. Villareal DT, Civitelli R, Chines A, Avioli LV. Subclinical vitamin D deficiency in postmenopausal women with low vertebral bone mass. J Clin Endocrinol Metab 1991;72:628–34.
35. Punnonen R, Salmi J, Tuimala R, Jarvinen M, Pystynen P. Vitamin D deficiency in women with femoral neck fracture. Maturitas 1986;8:291–5.
36. Holick MF. McCollum Award Lecture, 1994: vitamin D – new horizons for the 21st century. Am J Clin Nutr 1994;60:619–30.
37. Holick MF. Environmental factors that influence the cutaneous production of vitamin D. Am J Clin Nutr 1995;61(3 Suppl.):638–45S.
38. Kessenich CR, Rosen CJ. Vitamin D and bone status in elderly women. Orthop Nurs 1996;15:67–71.
39. Adachi JD, Bensen WG, Brown J *et al.* Intermittent etidronate therapy to prevent corticosteroid-induced osteoporosis. N Engl J Med 1997;337:382–7.
40. Adachi JD, Bensen WG, Anastassiades TP *et al.* Etidronate in the prevention of corticosteroid-induced osteoporosis: one year follow-up on calcium only. Arthritis Rheum 1998;41:S137.
41. Saag KG, Group G-IOIS. Alendronate for the prevention and treatment of glucocorticoid-induced osteoporosis. N Engl J Med 1998;339:292–9.
42. Gallacher SJ, Fenner JAK, Anderson K *et al.* Intravenous pamidronate in the treatment of osteoporosis associated with corticosteroid dependent lung disease: an open pilot study. Thorax 1992;47:932–6.
43. Boutsen Y, Jamart J, Esselinckx W, Stoffel M, Devogelaer J-P. Primary prevention of glucocorticoid-induced osteoporosis with intermittent intravenous pamidronate: a randomized trial. Calcif Tissue Int 1997;61:266–71.
44. Woitge HW, Pecherstorfer M, Li Y *et al.* Novel markers of bone resorption: clinical assessment and comparison with established urinary indices. J Bone Miner Res 1999;14:792–801.
45. Walsh LJ, Wong CA, Pringle M, Tattersfield AE. Use of oral corticosteroids in the community and the prevention of secondary osteoporosis: a cross sectional study. Br Med J 1996;313:344–6.

17
Steroid-induced osteonecrosis in inflammatory bowel disease: Canadian legal status

R. M. CARTER AND M. G. A. GRACE

ABSTRACT

The challenges of treating inflammatory bowel disease (IBD) with steroids has not only serious medical implications but also the potential for legal ramifications. There are a number of possible side-effects with steroid use, including the risk of avascular necrosis, or osteonecrosis (ON).

If the clinician treats an IBD patient with steroids and is sued, the legal principles of standard of care and informed consent are triggered. These common law principles form the basis of medical negligence actions against physicians and affect physicians sued in common law jurisdiction such as Canada, United States and Commonwealth countries. Allegations of medical negligence are predicated on assumptions that physicians in prescribing steroids for IBD may have breached the standard of care in relation to dosage, both in time and amount prescribed, and in failure to refer the patient for surgery in a timely fashion. Lack of informed consent is almost always an issue.

At least 10 lawsuits in Canada relating to steroid use in IBD have occurred since 1990 and the risk of legal actions against gastroenterologists in Canada has more than doubled since the 1980s. A recent (1999) Canadian court judgement against a gastroenterologist alleging an inappropriate prescribing of steroids for IBD that resulted in ON, provided a change in the stance of the courts. Emphasis was placed on standard of care, informed-consent status, timing of referral for surgery, and analysis employed by the court resulted in a favourable finding for the defendant gastroenterologist. This case provides a contrast to earlier judgements in favour of patients. In spite of the favourable finding for the gastroenterologist the court still concluded, based on evidence of orthopaedic surgeons and gastroenterologists, that a direct link existed between steroid use in treatment of IBD and development of ON.

INTRODUCTION

Use of steroid therapy in treatment of various medical conditions is perceived to be the potential cause of a variety of side effects. Osteonecrosis (ON) [often referred to as avascular necrosis] following steroid therapy has been cited in numerous medical treatments but it is still unexplained why only a limited number of these complications occur. It has been assumed in the medical community that occurrence of ON in inflammatory bowel disease (IBD) following steroid therapy is a result of the treatment rather than the disease or some other factor. Consequently the courts have been faced with medical experts automatically making this assumption, although there appears to be limited scientific support for this statement.

There are five reported legal decisions in Canada (although other actions are brought) concerning treatment of steroids in IBD cases which purportedly caused ON. There may be limited scientific evidence regarding whether treatment of IBD with steroids does carry with it the risk of ON[1]. Experts in the reported legal cases state as a given that a plaintiff who develops ON following treatment with steroids does so as a result of steroid therapy. In other words, there appears to be no consideration given that ON may be disease-based rather than steroid-induced. The purpose of this chapter is to demonstrate the ramifications of this premise being accepted as medical fact by the courts by examining the legal decisions, particularly in terms of standard of care and consent issues.

LEGAL PRINCIPLES

Consent

The common law is that plaintiffs must establish, on a balance of probabilities, that they were not informed of the risks of treatment and that the result would have been different had they been fully informed of the risks. The test as enunciated by the Supreme Court of Canada is an objective one. If the plaintiff is not informed of risks, the issue becomes whether a reasonable person, in the position of the plaintiff, would have declined the course of treatment if fully informed of the risks[2]. Even if the legal test was a subjective one, the issue is would this particular plaintiff, being fully informed of the risks of treatment, accept it.

In IBD, plaintiffs would have to be advised not only of risks inherent in steroid therapy, but also the possible alternatives and risks inherent in other treatments and in no treatment. Courts have accepted that surgery is regarded in the medical profession as a last resort in treatment of Crohn's disease.

In law a material risk is a significant risk that poses a real threat to the plaintiff's life, health or comfort. In considering whether a risk is material one must balance the severity of the potential result and the likelihood of its occurring. A risk which is a mere possibility is not a material risk unless, even though rare in occurrence, its consequences are serious.[3] On the other hand, if there is a significant chance of slight injury this too may be held to be material. Definition of a material risk depends on the specific facts of each case. Plaintiffs must be informed of all material risks associated with any form of treatment to enable them to make informed decisions whether to accept offered treatments[2,3]. Risk of development of ON is a very small one, with the rate of occurrence being one in many thousands of plaintiffs treated.[4]

The plaintiff must prove on a balance of probabilities that the gasteroenterologist (GI) failed to meet the standard of care reasonably expected of a normal and prudent GI at the time the plaintiff was treated. An honest and intelligent error in exercise of medical judgement does not amount to breach of the standard of care. A higher degree of skill is required for specialists such as GIs than for general practitioners (GPs)[5].

Medical experts are often called by lawyers for plaintiffs and defendants to give expert evidence at trial on the applicable standard of care at the time the plaintiff was treated. Typically, in cases involving GIs, each party would retain one or more GIs to give expert opinion.

Standard of care

The general clinical background and demographics of the plaintiffs in the reported legal cases are provided in Table 1. All five plaintiffs were treated with steroids. Three plaintiffs suffered from ulcerative colitis. One was diagnosed as having possible Crohn's disease but evidence showed he did not. One was believed to suffer from early colitis with possible proctitis which was later proven to be ulcerative colitis. The plaintiffs all developed ON of the femoral heads. Four plaintiffs had hip replacements (one also had shoulder joints replaced) while one plaintiff had not had hip surgery at the time of the trial.

As shown in Table 2, the plaintiffs alleged the defendant GIs either inappropriately prescribed steroids or, where steroid therapy was appropriate, the steroid dosage was too high. All plaintiffs alleged the defendant GIs failed to warn of dangers of steroid-induced ON.

All plaintiffs were treated with prednisone. Two plaintiffs were treated with adrenocorticotropic hormone (ACTH). Another was treated with Betnesol enemas and Solumedol (Table 3). The drug history has been drastically condensed for summary purposes. Detailed individual drug histories are not always provided in reported legal cases.

The awards ranged from Can$320 000 to Can$784 000. In cases 2 and 5, in which the GIs successfully defended themselves, the Court, following normal practice, awarded provisional damages (no money paid). Those are noted in parentheses in Table 4. As usual in medical malpractice actions, monetary awards are given not only to the plaintiff but may include spouses, children and the Provincial Health Care provider. In addition to monetary awards, costs and interest are normally awarded. In case 1 the plaintiff was awarded costs at trial, but at appeal the plaintiff and defendant had to bear their own costs. In case 2 the Court declined to award costs, which meant the defendant GI would not be able to recover costs of defending even though he won the action. In addition to the awards, there may be substantial legal costs which are not recoverable even if the physician wins the action.

Table 1 Demographic and clinical background

	Case 1	Case 2	Case 3	Case 4	Case 5
Age (years)	29	39	22	23	30
Gender	Male	Female	Male	Male	Male
Diagnosis	UC	UC	Possible Crohn's disease (disproven)	1. Early colitis 2. Proctitis (tentative) with Crohn's features 3. Proven UC	UC
History	Diarrhea with blood in stool	1/2 attacks of UC yearly, lasting 3 weeks to 3 months	1. Consumed chicken and had nausea, vomiting, diarrhoea. 2. Became worse after treatment by GP	1. Three flareups, worsening 2. Two years after diagnosis surgery showed UC	1. Felt bloated, had pain 2. Six months later continued cramps and rectal bleeding
Diagnosis/ surgery*	ON L–R hip and shoulders and replace hip and shoulder joints	ON L–R hips – no surgery	ON L–R hips – surgery	ON L–R hips – surgery	Early ON of R femur – no surgery
Location	British Columbia	British Columbia	Ontario	British Columbia	British Columbia

*L = left; R = right.

DISCUSSION

Consent

Case 1

A GI and GP were sued[4]. The plaintiff was not advised of ON complication from high doses of steroids taken over a long period of time. The judge felt the GI seemed indifferent to well-known side-effects such as osteoporosis and cataracts, and had no clear understanding why steroids had to be tapered. The judge rejected the argument of the GI that he was not obligated to warn the plaintiff of ON as it was a remote possibility. As both the GI and GP were 'neglectful' that ON could develop, the plaintiff did not have to prove he would have elected surgery if told of the possibility of ON by the defendants.

ON was a material risk that had to be disclosed to the plaintiff. The GI was negligent in not informing the plaintiff of the ON risk.

Table 2 Allegations against gastroenterologist

Case 1	Case 2	Case 3	Case 4	Case 5
Negligent in prescribing prolonged high prednisone doses	Negligent in prescribing and managing therapy	Negligent in diagnosing Crohn's disease and prescribing prednisone for possible Crohn's disease	Negligent in prescribing prolonged high doses of prednisone	Negligent in continuing prednisone/no surgery recommendation
Failed to inform of alternative treatment by surgery	Failed to warn of prednisone risks including ON	Failed to warn of risks of prednisone	Failed to warn of prednisone risks and delayed recommending surgery	Failed to disclose and warn of risks of prednisone

Table 3 Drug history

Case 1	Case 2	Case 3	Case 4	Case 5
Prednisone 40–60 mg on and off for 2 years	Salazopyrine for 9 years; ACTH 60–100 units/day for 25 days then prednisone tapered	Short course of prednisone (2 days?)	5 months prednisone from 40–50 mg day except 14 day ACTH	Prednisone and betnesol enemas for 2 months; solumedol 75–25 mg for 4 days

Case 2

Two GIs were sued.[6] The plaintiff testified defendants were reluctant to state what medications were administered. She stated she was on steroids for several weeks without her knowledge and, had she known, she would not have taken steroids. The evidence showed discussion and recorded evidence of the plaintiff's aversion to steroids. Neither defendant GI told the plaintiff of possible side-effects of steroids. The judge held the plaintiff did not give an informed consent but, had she been informed of risks, she would have accepted them.

Case 3

A GI was sued for misdiagnosing Crohn's disease in a young male and consequently prescribing steroids[2]. The plaintiff testified the defendant GI did not inform him of potential risks of prednisone. The defendant GI testified he always advised patients of side-effects and specifically told this plaintiff of certain side-effects including swelling, weight gain, possible facial fomas and stomach pains. The judge preferred evidence of the plaintiff and held the GI was negligent in not advising the plaintiff of the risks of steroids. The judge found steroid-induced ON was a rare but known complication of steroids.

Table 4 Awards ($)*

Category	Case 1	Case 2	Case 3	Case 4	Case 5
General damages	135 000	(75 000)	125 000	90 000	(50 000)
Past loss of income	66 000	(100 000)	110 000	150 000	(240 000)
Future income and earning capacity loss	150 000	(125 000)	413 000	135 000	(50 000)
Future care cost	100 000	(20 000)	55 000	30 000	0
Home modifications	0	(20 000)	0	0	0
Management fee	0	0	0	25 000	0
Special damages	0	0	2 400	0	(1 000)
Housekeeping	0	0	16 000	0	0
Spousal companionship loss	0	0	10 000	0	0
Children parental loss	0	0	40 000	0	0
Health Care Claim	0	0	13 000	0	0
Total	451 000	(340 000)	784 400	430 000	341 000
Interest	Yes	No	Yes	Yes	No
Costs	Trial – patient Appeal – patient/GI	No	Yes	Yes	Yes

Figures in parentheses are provisional.
*Figures approximate.

Case 4

A GI was sued[8]. Experts testified various risks of steroids should be told to patients but, because ON was considered a rare complication of steroid use in IBD treatment, ON might not be listed and explained as a specific risk. However, when surgery was recommended or had to be undertaken, and the patient was reluctant or unwilling to undergo surgery, the risk of ON from continued use of high-dosage steroids must be explained. The defendant GI testified it was not his practice to warn patients about the risk of developing ON as a result of steroids even though it was deemed to be a complication of steroids.

Experts testified, and it was accepted by the court, that a prudent GI would have recommended surgery no later than 6 weeks after unsuccessful treatment with steroids. In this case surgery should have been strongly urged to the plaintiff after 6 weeks of steroid therapy failed. The judge would not draw an inference that the plaintiff would not have undergone surgery if advised of steroid risks.

Case 5

A GI was sued[9]. The judge found the defendant did discuss risks of using steroids. All experts agreed patients are to be advised of risks of steroids. One defence expert testified she would advise patients of steroid risks after a few weeks of therapy. The Court held the defendant GI failed to meet the standard of care applicable in that the plaintiff was not warned of risks of steroids prior to these being prescribed.

DISCUSSION

Standard of care

Case 1

A rheumatologist called by the defendant GI testified long-term use of steroids might cause thinning of the bone and there was an indication ON was connected to steroids. Surgery should be considered. The GI called by the defendant GI practised with him. The expert GI for the plaintiff knew of ON risks for 20 years. The defendant GI did not monitor the steroid program and withdrawal of steroids, so there was a lack of follow-up. All experts agreed steroid therapy was the first choice for ulcerative colitis.

The judge ruled that the practice of a rheumatologist was different from that of a GI so his evidence was not helpful. The expert GI was biased in favour of the defendant GI. The expert GI was an 'apologist' for the defendant GI's conduct and not 'impartial'. This expert GI's evidence was rejected. The GI failed to meet the standard of care in not knowing or lacking concern about steroid dangers, prolonged use of steroids or providing information about a surgical option.

Expert evidence for the plaintiff and accepted by the judge was that steroids are 'very dangerous' and plaintiffs should be closely monitored for consumption and progress of the drug treatment. The judge rejected the evidence of the expert called for the GI when it conflicted with witnesses for the plaintiff. The judge found the GI failed to meet the standard of care, mainly in not knowing the dangers of prescribing steroids.

Case 2

Based on expert evidence the judge found there was a causal link between steroid treatment and ON, infections, diabetes and psychosis. Both dose levels and duration of treatment were 'well within' the generally accepted standard of care. The judge also accepted evidence of admitting nurses and attending physicians, and held the diagnosis of a severe attack and choice of ACTH were correct. Based on defence expert evidence and literature it was appropriate for the defendant to have continued high-dose steroid therapy after 2 weeks. The case was dismissed without costs.

Case 3

Based on expert evidence the judge found that treatment by the GI fell below the standard of care and skill reasonably expected of a specialist in GI when prescribing prednisone for non-IBD. The judge found the complication of ON of femoral heads with a short dose of prednisone is known but unusual. Even though the particular side-effects suffered by the plaintiff were not reasonably predictable it was foreseeable that damage might occur to the plaintiff's health and, as such, the defendant GI was liable.

Case 4

The expert evidence at trial was that the standard in GI was to treat IBD with high doses of steroids for no longer than 6 weeks before resorting to surgery or reducing maintenance steroid usage. An expert testified the standard of treatment for IBD was 40–60 mg/day of oral or intravenous steroids for 2–3 weeks to attempt remission. Steroids can be used for 2–3 weeks followed by another 3–4 weeks during which the dosage is tapered. If there is no improvement in 4 weeks other therapy should be employed. Use of steroids could continue in gradually reduced dosages for 2–3 further weeks while employing other conservative modes. Without a favourable result surgery was the recommended treatment unless the diagnosis was Crohn's disease, in which case many doses of steroids were justified because of the uncertainty that surgery would be curative.

The judge held that the defendant GIs breached the standard of a reasonable, competent GI of similar skill and experience by continuing to administer high doses of steroids after more than 6 weeks of therapy failed to induce remission of IBD.

Case 5

Expert evidence was that the medical knowledge at the time of this case indicated that risks of developing ON associated with use of steroids occurred when high dosages were consistently prescribed and used in excess of 40–60 mg per day for periods exceeding 6 weeks. That was not the situation in this case. It was perceived that total dosage was of significance, rather than length of time of dosing or daily dosing average.

The judge held the amount of steroids prescribed by the defendant in conjunction with what the defendant knew, or should have known, about a GP additionally prescribing steroids, came within acceptable levels of prescription given the standard of care. Medical treatment and not surgery is the first choice with IBD. Surgical removal of bowel portions and the restorative surgery that follows is the last resort of treatment.

SUMMARY

In all cases the judge held that patients must be advised of the risk of developing ON from taking steroids. Failure to advise a patient of steroid risks is negligence. If the plaintiff was advised, then the defendant was not held liable for prescribing steroids providing the standard of treatment was met. However, if the plaintiff was not advised the question to be answered by the judge was whether a reasonable plaintiff would have agreed to undergo steroid therapy if advised of the risks. In one of the five cases the judge found the plaintiff would have undergone treatment if advised of the risk of ON.

The standard of care issue is less contentious. There was usually a consensus on this point among those experts that the judges held in high regard. Overall there was a consistency in reasonable levels of dosing and timing that were proffered by experts from both sides.

Throughout all these cases it was automatically assumed by all doctors, experts from both sides and defendant GIs, that steroid therapy in IBD can cause ON. Consequently all judges took as a given that a relationship existed. What was never debated in these cases is whether scientific evidence exists to demonstrate a causal link between steroid administration and development of ON. Certainly from the literature the possible association is tenuous at best. A recent paper presents clear arguments and refutes the association at a number of levels[1]. The literature prior to this article gives a mixed picture at best[10–15].

What impact did this supposed causal link have on judges when their decision was made? This cannot be readily determined, but it seems likely that if no causal link exists then it is possible the legal outcomes would have been different, and some cases would never have reached trial. It is also likely that fewer cases would be initiated.

The courts are constrained by the background of the issues brought before them and testimony of experts. If experts are willing to assume or state unequivocally about cause and effect it is impossible for a judge to ignore this information. Consequent decisions that might stem from 'junk science' or assumptions that have not been tested are the responsibility of the medical and scientific community. With significant cost impacts and obvious stress to plaintiffs, defendants and their families it is incumbent on the medical and scientific community to provide clear and valid information.

References

1. Freeman HJ. Osteomyelitis and osteonecrosis in inflammatory bowel disease. Can J Gastroenterol 1997;11:601–6.
2. *Reibel v. Hughes* [1980] 2 S.C.R. 880.
3. *Hopp v. Lepp* [1980] 2 S.C.R. 192.
4. 50 B.C.L.R. 166, varied 10 B.C.L.R. (2d) 121 (C.A.).
5. *Crits v. Sylvester* [1956] O.R. 132, 1 D.L.R. (2d) 502 (C.A.), aff'd [1956] S.C.R. 99.
6. [1982] B.C.J. No. 918, (1986) 36 C.C.L.T. 150 (C.A.).
7. [1984] O.J. No. 430, (1986) 55 O.R. (2d) 10.
8. [1989] B.C.J. No. 1236, [1992] B.C.J. No. 704 (C.A.).
9. 85 A.C.W.S. (3d) 1185.
10. Brom B, Bank S, Marks IN, Cobb JJ. Periostitis, aseptic necrosis, and arthritis occurring in a plaintiff with Crohn's disease. Gastroenterology 1971;60:1106–9.
11. Shapiro SC, Rochskin FC, Newman AJ, Fletcher B, Halpin TC Jr. Multifocal osteonecrosis in adolescents with Crohn's disease: a complication of therapy? J Pediatr Gastroenterol Nutr 1985;4:502–6.
12. Vakil N, Sparberg M. Steroid related osteonecrosis in inflammatory bowel disease. Gastroenterology 1989;96:62–7.
13. Culp RW, Schaffer JL, Osterman AL, Bora FW. Kienbock's disease in a plaintiff with Crohn's enteritis treated with corticosteroids. J Hand Surg 1989;14A:294–6.
14. Nugent FW, Glaser D, Herilhy-Fernandez L. Crohn's colitis associated with granulomatous bone disease. N Engl J Med 1976;294:262–3.
15. Madsen PV, Andersen G. Multifocal osteonecrosis related to steroid treatment in a plaintiff with ulcerative colitis. Gut 1994;35:132–4.
16. Freeman HJ, Kwan WCP. Non-corticosteroid-associated osteonecrosis of the femoral heads in two plaintiffs with inflammatory bowel disease. N Engl J Med 1993;329:1314–16.

Section VI
Alternative therapy

Moderator: **F. Martin,** Montreal

18
Psychotherapy for inflammatory bowel disease: new prospects

R. G. MAUNDER

ABSTRACT

Psychotherapeutic approaches to inflammatory bowel disease (IBD) have come in two historical waves. In the first, psychoanalysis assumed a model of psychogenic aetiology and aimed for cure. This resulted in a literature that is clinically rich but very weak scientifically. The underlying assumptions resulted in stigma. A second wave aimed to improve coping and reduce the psychosocial consequences of IBD. This led to interventions such as stress management and relaxation which were tested in controlled trials with adequate results, but which lacked experiential depth. In this presentation two new psychotherapeutic approaches are described which build on the strengths of these approaches: psychological depth and empirical rigour, respectively.

Supportive–expressive (SE) group psychotherapy was originally described for women with metastatic breast cancer. An adaptation for use in IBD has been tested in four 20-week groups ($n=30$). The group discussion is grounded in major IBD concerns including uncertainty, personal control and burden on others, physician–patient relationship, medication concern and body image. The expressive aspect of SE refers to facing the challenges and limitations imposed by illness honestly, and expressing the feelings that result. The supportive aspect of SE refers to the emphasis on interpersonal support as a buffer against the negative psychosocial consequences of disease. Results demonstrate that among those who complete the group ($n=24$), improvement in maladaptive coping behaviours occurs concurrently with improvement in IBD-related quality of life in subjects who improve with therapy (67%). A second approach to psychotherapy follows from recent data suggesting that a personality trait which results in stress vulnerability (insecure attachment) may be relevant to disease course in a biologically identified subgroup of ulcerative colitis (UC) patients (those who do not produce antineutrophil cytoplasmic antibody, ANCA). A pilot study of 47 UC subjects found avoidant insecure attachment present in 58.6% of ANCA-absent subjects but in only 22.2% of ANCA+ subjects (chi square=5.95, $p=0.01$). The model of interaction between individual differences in stress response and biological subtypes of UC which predicted this finding is described. These data, pending replication, imply that screening of UC patients to identify stress-vulnerable individuals may be useful. The selective application of psychotherapy to modify an interpersonal style which increases stress vulnerability is discussed with respect to therapeutic technique and goals.

INTRODUCTION

This chapter presents two prospects for using psychotherapy as an adjunct to the medical and surgical treatment of ulcerative colitis (UC) and Crohn's disease (CD). These pilot projects build upon two historical applications of psychotherapy to inflammatory bowel disease (IBD). The first trend was to view psychological factors as a cause of IBD; the more recent trend has been to attend to the consequences of living with IBD.

Psychoanalysis was introduced as a treatment for UC in the 1930s following Murray's observation of an interaction of psychological factors and disease onset[1]. Assuming a psychogenic aetiology, psychoanalysis often aimed for cure. Over three decades, careful descriptions accumulated describing an interaction of personality and life events in the course of colitis in dozens or hundreds of patients[2]. However, the biases of the case-study method led to unsupported claims about the specificity of psychological factors to IBD and about the general applicability of findings in psychoanalytical subjects to all IBD patients[3]. Furthermore, a stigmatizing belief emerged that IBD is the result of psychological immaturity.

Nonetheless, careful investigation of environmental factors, including psychological factors, remains important to a multifactorial model of illness. Most people with IBD endorse the belief that stress and psychological factors play an important role in their illness[4]. Recent studies also support some role of psychological stress in inflammatory disease in general[5] and gastrointestinal inflammation in particular. For example, Collin's group has demonstrated that an acute inflammation of the gut can result in long-term changes in the gut's functional response to stress[6]. It is less clear whether or not stress promotes inflammation. The literature that has examined this question has produced inconsistent results, due in large part to methodological limitations[3], but probably also due to the wide variability in stress response in the general population[5].

As effective methods of treatment for IBD became available, a second wave of psychosocial interventions emerged which aimed to improve coping and buffer the consequences of IBD. Many forms of intervention that do not presuppose any psychopathology have been described[7]. In particular, stress management and relaxation training are widely applicable interventions that lend themselves to controlled trials using standardized interventions and objective outcome measures. Randomized, controlled trials have demonstrated the effectiveness of relaxation therapy for chronic pain associated with ulcerative colitis[8] and the short-term effectiveness of a supportive group for reducing anxiety[9]. More ambitiously, Milne and Joachim report subjects receiving stress management training had lower disease activity, measured by the Crohn's

Disease Activity Index, at outcome than a standard treatment control group[10]. Unfortunately the treatment group had greater disease activity than the control group at the study onset, so it cannot be ruled out that the result is due to regression to the mean. The application of cognitive–behavioural techniques to a mixed UC/CD population resulted in worse outcome in the treatment group than the waiting list control in another study[11].

Usefully, this focus on the psychosocial consequences of IBD has resulted in a reliable description of the concerns associated with IBD, and their relative importance. Empirical measurement provides the information required to develop psychosocial interventions that meet the specific needs of people with IBD. It is now clear, particularly from the work of Drossman in this area, that concern with illness uncertainty, medication effects and lack of energy are virtually universal in IBD[12]. Other concerns are of special importance in particular groups, such as feelings about the body, having children, and being alone in women[13], or a number of interpersonal and emotional concerns which are greater in people with IBD who seek psychological counselling[14].

This chapter describes two studies that extend these traditions. In the first, a novel hypothesis of a psychosomatic contribution to the course of IBD is tested. The second study explores a group therapy intervention that incorporates a contemporary understanding of disease concerns and coping to improve quality of life in IBD.

p-ANCA AND ATTACHMENT: A STUDY OF PSYCHOSOCIAL DISEASE RISK

The hypothesis that there is a psychological predisposition to IBD, which is both a necessary and sufficient condition, is false[3]. However, the hypothesis that certain psychological factors contribute to the pathophysiology of UC or CD is insufficiently tested. Two strategies have emerged that may lead to more investigative precision. First, there is wide variation in individual susceptibility to the physiological effects of stress[5]. This implies that it may be more fruitful to investigate the role of stress vulnerability than the role of stress *per se*. Second, the hypothesis of aetiological heterogeneity[15] suggests that, rather than seeking causal factors that are at work in all people with UC or CD, it may be more appropriate to identify aetiological subgroups.

At the intersection of these two strategies lies the hypothesis that we have tested. Namely, that there exists a group of people with a particular predisposition to UC or CD that includes stress-susceptible mechanisms, and that among this group those individuals who are most vulnerable to stress are at the highest risk of developing manifest illness. We have studied the distribution of attachment insecurity in UC. We hypothesized that insecure attachment provides a vulnerability to life stress that contributes to the development of UC in a certain subgroup, and that members of this subgroup are identified by the absence of perinuclear antineutrophil cytoplasmic antibody (p-ANCA).

Attachment style is an element of personality; specifically how an individual behaves in close interpersonal relationships at times of perceived threat. Attachment occurs in all mammals; it has been robustly preserved by evolution.

Attachment theory describes how individuals reduce real and perceived threats to safety by association to key people, such as parents and adult partners. About 60% of the general population have a secure pattern of attachment. An insecure pattern of attachment, consisting of anxious proximity-seeking or avoidant self-reliance, may predispose a person to experience more life stress and to a relative lack of the types of social relationship that buffer against stress. Of particular note, attachment insecurity is associated with increased vulnerability to the biological consequences of stress, such as lower basal cortisol levels and prolonged cortisol reactivity to acute stress[16].

While attachment insecurity is linked with an increased stress response, acute and chronic stress are in turn associated with alterations in the regulation of a number of molecules that are implicated in the inflammatory cascade in IBD. For example, substance P, which has a number of proinflammatory responsibilities[17], is a critical regulator of core attachment behaviours such as infant vocalizations in response to maternal separation[18], and the aggressive response to territorial threat[19].

The second feature of the hypothesis is that ANCA marks the division between stress-responsive UC and stress-neutral UC. This speculative connection emerged from a synthesis of existing literature that suggests that:

1.   Disruption of close social relationships in primates is a good model of human attachment insecurity[20].
2.   Disruption of social relationships may contribute to the high rate of colitis in captive cottontop tamarins[21].
3.   Cottontop tamarin colitis is a good model of human UC[22].
4.   Captive cottontop tamarins with colitis do not produce p-ANCA[23].

It is not assumed that ANCA marks a genetic group; only that whatever causal factor(s) are contributing to UC, ANCA is marking a path that is relatively neutral to stress. This could be the case even if ANCA were, for example, a marker of an aetiological path with earlier onset in which there is less opportunity for stress to exert any significant effect[24].

The entry criteria for this study were a confirmed diagnosis of UC and previous testing for ANCA by immunofluorescence. Of 108 potential subjects, 47 completed the self-report mail questionnaire. Attachment was measured with the Reciprocal Attachment Questionnaire[25]. Subjects are asked to describe attitudes towards their partner or other significant figure such as 'I expect her to take care of her own problems' (avoidant insecure attachment) or 'I can't get on with my own work if he has a problem' (anxious insecure attachment).

Avoidant insecure attachment was present in 58.6% of the 28 ANCA-absent subjects but in only 22.2% of the 19 ANCA+ subjects (chi-square=5.95, $p<0.02$). There was no similar difference between groups with respect to anxious insecure attachment. Although the actual rates of prevalence depend on the cut-offs used for this instrument, which are not well established, the rates we are reporting in the p-ANCA subgroup are in excess of the prevalence of avoidant attachment in the general population, which tends to run between 10% and 15%[26].

The avoidant attachment style includes a number of traits that are highly valued in our culture, such as independence, self-reliance and competitiveness[27]. On the other hand avoidant individuals are unlikely to seek help, tend to minimize their acknowledgement of vulnerabilities, and will tend not to have a wide social support network. Interestingly, our finding that avoidant attachment, but not anxious attachment, is associated with ANCA-negative UC is consistent with findings from other illnesses. Insecure attachment has been associated with chronic disease of childhood including cystic fibrosis[28], epilepsy[29], and asthma[30]. When the subtypes of insecurity are distinguished, avoidant insecurity but not anxious insecurity is associated with congenital heart disease in toddlers[31], with physical symptoms in university students[32], and with non-compliance in diabetes[33].

If the results of the p-ANCA and attachment study are confirmed by replication, then a challenge will be posed for psychotherapy – to design interventions that address avoidant attachment in the minority of UC patients who may be at particular risk. Two strategies would require empirical evaluation. One strategy would aim to alter the trait, as has been done in the somewhat similar link between Type A personality and heart disease. Alternatively one can accept the attachment style and make use of the strengths of avoidant behaviour, autonomy and control, to improve rather than impair long-term health.

SUPPORTIVE–EXPRESSIVE GROUP PSYCHOTHERAPY FOR IBD

In choosing how to provide psychosocial support in the course of IBD, it is important to understand an individual's stage of psychological adaptation. We have proposed a model of normal coping in IBD which describes a triad of illness challenges: uncertainty about the illness, imposed losses and limitations, and more enduring suffering which results from uncertainty, loss and from the direct effects of illness[7]. The psychosocial interventions that have been tested in clinical trials in IBD have tended to focus on the earlier challenges– interventions such as relaxation therapy, various forms of bibliotherapy, and stress management. Recently we completed a pilot study of an intervention that also targets the non-psychiatrically ill person with IBD, but focuses more on persistent suffering, irreducible uncertainty, and challenges to personal systems of meaning and value.

Supportive–expressive (SE) group psychotherapy was originally described as a treatment for women with metastatic breast cancer[34], and has since been adapted for other medically ill populations.

In the adaptation of SE for IBD, a group of six to 10 people with UC or CD meets weekly for 20 weeks for a discussion of major IBD concerns including uncertainty, personal control and burden on others, physician–patient relationship, medication concern and body image. The expressive aspect of SE refers to facing the challenges and limitations imposed by illness honestly, and expressing the feelings that result. The supportive aspect of SE refers to its emphasis on interpersonal support as a buffer against the consequences of disease.

In a pilot trial of SE for four groups ($n-30$), 24 people completed the group, and of these 12 of 19 for whom there are complete data showed an improvement in IBD-related quality of life (measured by IBDQ[35]) over the course of the intervention.

Of potentially greater interest, changes in patterns of coping with IBD were observed in those subjects whose quality of life improved which were not observed in subjects whose quality of life did not improve. A cluster of three behavioural coping patterns (self-blame, excessive self-control, and escape-avoidance), which are associated with poor qualitative outcome from IBD surgery[36], were higher at the onset of SE therapy in subjects whose quality of life subsequently improved compared than in those who showed no improvement over therapy (Figure 1). Over the course of therapy improvers reported a simultaneous reduction in maladaptive coping, whereas maladaptive coping in non-improvers was stable (Figure 2).

The IBD-specific concerns that were most important to our group were a mix of those that are very important to most people with IBD (illness uncertainty and fatigue) and those that are of greater concern in people who seek counselling (financial difficulties and pain). It is interesting to note that concern over lost potential was highly prevalent in our group. This is not consistent with other populations that have been studied, but it is a very good fit with the existential roots of SE therapy.

SE group psychotherapy for IBD presents a new possibility for the supportive treatment of the psychosocial consequences of chronic illness that has a number of clinical strengths. First, SE therapy has the potential to offer greater psychological depth and greater specificity for the particular concerns related to IBD than can be offered by more generic supportive interventions such as relaxation therapy and stress management. At the same time, SE therapy is

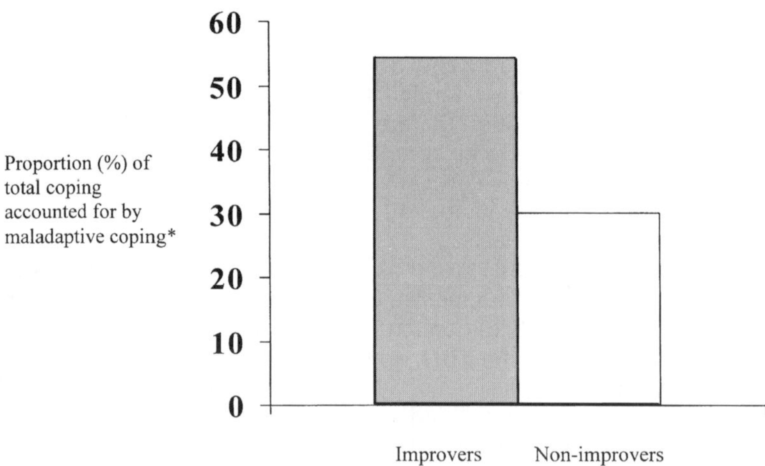

Figure 1 Difference at start of therapy in use of maladaptive coping* between subjects whose quality of life improves with therapy and subjects whose quality of life does not improve. *Maladaptive coping is the sum of ways of coping relative scores for escape-avoidance, taking responsibility and self-control as a proportion of total coping. The scales that have not been associated with poor quality of life in IBD are seeking support, problem solving, positive reappraisal, distancing and confrontation

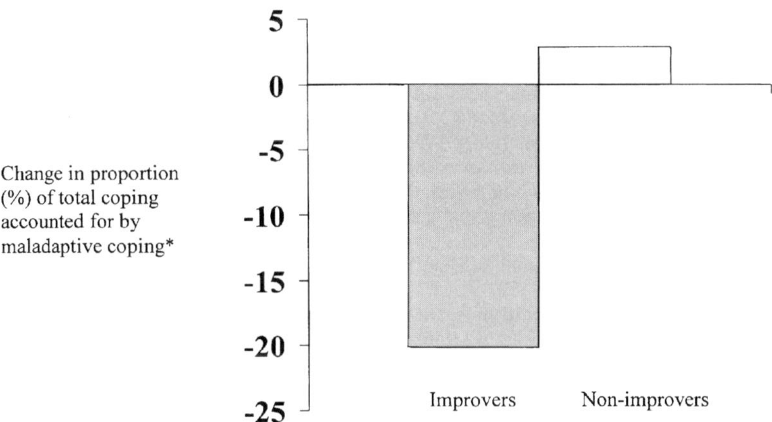

Figure 2 Change from start to end of group psychotherapy in use of maladaptive coping* in subjects whose quality of life improves with therapy and subjects whose quality of life does not improve. *Maladaptive coping is sum of Ways of Coping relative scores for escape-avoidance, taking responsibility and self-control as a proportion of total coping. The scales that have not been associated with poor quality of life in IBD are seeking support, problem solving, positive reappraisal, distancing and confrontation

designed to be tested in clinical trials, through its use of therapy manuals and sessions observable on videotape. Further research on the adaptation of SE to IBD is required, particularly a randomized controlled clinical trial, and efforts to determine the optimal frequency and duration of treatment.

DISCUSSION

The studies reviewed here briefly represent the early stage of development of a programme of psychiatric research into the role of psychotherapy in IBD. The conclusions that can be drawn from each, as described above, are tentative because of the methodological limitations of pilot work. This caution applies especially to the p-ANCA study that is based on a highly speculative hypothesis. Nonetheless, each study has been designed to allow for careful empirical testing. The results are presented in the hope of promoting discussion about the role of psychotherapy in IBD and generating enthusiasm to pursue the careful empirical investigation that is required to move the study of psychotherapy for IBD forward. Such study is important to a field of investigation that may still be in its infancy in spite of 60 years of intermittent attention.

References

1. Murray CD. A brief psychological analysis of a patient with ulcerative colitis. J Nerv Ment Dis 1930;72:617–27.
2. Engel GL. Studies of ulcerative colitis. 2. The nature of the somatic processes asnd the adequacy of psychosomatic hypotheses. Am J Med 1954;16:416–33.
3. North CS, Clouse RE, Spitznagel EL, Alpers DH. The relation of ulcerative colitis to psychiatric factors: a review of findings and methods. Am J Psychiatry 1990;147:974–81.

4. Moser G, Maeir-Dobersberger T, Vogelsang H, Lochs H. Inflammatory bowel disease: patients' beliefs about the etiology of their disease – a controlled study. Psychosom Med 1993;55:131.

5. Chrousos GP, Gold PW. The concepts of stress and stress system disorders. Overview of physical and behavioral homeostasis. J Am Med Assoc 1992;267:1244–52.

6. Collins SM, McHugh K, Jacobson K *et al*. Previous inflammation alters the response of the rat colon to stress. Gastroenterology 1996;111:1509–15.

7. Maunder RG, Esplen MJ. Facilitating adjustment to inflammatory bowel disease: a model of psychosocial intervention in non-psychiatric patients. Psychother Psychosom 1999;68:230–40.

8. Shaw L, Ehrlich A. Relaxation training as a treatment for chronic pain caused by ulcerative colitis. Pain 1987;29:287–93.

9. Freyberger H, Müller-Wielaud K. Combined internal and psychosomatic therapy in colitis ulcerosa. Med Klin 1966;61:228.

10. Milne B, Joachim G, Niedhardt J. A stress management programme for inflammatory bowel disease patients. J Adv Nurs 1986;11:561–7.

11. Schwarz SP, Blanchard EB. Evaluation of a psychological treatment for inflammatory bowel disease. Behav Res Ther 1991;29:167–77.

12. Drossman DA. Psychosocial factors in ulcerative colitis and Crohn's disease. In: Kirsner JB, Shorter RG, editors. Inflammatory Bowel Disease. Baltimore; MD: Williams & Wilkins; 1995:492–513.

13. Maunder R, Toner B, de Rooy E, Moscovitz D. The influence of gender and disease on illness-related concerns in inflammatory bowel disease. Can J Gastroenterol 1999;13:728–32.

14. Maunder RG, de Rooy E, Toner B *et al*. Health-related concerns of people who receive psychological support for inflammatory bowel disease. Can J Gastroenterol 1997;11:681–5.

15. Yang H, Rotter JI. Genetic aspects of idiopathic inflammatory bowel disease. In: Kirsner JB, Shorter RG, editors. Inflammatory Bowel Disease. Baltimore, MD: Williams & Wilkins; 1995:301–31.

16. Luecken LJ. Childhood attachment and loss experiences affect adult cardiovascular and cortisol function. Psychosom Med 1998;60:765–72.

17. Ottaway CA, Stanisz AM. Neural–immune interactions in the intestine: implications for inflammatory bowel disease. In: Kirsner JB, Shorter RG, editors. Inflammatory Bowel Disease. Baltimore, MD: Williams & Wilkins; 1995:281–300.

18. Kramer MS, Cutler N, Feighner J *et al*. Distinct mechanism for antidepressant activity by blockade of central substance P receptors. Science 1998;281:1640–5.

19. De Felipe C, Herrero JF, O'Brien JA *et al*. Altered nociception, analgesia and aggression in mice lacking the receptor for substance P. Nature 1998;392:394–7.

20. The Psychobiology of Attachment and Separation. Reite M, Field T, editors. Behavioral Biology. 1985. Orlando, FL: Academic Press.

21. Wood JD, Peck OC, Tefend KS *et al*. Colitis and colon cancer in cotton-top tamarins (*Saguinus oedipus oedipus*) living wild in their natural habitat. Dig Dis Sci 1998;43:1443–53.

22. Fedorak RN. Naturally occurring and experimental models of inflammatory bowel disease. In: Kirsner JB, Shorter RG, editors. Inflammatory Bowel Disease. Baltimore, MD: Williams & Wilkins; 1995:71–95.

23. Targan SR, Landers CJ, King NW, Podolsky DJ, Shanahan F. Ulcerative colitis-linked antineutrophil cytoplasmic antibody in the cotton-top tamarin model of colitis. Gastroenterology 1992;102:1493–8.

24. Maunder R, Lancee WJ, Greenberg GR, Hunter JJ. Avoidant insecurity and later age of ulcerative colitis onset in a subgroup without ANCA antibodies. Gastroenterology 1999;116:A772.

25. West ML, Sheldon-Kellor AE. Patterns of Relating: an Adult Attachment Perspective. New York: Guilford Press; 1994.

26. Mickelson KD, Kessler RC, Shaver PR. Adult attachment in a nationally representative sample. J Pers Soc Psychol 1997;73:1092–106.

27. Klohnen EC, John OP. Working models of attachment: a theory-based prototype approach. In: Simpson JA, Rholes WS, editors. Attachment Theory and Close Relationships. New York: Guilford; 1998;115–40.

28. Goldberg S, Gotowiec A, Simmons RJ. Infant–mother attachment and behavior problems in healthy and chronically ill preschoolers. Devel Psychopathol 1995;7:267–82.

29. Marvin RS, Pianta RC. Mother's reaction to their child's diagnosis: relations with security of attachment. J Clin Child Psychol 1996;25:436–45.
30. Mrazek DA, Casey B, Anderson I. Insecure attachment in severely asthmatic preschool children: Is it a risk factor? J Am Acad Child Adolesc Psychiatry 1987;26:516–20.
31. Goldberg S, Simmons RJ, Newman J, Campbell K, Fowler RS. Congenital heart disease, parental stress and infant–mother relationships. J Pediatr 1991;119:661–6.
32. Kotler T, Buzwell S, Romeo Y, Bowland J. Avoidant attachment as a risk factor for health. Br J Med Psychol 1994;67:237–45.
33. Ciechanowski P, Katon W, Hirsch I. Attachment style and adherence in the diabetic patient. Psychosom Med 1999;61:110.
34. Spiegel D, Bloom JR, Yalom I. Group support for patients with metastatic breast cancer. Arch Gen Psychiatry 1981;38:527–33.
35. Irvine EJ, Feagan B, Rochon J *et al*. Quality of life: a valid and reliable measure of therapeutic efficacy in the treatment of inflammatory bowel disease. Canadian Crohn's Relapse Prevention Trial Study Group. Gastroenterology 1994;106:287–96.
36. Maunder RG, Moskovitz DN, Cohen Z, McLeod RS, MacRae H. Escape-avoidance, self-control and accepting responsibility are negatively associated with quality of life outcome of surgery for IBD. Gastroenterology 1999;116:A772.

19
The use of complementary and alternative medicine by patients with inflammatory bowel disease

R. J. HILSDEN AND M. J. VERHOEF

ABSTRACT

Given the worldwide increase in the use of complementary and alternative medicine (CAM), it is not surprising that patients with inflammatory bowel disease (IBD) commonly use these therapies. Studies have shown that one-third to one-half of patients are currently using or have used CAM, depending on the time interval examined and the therapies considered in the study. Patients often use multiple therapies concurrently and usually use them in conjunction with, rather than in place of, conventional medicine. Therapies used by patients depend on what is locally available to them, but often include vitamin and mineral supplements, herbal products (*Aloe vera*, slippery elm, cat's claw) and dietary manipulations. In some parts of the world patients may be more likely to use homeopathy or traditional Chinese medicine.

Patients with IBD often turn to CAM when they find conventional medicines fail them, either by being ineffective or causing unacceptable side-effects. Patients may also use CAM if they hold health beliefs that are more in keeping with the principles of CAM (holism, naturalism, and spiritualism) rather than those of conventional medicine.

The World Wide Web is now an important supplement to other common information sources about CAM available to patients. Although access to information may be improved, valid concerns exist about the accuracy and completeness of the available information, especially in terms of safety and efficacy. Physicians are especially concerned by the lack of well-conducted scientific studies. Many patients also recognize these concerns, but are unwilling to discuss CAM with their physicians. In our study 38% did not disclose their CAM use, often because they viewed their physician as being either uninformed or intolerant.

Patients are increasingly taking a more active role in health-care decision-making and may seek out and use CAM even if their physician advises against it. However, it is important for physicians to discuss the use of CAM with their patients. First, a patient's desire to use CAM may indicate dissatisfaction with current medical care, which may be remediable. Second, unless the physician is aware of CAM use, any effects, either good or bad, resulting from them may be falsely attributed to the conventional medicine. Third, the patient's desire to use a specific CAM may result from overly optimistic representations of its benefits and safety. Therefore, physicians caring for patients with IBD should be able to provide knowledgeable and non-judgemental counselling about CAM to their patients.

INTRODUCTION

The use of complementary and alternative medicine (CAM) is common among the general population, especially among those with chronic disease[1–3]. Therefore, it is not surprising that patients with inflammatory bowel disease (IBD) also commonly use CAM[4]. This chapter will address several key questions about IBD patients' use of CAM, describing what is known and indicating areas where further work is required.

WHAT IS CAM?

One of the common difficulties in conducting studies on CAM is defining what it is and what practices it encompasses. Other terms that have been used include unconventional medicine, unorthodox medicine, unproven therapies, quackery, folk medicine, holistic medicine and alternative medicine. We have chosen to use the term CAM for several reasons. First, it is purely descriptive rather than implying any form of judgement about the therapies. Second, it does not suggest what types of therapies should or should not be included. Finally, it is the term adopted by the National Institutes of Health for the National Center for Complementary and Alternative Medicine (NCCAM).

Different definitions have been proposed of what CAM is. Eisenberg's definition is commonly used; it defines CAM as 'medical interventions not taught widely at U.S. medical schools or generally available at U.S. hospitals'[1]. The problem with this and many other definitions is that it is 'U.S.-centric' and that it defines CAM by what it is not, rather than by what it is. The very diversity of practices and beliefs encompassed by CAM makes creating a uniform, clear and specific definition difficult. CAM includes alternative medical systems (homeopathy, acupuncture, Ayurveda), products derived from nature (phytotherapy), orthomolecular medicine (high-dose vitamin C, coenzyme Q10), pharmacological interventions (antineoplastons), manipulative practices (chiropractic, craniosacral therapy) and procedures and devices (bioresonance). For some practices–such as prayer, diet changes, and exercise – it can be difficult to determine whether they should be considered lifestyle choices or CAM.

Table 1 Forms of CAM by patients with IBD (%).

	Calgary, Canada[4]	Winnipeg, Canada[3]	Los Angeles, USA[3]	Cork[3]	Sweden[3]	Austria[6]
Time period	Current use	Ever used	Ever used	Ever used	Ever used	Ever used
Overall	33	57	68	31	32	46.6
Homeopathy	3	5	8	5	7	45
Acupuncture	1	3	12	5	7	8
Massage/relaxation	7/NI	16/18	15/12	5/3	2/2	6
Chiropractic	7	15	15	5	7	NI
Herbal therapies	13	5	8	5	0	NI
Special diets	5	NI	NI	NI	NI	39
Exercise	NI	30	41	3	21	NI
Prayer	NI	20	25	17	2	NI

NI: Not included.

HOW COMMON IS CAM USE IN IBD?

There is growing evidence that the use of CAM is very common by patients with IBD (Table 1). In general these studies tell us about patients attending specialty gastrointestinal clinics and, therefore, their findings may not be generalizable to all patients. Patients attending gastrointestinal clinics are probably sicker and more comfortable within a Western medical framework than patients not attending these clinics. These studies are also difficult to compare because they have used different definitions of what constitutes CAM, and have examined use over different time periods. However, it appears that approximately one-half of patients have tried CAM and one-third are currently using it. Because these studies have examined clinic patients, it is very difficult to determine what proportion of patients have abandoned Western medicine for CAM, but it is probably quite small[1,5].

WHY DO PATIENTS TURN TO CAM?

Understanding health behaviours is complicated by the vast array of factors that influence them, including the patient's health beliefs, culture, previous experiences, knowledge and preferences. When considering patients with IBD, we are especially interested in whether there are particular aspects of the disease or its treatment that lead them to use CAM. If we could identify a common factor, such as dissatisfaction with conventional treatment, it could indicate an area where gastroenterologists could endeavour to alter or improve patient care. It is also important to recognize that patients may use CAM not only for their IBD but also for other medical problems, or for general disease prevention and health promotion. We found that one-half of the 33% of Calgary IBD patients currently using CAM were using it for their IBD[4], although patients do not always make a clear distinction.

We found that the most common reasons cited by patients for turning to CAM were either the lack of effect or the side-effects of conventional medical treatments[4]. Consistent with this was the finding that longer duration of disease and prior history of intravenous steroid use and surgery was associated with the use of CAM. Moser *et al.*, in their study of patients in Austria, also found that duration of disease was longer in CAM users[6]. Rawsthorne *et al.*, in a multicentre study, found users were characterized by being dissatisfied with conventional medicine, although these workers did not find an association with duration of disease. In our study we conducted several in-depth interviews with CAM users and, in these, the importance of the side-effects of conventional therapies in a patient's decision to use CAM was even more strongly emphasized. For example one participant said, 'It got to the point where I couldn't really handle the side effects, they're brutal. So that's why I kind of looked for complementary medicines.'[4]

Moser *et al.* determined that CAM users were more concerned about feeling out of control, being treated as different and having surgery than did non-users[6]. In our interviews with patients the importance of feeling in control of their health and treatment was also a common theme. Therefore, it appears that the use of CAM is one way in which patients try to assume an active and controlling role in their health care rather than playing a passive role as encouraged by Western medicine.

Factors such as gender, age and disease diagnosis have not been associated with CAM use in several studies of IBD patients[3,4,6]. The influence of health beliefs has not been adequately addressed because of the limited patient populations studied.

WHAT FORMS OF CAM DO IBD PATIENTS COMMONLY USE?

Table 1 shows the most commonly reported therapies from three surveys. Not surprisingly, common therapies vary between different sites, probably reflecting what is locally available and cultural preferences and which therapies were included in the questionnaire. Commonly used herbal therapies include ginseng, cat's claw, slippery elm and *Aloe vera*[4]. Differences between studies will also be affected by what was included in the questionnaire. One of the most important and consistent findings is that many patients use multiple therapies concurrently. For example, 63% of Calgary IBD patients were using more than one type and 22% were using four or more therapies[4].

DO PATIENTS DISCUSS CAM USE WITH THEIR PHYSICIANS?

Nearly all articles about CAM recommend that physicians must be able to counsel patients about CAM use. However, for this to occur, patients first must be willing to disclose and discuss CAM use with their doctor. We found that only 62% of patients reported telling their doctor about their CAM use. During patient interviews, two factors explaining patients' reluctance to disclose this emerged. First was the belief that the physician would reject out of hand the use of CAM. The second was that patients viewed their physicians as uninformed about CAM and that therefore there would be no value in discussing it with them. As one patient said when asked whether she had discussed CAM use with her doctors, 'No, I don't think they really know that much about it and I don't really see the point. I don't think they would really be that interested.'[4] This is unfortunate because we have found that patients with IBD rated information about CAM as one of their greatest information needs[7]. Patients have increasing access to information about CAM, but much of this is generated by CAM providers and often provides an uncritical and overly optimistic opinion of a treatment's benefits and safety.

HOW EFFECTIVE AND SAFE IS CAM?

There are insufficient data on the efficacy and safety of the various forms of CAM. There are very few well-conducted, scientifically valid studies. Most of the evidence supporting the benefits of CAM is in the form of testimonials and case series, where the risk of bias is high. Physicians may also have trouble obtaining useful information on CAM because much of it is published in journals they may not be familiar with, that are not written in English or that are not included in common indices, such as Medline.

At the present time there is no strong evidence supporting any form of CAM for the treatment of IBD, although several therapies have shown some promise in randomized controlled trials or large cases series or when tested in animal models[8–10]. In two surveys we have conducted we have asked patients to rate their satisfaction with CAM for their IBD on a five-point scale, with 1 being not at all satisfied and 5 being very satisfied. Only 32% and 41% of patients rated their satisfaction as at least a 4[4,11]. Therefore, despite the common use of CAM, overall satisfaction with it for the treatment of IBD is not high. Consistent with this is our observation that IBD patients frequently change from one therapy to another.

Patients could potentially be harmed through the use of CAM in several ways. First, patients could suffer an adverse event directly related to the therapy. Second, delaying the use of an effective medical intervention could harm patients. Third, patients could experience 'financial harm' because of the costs associated with CAM. And fourth, patients could suffer from an interaction between their conventional medicines and a complementary one. In general, the risk of suffering a direct adverse event from the therapies commonly reported by IBD patients is probably low. We are unaware of any reported adverse effect due to CAM in a patient with IBD. However, patients should be aware about the possibility of adulterated herbal preparations, the risk of serious nutritional deficiencies with rigid and restrictive diets, and the special concern about pregnant women using any potentially pharmacologically active substance.

Because IBD is a chronic and rarely life-threatening condition, modest delays in seeking medical attention are unlikely to result in serious harm, except in the case of severe, fulminant disease. Several drug–CAM interactions are well documented[12,13]. For example, cat's claw is said to potentiate the effects of antihypertensive medications and anticoagulants[13]. Unfortunately, many books on CAM directed at the public do not alert the patient to this possibility. There is essentially no good information readily available on the potential for CAM interactions with the potent immunosuppressants that many IBD patients use.

HOW TO COUNSEL PATIENTS ABOUT CAM USE

All physicians should read Dr David Eisenberg's excellent article on advising patients who seek CAM[14]. We believe that it is important for the physician to ask IBD patients about CAM use not only because of potential safety concerns but because the patient's use of CAM may indicate some dissatisfaction with conventional treatment that could be corrected. Because patients are reluctant to disclose their CAM use with their doctors, it is critical that the physicians ask their patients. However, this must be done in a non-judgemental fashion, to facilitate disclosure. In patients who are using or who are interested in using CAM, the next step should be to explore the patient's perception of what is good and bad about the form of CAM he/she is interested in, and what, if anything, about their conventional treatment is leading that person to consider CAM.

For a physician to effectively advise and inform a patient about CAM, knowledge of the different forms of CAM is required. However, given the diversity of practices and therapies, it is not possible for a typical physician to be familiar with all types. There are several useful references on CAM that provide detailed descriptions of therapies including what is known (and not known) about their efficacy and safety[13,15,16]. Unfortunately, because IBD is relatively uncommon, reference and lay books usually do not specifically address its treatment. Therefore, comprehensive reviews of therapies commonly used for IBD are required.

SUMMARY

In summary, patients with IBD commonly use complementary and alternative therapies. It is important for the physician to be aware of a patient's use of CAM and the nature, benefits and risks of commonly used therapies so that they can effectively counsel patients.

References

1. Eisenberg DM, Kessler RC, Foster C, Norlock FE, Calkins DR, Delbanco TL. Unconventional medicine in the United States. Prevalence, costs, and patterns of use. N Engl J Med 1993;328:246–52.
2. Astin JA. Why patients use alternative medicine – results of a national study. J Am Med Assoc 1998;279:1548–53.
3. Rawsthorne P, Shanahan F, Cronin NC et al. An international survey of the use and attitudes regarding alternative medicine by patients with inflammatory bowel disease. Am J Gastroenterol 1999;94:1298–303.
4. Hilsden RJ, Scott CM, Verhoef MJ. Complementary medicine use by patients with inflammatory bowel disease. Am J Gastroenterol 1998;93:697–701.
5. Druss BG, Rosenheck RA. Association between use of unconventional therapies and conventional medical services. J Am Med Assoc 1999;282:651–6.

6. Moser G, Tillinger W, Sachs G *et al*. Relationship between the use of unconventional therapies and disease-related concerns: a study of patients with inflammatory bowel disease. J Psychosom Res 1996;40:503–9.

7. Hilsden RJ, Dunn C, Patten S, Scott CM, Verhoef MJ. Information needs and seeking behaviors of patients with inflammatory bowel disease. Gastroenterology 1998;114:A995 (abstract).

8. Hilsden RJ, Verhoef MJ. Complementary and alternative medicine: evaluating its effectiveness in inflammatory bowel disease. Inflam Bowel Dis 1998;4:318–23.

9. Carty E, Ballinger A, Azooz O, Feakins RM, Rampton DS. Does topical *Aloe vera* reduce the severity of trinitrobenzene sulphonic acid (TNBS) colitis in rats? Gastroenterology 1998;114:A948 (abstract).

10. Sadoval M, Mannick EE, Mishra J, Sadowska-Krowicka H, Clark DA, Miller MJS. Cat's claw (*Uncaria tomentosa*) protects against oxidative stress and indomethacin-induced intestinal inflammation. Gastroenterology 1997;112:A1081 (abstract).

11. Hilsden RJ, Meddings JB, Verhoef MJ. Complementary and alternative medicine use by patients with inflammatory bowel disease: an internet survey. Can J Gastroenterol 1999; 13:327–32.

12. Crone CC, Wise TN. Use of herbal medicines among consultation–liaison populations. Psychosomatics 1998;39:3–13.

13. Fetrow CW, Avila JR. Professional's Handbook of Complementary and Alternative Medicine. Springhouse: Springhouse Corporation, 1999.

14. Eisenberg DM. Advising patients who seek alternative medical therapies. Ann Intern Med 1997;127:61–9.

15. Bettschart R, Glaeske G, Langbein K, Saller R, Skalnik C. The Complete Book of Symptoms and Treatments. Boston MA: Element Books; 1998.

16. Peirce A. The American Pharmaceutical Association Practical Guide to Natural Medicines. New York: William Morrow; 1999.

20
Gut inflammation: is there a role for herbal medicines?

M. J. S. MILLER

ABSTRACT

There is increasing interest in the role of herbal medicine as a complementary approach to therapeutics, including the treatment of gut inflammation. In the developing world this is born of fiscal necessity as Western medicines are beyond the financial reach of the populace. In the developed world there has been a renewed interest in traditional forms of medicine. However, it is often unclear as to how these herbal medicines work. Recently, we have directed our research in a manner that bridges the information gap. The goals are to provide the basic data as to how and when herbal medicines work.

By way of example, three herbal medicines will be discussed: genistein, an example of a soy-derived phyto-oestrogen isoflavone, and two South American herbs – cat's claw (*Uncaria tomentosa*) and Sangre de grado (*Croton lechleri*). Administration of genistein (0.1 mg/kg, subcutaneously) resulted in a mild reduction in guinea pig ileitis induced by the hapten trinitrobenzenesulphonic acid (TNBS). This anti-inflammatory response was associated with a reduction in granulocyte infiltration, nitrite production and nitrotyrosine formation; effects which were lost, paradoxically, with increasing doses. Inhibition of nitric oxide (NO) production in cultured macrophages, by genistein, was supportive of its proposed action as an inhibitor of signal transduction through protein kinase inhibition. Cat's claw is a vine, from the bark of which a tea is made. Ethnomedically, cat's claw is used for the treatment of arthritis and gut inflammation. We found that cat's claw was an effective inhibitor of transcription by preventing the activation of the transcription factor, NF-κB. Inhibition of gene expression was confirmed *in vitro* and *in vivo*, in models of non-steroidal anti-inflammatory drug (NSAID)-induced gastritis and enteropathy. In gastritis, cat's claw negated the induction of apoptosis and the expression of tumour necrosis factor-α (TNF-α) by epithelia. In enteropathy, cat's claw restored small intestinal morphology and greatly reduced the mucosal inflammation. Sangre de grado, an Amazonian tree sap, was evaluated in a model of gastric ulceration and in Ussing chambers for its antisecretory actions. Sangre de grado, diluted (1:1000 to 1:10 000) in the drinking water, promoted the healing of gastric ulcers, reduced the expression of proinflammatory cytokines, and decreased ulcer colonization. Antisecretory effects were evident only against activation of sensory afferent activation (capsaicin); cholinergic responses were unaffected.

In conclusion, these studies highlight the potential of herbal medicines as therapeutic options for the treatment of gut inflammation. More research, particularly clinical investigations, is required to place these options into perspective.

INTRODUCTION

There is an increase in awareness and consumption of herbal medicines in the USA, and throughout the Western world. Complementary medicine has garnered the cover of *Time* magazine and the *Journal of the American Medical Association*, as well as attracting the major pharmaceutical companies' interests. Estimates vary, but it is likely that >30% of all patients seeking care from physicians are also taking some form of complementary medicine. 'Alternative medicine' is a term that is also coined but 'complementary medicine' is a more accurate description of its use and intent. This topic includes the use of acupuncture, aromatherapy, dietary supplements, holistic medicine as well as herbal medicine. However, for the purpose of this discussion we will concentrate on herbal medicines.

The major issues that health-care practitioners raise in regards to herbal medicines are: (1) safety and toxicity, (2) efficacy, (3) mechanisms of action, (4) drug interactions. Often it is difficult to translate the body of knowledge and experience with herbal medicines into a language and form that satisfies these concerns. Clearly, if Western health-care practitioners are to make informed and intelligent decisions as to how these herbal medicines are to be used, then there needs to be research focused on translating this information into a form that fosters accessible comparisons with standard pharmaceuticals. By way of example we will describe the effects of three different herbal medicines, in order to approach the questions of efficacy and mechanisms of action.

SAFETY AND TOXICITY

Without the benefit of the Federal Drug Admistration (FDA) approval process, and the lengthy clinical trials and data collection, most herbal medicines or dietary supplements do not possess the hard data to advocate their safety and acceptable toxicity. Does this mean that they are not safe, or that they are potentially harmful? In the vast majority of cases herbal medicines are remarkably safe. Deaths due to the intake of herbal medicines are remarkably low (16 in the USA last year); far below that noted with pharmaceuticals. In actuality the toxicity that is present is often due to inappropriate production or contaminants (heavy metals). Toxicity due to the medicinal substance itself is quite rare, and usually associated with excessive consumption, e.g. stimulants. By comparison the new COX-2 inhibitors have been associated with lethality due to gastrointestinal complications within the first months on the market.

The dietary supplement industry is aware that improvements need to be made in assuring the public that the products are free of contaminants, but we must be cautious and place such events in their proper perspective. The public appreciates that herbal medicines have a better safety record than pharmaceuticals, despite the inability to produce FDA-style data to affirm this conclusion. The combination of chemicals present in a natural medicine are often touted as a means to reduce toxicity as well as improved efficacy, although direct proof of this concept is generally lacking.

EFFICACY AND MECHANISMS OF ACTION

Given that there is a clear lack of clinical trials comparing herbal medicines to pharmaceuticals it is often difficult to ascertain if the herbal medicines are efficacious. Generally, we regard herbal medicines as having mild effects; perhaps better suited to the maintenance of disease remission or a healthy lifestyle than to treat a major, debilitating condition such as inflammatory bowel disease (IBD). Certainly the apparent reduction in toxicity is compatible with a mild action. What, then, is the role of herbal medicines in gut inflammation?

Examples may be the best way to address this issue. In our research we have tried to address the issue of efficacy in animal models, and mechanisms of action *in vitro* as well as *in vivo*.

GENISTEIN

Genistein is a phyto-oestrogen, isoflavone, that is commonly derived from soy. Thus, it can either be obtained as a dietary source or purchased in capsule form. Pharmacologically, genistein is used as an inhibitor of tyrosine kinase activity, affecting signal transduction[1]. We examined its ability to modify gut inflammation in the guinea pig TNBS ileitis model of IBD. Genistein was an effective suppressor of gut inflammation but it possessed an unusual dose–response curve, in that efficacy was reduced with increasing doses[2]. We have seen this pattern with other anti-inflammatory therapies, e.g. interleukin 10 (IL-10)[3]. Concomitant with genistein's *in vivo* anti-inflammatory actions was a reduction in nitrite levels in the ileal lumen, with the same dose–response pattern. As nitrite levels reflect the expression of inducible NO synthase expression, this reduction in NO synthesis was indicative of an action of genistein at the transcriptional level. *In vitro*, genistein was also able to protect macrophages from apoptosis following activation by lipopolysaccharide (LPS). This may be through a shared mechanism or additional pathways. We do not often think of dietary factors regulating gene expression and thereby disease, but it is a possibility that we should entertain more often. Usually, dietary factors influencing gut inflammation are evaluated in terms of their antigenic potential rather than inherent biological actions. Whether dietary factors such as soy-derived genistein plays a role in the reduced incidence of IBD in Asians remains to be determined, but cultural differences certainly extend beyond genetics.

CAT'S CLAW

Cat's claw, or *Uña de gato*, is a vine indigenous to the rainforests of South America. Ethnomedically it is taken in the form of a tea, which is made from its bark. Cat's claw, whose name is derived by the characteristic claw-like interpetiolar stipule, is used in chronic inflammation, e.g. arthritis, gastritis and colitis. Despite it being the most widely used South American herbal medicine in the Western world (after cocaine), its mechanism of action has remained elusive until recently.

We administered cat's claw in a form consistent with its ethnomedical use, as a tea in the drinking water, to rats with indomethacin-induced enteropathy. This model mimics the intestinal damage induced by NSAIDs and has strong similarities to IBD. Bile and bacterial proliferation are key components of mucosal injury. At concentrations consistent with traditional consumption (10 mg bark/ml water) this tea almost completely suppressed intestinal injury in this model, and prevented the hepatic expression of metallothionein, an antioxidant acute-phase protein[4]. In indomethacin-induced acute gastritis cat's claw was also effective, but only when given as a pretreatment[5]. In gastritis, cat's claw prevented the induction of epithelial apoptosis and the expression of TNF-α. Further evidence that cat's claw works by preventing the expression of proinflammatory genes was obtained in cultured macrophages, using inducible NO synthase as the prototypical gene. Suppression of gene expression by cat's claw was due to its ability to prevent the activation of the transcription factor NF-κB by LPS. NF-κB has been a highly sought after therapeutic target by the pharmaceutical industry, whether it be by pharmacological means or antisense technology[6]. While these data with cat's claw offer proof of concept for the choice of NF-κB suppression as a therapeutic approach, it is interesting to note that it was achieved with a simple aqueous extraction of the bark from a vine from the rainforest. This is not drug discovery based on random screening. This herbal medicine has been used for this specific purpose for centuries; all we have done is perform studies to confirm that it is effective and by what means it achieves benefit. In that regard our research is more of a translation of knowledge than a true discovery.

In the USA cat's claw is often sold in a form that is standardized for oxindole alkaloids, the proposed active components[7]; however, oxindole alkaloids possess proinflammatory properties as opposed to anti-inflammatory characteristics of the whole herb. Specifically, oxindole and pentacyclic alkaloids stimulate phagocytosis[8] and IL-6 production in alveolar macrophages[9]. The misinterpretation that oxindole alkaloids are the active chemicals of cat's claw arose from a series of patents initiated by a journalist, and were without regard for the medicinal applications. Thus, cat's claw has been mislabelled as an immunostimulatory herbal medicine, whereas our data clearly show that it is anti-inflammatory and returns elevated cytokine levels to homeostasis by a suppression of transcription. This highlights the type of problems that exist in the herbal medicine field and the potential for mass confusion.

SANGRE DE GRADO

Sangre de grado is a viscous, red tree sap that is derived from various *Croton* species indigenous to the Amazon River basin[10]. Ethnomedically it is used topically for the treatment of cuts, wounds, insect bites/stings, plant reactions and burns. Sangre de grado is also taken orally, in highly dilute form, for serious gastrointestinal distress, including ulcers and diarrhoea[11]. Sangre de grado is an antibacterial agent (bactericidal and bacteriostatic), although its efficacy diminishes greatly with dilution[12,13]. An extract has been in Phase III trials for the treatment of diarrhoea associated with HIV infection (SP-303, Shaman Pharmaceuticals). We have evaluated the ulcer-healing properties of sangre de grado using an acetic acid model whose repair is known to be dependent on the number and form of bacteria present in the ulcer bed[14].

We found that sangre de grado at dilutions as great as 1:10 000 resulted in gastric ulcer healing, diminished bacterial content in the ulcer bed, and reduced inflammation (myeloperoxidase activity). Concomitant with the anti-inflammatory effects of sangre de grado was a diminished gene expression of proinflammatory mediators or enzymes, e.g., IL-1, IL-6, TNF-α, iNOS and COX-2. Expression of COX-1 was unaltered by gastric ulceration and not affected by sange de grado. The anti-inflammatory effects may be mediated by the antibacterial actions of sangre de grado but other factors are also likely to be involved, as antibiotic treatment alone did not reduce myeloperoxidase activity in the ulcer[14].

The apparent anti-diarrhoeal actions of sangre de grado are not well known but result from an action on sensory afferents. Unpublished data in Ussing chambers using rat colon suggest that cholinergic responses are unaffected. However, vasodilation of rat mesenteric arteries in response to calcitonin gene-related peptide (CGRP) was attenuated by sangre de grado. Similarly in rat paw oedema studies sangre de grado driven by sensory afferents and CGRP was greatly attenuated by dilute sangre de grado (unpublished data). Thus it is likely that the anti-diarrhoeal actions of sangre de grado are due to its ability to modify sensory afferent mechanisms, particularly those involving CGRP. While it is unclear if herbal medicines have any role in the treatment of gut inflammation in the Western world, it remains intriguing that it may have utility for patients with resistant strains of *Helicobacter pylori*. In addition, sangre de grado may offer some relief to IBD patients with copious diarrhoea, similar to the trials for AIDS. In the developing world, where pharmaceuticals are beyond the financial means of the general population, herbal medicines such as sangre de grado are the only means of controlling disorders and disease.

SUMMARY

Lack of information and poor science plagues the herbal medicine field. The data that have been published are often subject to profound over-interpretation. Published studies in the herbal medicine field are often regarded to be gospel, in contrast to the traditional conservative approach given to pharmaceuticals, which requires procedures of re-evaluation, challenge and confirmation. Consequently, the herbal medicinal information is often conflicting, murky and misinterpreted. For example, cat's claw is one of several herbal medicines that the Federal Trade Commission has targeted for excessive claims by overzealous retailers and manufacturers. Clearly poor science and inappropriate claims harm the industry and its credibility, and serve to cause confusion among the public and health-care providers.

This scenario can compromise the use and trust of credible herbal medicines. The use of cat's claw has declined in recent years, partly as a result of this problem. Nevertheless, we contend that cat's claw is indeed an excellent anti-inflammatory agent with utility in gut inflammation, and a strong candidate as an adjunct therapeutic agent in IBD. The mechanism of action supports that contention. However, clearly more data and strong science are required to provide a foundation of information. It is from this base that the public and physicians can make an informed and intelligent decision as to the potential utility of herbal medicines in the management of disorders or disease processes. It is highly likely that the use of herbal medicines will continue to increase. Now is not the time to ignore this component of health-care delivery. Rather, here is an opportunity to evaluate the possibilities and potential of such herbal medicines, and where appropriate advocate their use in an informed setting.

References

1. Dong Z, Qi X, Xie K, Fidler IJ. Protein tyrosine kinase inhibitors decrease induction of nitric oxide synthase activity in lipopolysaccharide-responsive and lipopolysaccharide-nonresponsive murine macrophages. J Immunol 1995;151:2717–24.
2. Sadowska-Krowicka H, Mannick EE, Oliver PD *et al*. Genistein and gut inflammation: role of nitric oxide. Proc Soc Exp Biol Med 1998;217:351–57.
3. Ribbons KA, Thompson JH, Liu X, Pennline K, Clark DA, Miller MJS. Anti-inflammatory properties of interleukin-10 administration in TNBS-induced colitis. Eur J Pharmacol 1997;323:245–54.
4. Sandoval-Chacon M, Thompson JH, Liu X *et al*. Anti-inflammatory actions of cat's claw: the role of NF-κB. Aliment Pharmacol Ther 1998;12:1279–89.
5. Miller MJS, Zhang X-J, Lao X-J, Trentacosti AM, Sandoval M. Cat's claw attenuates the expression of TNFα, apoptosis and gastric injury caused by acute indomethacin administration. (Submitted).
6. Abraham E. Alterations in transcriptional regulation of proinflammatory and immunoregulatory cytokine expression by hemorrhage, injury, and critical illness. New Horizons 1996;4:184–93.
7. Keplinger K, Laus G, Wurm M, Dierich MP, Teppner H. *Uncaria tomentosa* (Willd.) DC. – ethnomedical use and new pharmacological, toxicological and botanical results. J Ethnopharmacol 1999;64:23–34.
8. Keplinger K, Wagner H, Kreutzkamp B. Oxindole alkaloids having properties stimulating the immunologic system and preparation containing the same. United States Patent No. 4,844,901, 4 July 1989.
9. Lemaire I, Assinewe V, Cano P, Awang DVC, Arnason JT. Stimulation of interleukin-1 and -6 production by the neotropical liana, *Uncaria tomentosa* (una de gato). J Ethnopharmacol 1999;64:109–15.
10. Duke J, Vasquez R. Amazonian Ethnobotanical Dictionary. Boca Raton, FL: CRC Press; 1994.
11. Schultes RE, Raffauf The Healing Forest. Medicinal and Toxic Plants of the Northwest Amazonia, R.F. Portland, OR: Dioscorides Press; 1990.
12. Phillipson JD. A matter of some sensitivity. Phytochemistry 1995;38:1319–43.
13. Chen ZP, Cai Y, Phillipson JD. Studies on the anti-tumour, anti-bacterial, and wound-healing properties of dragon's blood. Planta Med 1994;60:541–5.
14. Elliot SN, Buret A, McKnight W, Miller MJS, Wallace JL. Bacteria rapidly colonize and delay the healing of gastric ulcers in rats. Am J Physiol 1998;275:G425–32.

21
The role of nutrition in the treatment of inflammatory bowel disease

M. A. GASSULL

ABSTRACT

Nutritional management was seen as a possible therapeutic tool in imflammatory bowel disease (IBD) due to various clinical observations:

1. The fact that some foodstuffs may act as antigen-triggering symptoms, especially in Crohn's disease, which has prompted the use of exclusion diets. These have been shown to be of some use in a small percentage of patients. On the other hand, it has not been demonstrated that the reintroduction of the offending foods after a disease bout would induce disease relapse.
2. Nutritional deficiencies (macronutrients, micronutrients), frequent in these patients, may favour disease self-perpetuation, because of impairment of tissue repair and intestinal mucosal barrier, defective defence against free-radical damage and lipid peroxidation, as well as potential increase in mucosal dysplasia (folate). Although theoretically possible, there are no clinical trials showing the potential benefit of supplementing these patients with antioxidant micronutrients, either in inducing remission or in preventing relapse of the disease. However, this aspect merits proper investigation.
3. Some common severe long-term complications, such as growth and sexual development failure (children and adolescents) and osteopenia (children and adults) are not only related to the disease itself or its treatment (steroids), but also strongly linked to the presence of malnutrition.
4. Nutritional habits of some communities have been associated with low incidence of ulcerative colitis (UC) and Crohn's disease (CD), suggesting that some components of these diets may favour a modulation of the inflammatory response. These have been postulated to be related to changes in lipid composition in the membranes of the immune-competent cells which, in turn, may influence eicosanoid and cytokine release.

5. The insufficient amount of products of colonic metabolism of unabsorbed carbohydrates (butyrate) or its defective oxidation by colonocytes, has been related to the pathogenesis of UC and pouchitis.
6. Enteral formula diets, used as a unique or partial daily nutrition source, have been used as primary therapy in CD as an alternative to steroids in an attempt to avoid its severe side-effects.

The nutritional approach to IBD treatment has a common target: to avoid the use of steroids or other immunosuppressive drugs, by influencing metabolic routes involved in the inflammatory response.

There is no evidence that either parenteral (TPN) or enteral (TEN) nutrition had any primary therapeutic effect on the outcome of patients with acute severe UC. However, these studies show that 'bowel rest' using TPN showed no advantage in the treatment of these patients. In addition, those acutely ill patients given TEN (no bowel rest) needing colectomy because of steroid unresponsiveness suffered significantly fewer complications related to surgery as compared to those who received TPN.

The nutritional approach to the maintenance treatment of UC has been highlighted in recent paper showing that the relapse rate of quiescent UC treated with soluble dietary fibre (*Plantago ovata* seeds) was not different from that of patients given 5-aminosalicylic acid (5-ASA). Patients on fibre produced more butyrate in the colon (as measured by stool analysis) than those on 5-ASA. These nutritional approaches to maintenance therapy of UC further support the role of butyrate in the pathogenesis of the disease.

Greatest interest in the nutritional approach in IBD has centred on the possibility of using chemically defined enteral formula diets as primary treatment in CD. The first approach was made with the concept that introducing amino acids (elemental diets), instead of intact proteins (polymeric diets) in the gut lumen would decrease the intestinal antigenic load, which in turn would diminish the chances of triggering or maintaining the abnormal or up-regulated inflammatory bowel response. Randomized controlled trials in steroid-dependent CD, although with small a number of patients, showed that elemental diets achieved a similar remission rate to corticosteroids. However, further studies have shown that some, but not all, polymeric diets, used as a unique treatment, can also induce remission in active CD. In a meta-analysis performed to ascertain the effectiveness of enteral nutrition as compared to steroids, steroid-induced remission was shown in 80% of cases whereas with enteral nutrition (including all type of diets) the figures were 60–65%.

However, these percentages are 2–3 times those of the placebo used in randomized controlled trials (20–30%). This means that the response rate may be related to the composition of the diet, to a specific subgroup of patients (age, sex, race), disease location, the severity of the attack, the possible effect of previous treatments, etc. Studies are being carried out to address these possibilities.

With the data in our hands, it can be said that enteral nutrition, as a unique treatment in CD, is especially effective in children and adolescents (a population that should be especially protected from steroid side-effects), in moderate first and subsequent attacks, and possibly as maintenance treatment in clinically inactive disease. In addition, enteral (or in some cases parenteral) nutrition should be used as adjuvant therapy to prevent or reverse nutritional deficiencies whatever primary treatment is used.

INTRODUCTION

Steroids are the most used and effective treatment in acute attacks of inflammatory bowel disease (IBD). When administered at the appropriate doses the rate of remission in these cases ranges from 60% to 80% in most series[1-5]. Because of their high efficiency and low price, steroids, in this situation, could be considered one of the best examples for cost-effectiveness in health management. However, steroids have many side-effects, some most apparent because of the aesthetic consequences on the individual[5,6]. Although the aesthetic side-effects tend to disappear when treatment is discontinued, steroids are not a well-accepted therapy, mainly by adolescents and youngsters with IBD, especially when they have already experienced this treatment once or twice. In addition steroids may produce very severe metabolic side-effects[7-10]; some of them influence the future life of patients, such as growth and sexual development retardation[11] and osteopenia. The latter may develop quite early (within a week) when therapeutic doses of steroids are administered and may be reversible if the treatment course is short (3–4 weeks). However, prolonged treatments, even when administered at low doses (such as 10 mg per day for 7 months or 5.6 mg per day for 1 year) produce an irreversible and important bone mass loss[12-22]. This is an important point to be taken into account when planning treatments in children, older people and also in adults, since they are in the most productive and enjoyable parts of their lives. Steroids may also be dangerous when administered to patients with undiagnosed abdominal abscess[5,23].

Because up to 50% of patients may develop steroid dependence[24], other treatments have been used or are being introduced to avoid steroid side-effects. However most of these treatments, mainly immunosupressors, also have potentially severe side-effects[25-35]. All these reasons prompted the search for new less aggressive treatments.

The rationale for using nutrition as therapy in IBD was:

1. The evidence of protein–energy malnutrition and the detection of vitamin, mineral and trace element deficiencies of mulfactorial origin in these patients[36-40]. These may influence disease outcome, especially in children in whom, in addition to steroids, nutritional deficiencies are involved in growth and sexual development retardation[9,11]. In adults steroids may increase the need for surgical treatment[36] or increase the rate of surgical complications[41].
2. Exclusion diets have been used as therapy in CD[42], although their usefulness has been challenged, since the reintroduction of the offending foods after a disease bout did not always induce disease relapse.
3. The lack of butyrate in the colon, or its defective oxidation by colonocytes, has been involved in the pathogenesis of UC and pouchitis[43-48]. Fermentable fibre (*Plantago ovata* seeds), a substrate for butyrate

production in the colon, has been as effective as 5-ASA in preventing relapse in quiescent UC[49].

4. Neither parenteral nor enteral nutrition, when used as adjuvant therapy to the steroid treatment, had any primary therapeutic effect on the outcome of patients with acute severe UC. However, those patients receiving enteral nutrition, when operated, had fewer surgically related complications than those on parenteral nutrition[41].

5. Studies carried out in Greenland Eskimos suggested that their nutritional habits were associated with a low incidence of UC and CD and other immune-based conditions. The idea is that some of the components of such diets, especially fat, may favour a modulation of the inflammatory response[50,51] through changes produced in the membranes of the immune-competent cells which, in turn, may influence, chemotaxis as well as eicosanoid, adhesion molecules and cytokine release[52–57]. *In-vitro* and *in-vivo*[52,58–60] studies support this hypothesis. Various trials have been performed to prove this hypothesis in patients with UC and CD, with different preparations of n-3 long-chain polyunsaturated fatty acids, in active or quiescent disease. Most of them[61–68], except one[69] showed negative results. Most of the published clinical trials have defects in the design (crossover), use of a potentially active placebo or a possibly not-well-absorbed n-3 PUFA preparation, or the groups studied are too heterogeneous. All these facts have made it impossible to obtain reliable information about the potential use of n-3-rich marine oils in the treatment of IBD.

6. The possibility of using chemically defined enteral formula diets as primary treatment in CD has been pursued in the past 20 years. The initial idea was that using amino acids (elemental diets), instead of intact proteins (polymeric diets) as a nitrogen source would decrease the intestinal antigenic load. This, in turn would diminish the chances of triggering or maintaining the abnormal or up-regulated inflammatory bowel response[70]. In addition it has been reported that elemental diets decrease intestinal permeability in CD[71] and diminish the excretion of proinflammatory cytokines in the stools in these patients[72].

Randomized controlled trials, although with a small number of patients, showed very consistently that most (not all) elemental diets achieved similar remission rates to that of corticosteroids, both in children and adults[70,73–88]. Studies have also shown that some, but not all, polymeric diets, when used as a unique treatment, can also induce remission in active CD[76,77,80,81,89–93].

The contradictory results in some of the published trials, in addition to the fact that most of them were carried out with a small sample of patients, prompted the performance of a meta-analysis to ascertain the effectiveness of enteral nutrition as compared to steroids[94]. It was shown that steroids induced remission in 80% of cases whereas this occurred in about 60% of patients treated with enteral nutrition (including all type of diets). However, the percentage of remission with the enteral diets is 2–3 times that obtained with placebo in early therapeutic trials in CD (20–30%). This strongly suggests that, at least in some groups of patients, enteral nutrition may be of primary therapeutic value.

The possibility that the amount and type of the fat source would account for the therapeutic effect of enteral nutrition in CD was first pointed out by Fernandez-Bañares *et al.* in 1994[95]. This hypothesis suggested that the fatty acids contained in the lipid source used, and the quantity administered in the formula diet, may produce changes in the composition of the membrane phospholipids of the immune-competent cells.

Middleton *et al.*[85], in 1995, performed a meta-analysis relating the remission rate and the composition of the formula diets used as primary treatment in patients with CD. They pointed out that the response rate obtained with enteral nutrition was inversely correlated with the amount of long-chain triglycerides present in the enteral formula.

More recently Hiwatashi[84], in Japan, also found that elemental diets with low fat content are associated with the highest remission rate when administered as a primary treatment in active CD. He hypothesized that, in addition to the low antigenic effect produced by the amino-acid mixture, the low fat content will reduce intestinal motility, thus favouring an 'effective bowel rest'.

Factors related to the characteristics of the patients or the disease, such as age, sex, race, disease location, severity of the attack, possible effect of previous treatments, etc., may define specific subgroups of patients that may respond to enteral nutrition. As many as 72–85% of children with active CD respond to elemental diets, especially those with small bowel and ileocolonic disease[96].

There are interesting data regarding the role of enteral nutrition as long-term maintenance treatment in CD. Hiwatashi[84], has reported retrospective data including 410 CD patients. Three-hundred and twenty-two received nocturnal elemental diets at home, as a complement of a diet with low-fat foods. The control group were patients receiving drugs (mainly sulphasalazine). Both the cumulative probability of remission and non-hospitalization at 3000 days were significantly higher in the home enteral nutrition group than in the group of patients treated with drugs. Similar results were reported by Koga *et al.*[97] using polymeric instead of elemental diets. Both reports stress the fact that the larger the amount of calories administered daily (between 1200 and 1600) to these patients the greater the possibility of maintaining remission.

Wilchanski *et al.*[96] reported that children with CD who continued with nocturnal supplementary enteral nutrition with an elemental or semi-elemental liquid diet, after resuming a normal diet, remained well longer than those who discontinued nocturnal supplements completely after achieving remission. In addition height velocity for growing was significantly greater in those children receiving supplementary nocturnal enteral nutrition than in those of the control group.

In summary, with all the objective data shown, it can be said:

1. Artificial nutrition does not influence disease outcome in UC, although enteral nutrition diminishes the rate of complications in those patients requiring colectomy.

2. Enteral nutrition, rather than steroids, should be the first treatment to be used in children and adolescents with CD since, in addition to the observed clinical, biological and endoscopic anti-inflammatory effect[98], this will prevent or minimize growth failure, sexual development delay and osteopenia. This regime should also be used in high–moderate attacks.

3. Enteral nutrition should be tried as first-choice treatment in mild and moderate attacks, to prevent the loss of bone mass in older patients and also in adult cases, since there is a strong possibility that they may have received various long-term treatments with glucocorticoids during their life.

4. This therapeutic approach is also a safe way of preventing complications due to steroids when there might be an undiagnosed abdominal abscess.

5. Enteral nutrition should be used as maintenance treatment in children. In this case, in addition to keeping the disease in remission, the regimen ensures that the child maintains or catches up on linear growth. In adults, nocturnal enteral nutrition as a complement of a low-fat diet, has also been shown to be a useful tool in maintaining disease remission.

The recommended type of diet to be used in these patients, according to the actual knowledge, would be elemental, oligopeptide or polymeric diets with low fat content. There is still insufficient data regarding the type of lipids to be used in such cases.

References

1. Truelove SC, Witts LJ. Cortisone and corticotrophin in ulcerative colitis. Br Med J 1959;1:387–94.
2. Truelove SC, Jewell DP. Intensive intravenous regimen for severe attacks of ulcerative colitis. Lancet 1974;1:1067–70.
3. Meyers S, Sachar DB, Goldberg JD, Janowitz HD. Corticotropin versus hydrocortisone in the intravenous treatment of ulcerative colitis. A prospective, randomized, double blind clinical trial. Gastroenterology 1983;85:351–7.
4. Margolin ML, Krumholz MP, Fochios SE, Korelitz BI. Clinical trials in ulcerative colitis. II: Historical view. Am J Gastroenterol 1988;83:227–43.
5. Malchow H, Eve K, Brandes JW *et al*. European Cooperative Crohn's Disease Study (ECCDS). Result of drug treatment. Gastroenterology 1984;86:249–66.
6. Lennard-Jones JE. Corticosteroids and immunosuppressive drugs. In: Agnostides AA, Hodgson HJF, Kirsner JB, editors. Inflammatory Bowel Disease. London: Chapman & Hall; 1991:275–86.
7. Spencer JA, Kirsner JB, Mlynaryk P, Reed P, Palmer WL. Immediate and prolonged therapeutic effects of corticotrophin and adrenal steroids in ulcerative colitis: observations in 340 cases for periods up to 10 years. Gastroenterology. 1962;42:113–28.
8. Sparsberg N, Kirsner JB. Long-term corticosteroid therapy for regional enteritis: an analysis of 58 courses in 54 patients. Am J Dig Dis 1966;1:865–80.
9. Winter HS. Special consideration in pediatric inflammatory bowel disease. In: Targan SR, Shanahan F, editors. Inflammatory Bowel Disease: from Bench to Bedside. Baltimore, MD: Williams & Wilkins; 1994:701–10.
10. Williams GH, Dluhy G. Disease of the adrenal cortex. In: Fauci AS, Brawnwald E, Isselbacher KJ, *et al*., editors. Harrison's Principles of Internal Medicine, 14th edn. New York: Mcgraw-Hill; 1998:2035–60.
11. Grifits AM, Nguyen P, Smith C, MacMillan H, Sherman PM. Growth and clinical course of children with Crohn's disease. Gut 1993;34:939–43.
12. Canalis E. Mechanisms of glucocorticoid action in bone implications to corticosteroid-induced osteoporosis. J Clin Endocrinol Metab 1996;81:3441–7.
13. Adinoff AD, Hollister R. Steroid-induced fractures and bone loss in patients with asthma. N Engl J Med 1983;309:265–8.

14. Schoon EJ, Wolffenbuttel BHR, Stockbrügger RW. Osteoporosis as a risk in inflammatory bowel disease. Drugs Today 1999;35 (Suppl. A):17–28.
15. Hodsman AB, Toogood JH, Jennings B et al. Differential effect of inhaled budesonide and oral prednisone in serum osteocalcin. J Clin Endocrinol Metabo. 1991;72:530–40.
16. Lo Cascio V, Bonicci E, Imbimbo B et al. Bone loss after glucocorticoid therapy. Calcif Tissue Int 1984;36:435–8.
17. Buckley LM, Leib ES, Caetularo KS et al. Calcium and vitamin D3 supplementation prevents bone loss in the spine secondary to low-dose corticosteroids in patients with rheumatoid arthritis. Ann Intern Med 1996;125: 961–8.
18. Valentine JF, Sninsky CA. Prevention and treatment of osteoporosis in patients with inflammatory bowel disease. Am J Gastroenterol 1999;94:878–83.
19. Gokhale R, Favus MJ, Karrison T, Sutton MM, Rich B, Kirschner B. Bone mineral density assessment in children with inflammatory bowel disease. Gastroenterology 1988;114:902–11.
20. Cowan FJ, Parker DR, Jenkins HR. Osteopenia in Crohn's disease. Gut. 1995;73:225–56.
21. Semeao EJ, Stallings VA, Peck SN, Picolli DA. Vertebral compression fractures in pediatric patients with Crohn's disease. Gastroenterology 1997;112:1710–13.
22. Vakil N, Sparberg M. Steroid-related osteonecrosis in inflammatory bowel disease. Gastroenterology 1989;96:62–7.
23. Andus T, Targan SR. Glucocorticoids. In: Targan SR, Shanahan F, editors. Inflammatory Bowel Disease: from Bench to Bedside. Baltimore, MD: Williams & Wilkins; 1994:487–502.
24. Munkholm P, Langholz E, Davidsen M, Binder V. Frequency of glucocorticoid resistance and dependency in Crohn's disease. Gut 1994;35:360–2.
25. Connell WR, Kamm MA, Ritchie JK, Lennard-Jones JE. Bone marrow toxicity caused by azathioprine in inflammatory bowel disease; 27 years of experience. Gut 1993;34:1081–5.
26. Carbonel F, Boruchowicz A, Duclos B et al. Intravenous cyclosporine in attacks of ulcerative colitis; short and long-term responses. Dig Dis Sci 1996;41:2471–6.
27. Stack WA, Long RG, Hawkey CJ. Short-and long-term outcome of patients treated with cyclosporin for severe acute ulcerative colitis. Aliment Pharmacol Ther 1998;12:973–8.
28. Stange EF, Modigliani R, Pena AS, Wood AJ, Feutren G, Smith PR and the European Group of Crohn's Disease. European trial of cyclosporine in chronic active Crohn's disease. Gastroenterology 1995;109:774–82.
29. Fernandez-Banares F, Bertran X, Esteve-Comas M, Cabre E, Menacho M, Gassull MA. Azathioprine is useful in the long-term maintaining remission induced by i.v. cyclosporin in severe steroid-refractory ulcerative colitis. Am J Gastroenterol 1996;91:2498–9.
30. West SG. Methotrexate hepatotoxicity. Rheum Dis Clin N Am 1997;23:883–915.
31. Cannon GW. Methotrexate pulmonary toxicity. Rheum Dis Clin N Am 1997;23:917–37.
32. McKendry RJ. The remarkable spectrum of methotrexate toxicities. Rheum Dis Clin N Am 1997;23:939–54.
33. Neurath MF, Wanitschke R, Peters M, Krummenauer F, Meyer zum Büschenfelde KH, Schlaak JF. Randomized trial of mycophenolate mofetil versus azathioprine for treatment of chronic active Crohn's disease. Gut 1999;44:625–8.
34. Fellermann K, Ludwig D, Stahl M, David-Walek T, Stange EF. Steroid unresponsive acute attacks of inflammatory bowel disease: immunomodulation by Tacrolimus (FK 506). Am J Gastroenterol 1998;93:1860–6.
35. Anonymous. Infliximab (Remicade) for CD. Med Lett Drugs Ther 1999;41:19–20.
36. Gassull MA, Abad A, Cabre E, Gonzalez-Huix F, Giné JJ, Dolz.C. Enteral tube feeding in inflammatory bowel disease. Gut 1987;27 (Suppl.): 76–80.
37. Cabre E, Fernandez-Banares F, Esteve M, Gassull MA. Micronutrients in inflammatory bowel disease. J Clin Nutr Gastroenterol 1989;4:100–2.
38. Fernandez Banares F, Abad Lacruz A, Xiol X et al. Vitamin status in patients with inflammatory bowel disease. Am J Gastroenterol 1989;84:744–8.
39. Fernandez Banares F, Mingorance MD, Esteve M et al. Serum zinc, copper and selenium levels in inflammatory bowel disease. Am J Gastroenterol 1990;85:1584–9
40. Abad-Lacruz A, Fernandez-Banares F, Cabre E et al. The effect of total enteral tube feeding on the vitamin status of malnourished patients with inflammatory bowel bisease. Int J Vit Nutr Res 1988;58:428–35.
41. Gonzalez-Huix, Esteve M, Abad A et al. Enteral vs parenteral nutrition as adjunct therapy in acute ulcerative colitis. A prospective randomized study. Am J Gastroenterol 1993;88:227–32.

42. Alun Jones V, Dickinson RJ, Workman E, Wilson AJ, Freeman AH, Hunter JU. Crohn's disease: maintenance of remission by diet. Lancet 1985;2:177–80.

43. Rombeau JL, Kripke SA. Metabolic effects of short-chain fatty acids. J Parent Ent Nutr 1990;14 (Suppl.):181–5S.

44. Royall D, Wolever TMS, Jeejeebhoy KN. Clinical significance of colonic fermentation. Am J Gastroenterol 1990;85:1307–12.

45. Scheppach W. Effects of short-chain fatty acids on gut morphology and function. Gut 1994;35:S35–8.

46. Vernia P, Cittadini M, Caprilli R, Torsoli A. Topical treatment of refractory distal ulcerative colitis with 5-ASA and sodium butyrate. Dig Dis Sci 1995;40:305–7.

47. Roediger WEW, Duncan A, Kapanidis O, Millard S. Reducing sulfur compounds of the colon impair colonocyte nutrition: implications for ulcerative colitis. Gastroenterology 1993;104:802–9.

48. Roediger WEW, Duncan A, Kapanidis O, Millard S. Sulphide impairment of butyrate oxidation in rat colonocytes: a biochemical basis for ulcerative colitis? Clin Sci 1993;85:623–7.

49. Fernandez-Bañares F, Hinojosa J, Sanchez-Lombraña JL *et al*. Randomized clinical trial of *Plantago ovata* seeds (dietary fiber) as compared with masalamine in maintaining remission in ulcerative colitis. Am J Gastroenterol 1999;94:427–33.

50. Kromann N, Green A. Epidemiological studies in the Upernavik district, Greenland. Acta Med Scand 1980;208:401–6.

51. Bang H, Dyerberg J, Hjorne N. The composition of food consumed by Greenland Eskimos. Acta Med Scand 1976;200:69–73.

52. De Caterina, R, Cybulsky MI, Clinton SK, Gimbrone M, Libby P. The omega-3 fatty acid docosahexanoate reduces cytokine-induced expression of proatherogenic and proinflammatory proteins in human endothelial cells. Arterioscler Thromb 1994;14:1829–36.

53. Lee T, Hoover R, Williams J *et al*. Effect of dietary enrichment with eicosapentaenoic and docosanexaenoic acids on *in vivo* neutrophil and monocyte leucotriene generation and neutrophil function. N Engl J Med 1985;312:1217–24.

54. Cybulsky M, Grimbone MJ. Endothelial expression of a mononuclear leukocyte adhesion molecule during atherogenesis. Science 1991;251:788–91.

55. De Caterina R, Libby P. Control of endothelial leucocyte adhesion molecules by fatty acids. Lipids 1996;31 (Suppl):S57–63.

56. Yeh SL, Chang KY, Huang C, Chen WJ. Effect of n-3 and n-6 fatty acids on plasma eicosanoid and liver antioxidant enzymes in rats receiving total parenteral nutrition. Nutrition 1997;13:32–6.

57. Kinsella LE. Lipids, membrane receptors and enzymes: effects of dietary fatty acids. J Parent Ent Nutr 1990;14:200–7S.

58. De Caterina R, Libby P. Control of endothelial leucocyte adhesion molecules by fatty acids. Lipids 1996;31 (Suppl.):S57–63.

59. Yeh SL, Chang KY, Huang C, Chen WJ. Effect of n-3 and n-6 fatty acids on plasma eicosanoid and liver antioxidant enzymes in rats receiving total parenteral nutrition. Nutrition 1997;13:32–6.

60. Kinsella LE. Lipids, membrane receptors and enzymes: effects of dietary fatty acids. J Parent Ent Nutr 1990;14:200–17S.

61. Lorenz R, Weber PC, Szimnau P, Heldwein W, Strasser T, Oeschke K. Supplementation with n-3 fatty acids from fish oil in chronic inflammatory bowel disease: a randomized, placebo-controlled, double-blind cross-over trial. J Intern Med Suppl 1998;225:225–32.

62. Salomon P, Kornbluth AA, Janowitz HD. Treatment of ulcerative colitis with fish oil ω-3 omega fatty acid: an open trial? Clin Gastroenterol 1990;12:157–61.

63. Aslan A. Fish oil fatty acid supplementation in ulcerative colitis: a double blind, placebo-controlled, crossover study. Am J Gastroenterol 1992;87:432–7.

64. Hawthorne AB. Treatment of ulcerative colitis with fish oil supplementation: a prospective 12-month randomised controlled trial. Gut. 1992;33:922–8.

65. Stenson WF. Dietary supplements with fish oil in ulcerative colitis. Ann Intern Med 1992;116:609–14.

66. Greenfield SM. A randomized controlled study of evening primrose oil and fish oil in ulcerative colitis. Aliment Pharmacol Ther 1993;7:159–66.

67. Loesche K, Uberschaer B, Pietsch A *et al*. n-3 Fatty acids only delay early relapse of ulcerative colitis in remission. Dig Dis Sci 1996;41:2087–94.

68. Lorenz-Meyer H, Bauer P, Nicolay C *et al.* Omega-3 fatty acids and low carbohydrate diet for maintenance of remission in Crohn's disease – a randomized controlled multicenter clinical trial. Scand J Gastroenterol 1996;31:778–85.
69. Belluzzi A, Brignola C, Campieri M, Pera A, Boschi S, Miglioli M. Effect of an enteric-coated fish-oil preparation on relapses in Crohn's disease. N Engl J Med 1996;334:1557–60.
70. O'Morain C, Segal AW, Levi AJ. Elemental diet as primary treatment of acute Crohn's disease: a controlled study. Br Med J 1984;228:1859–62.
71. Teahon K, Smethurst P, Pearson M *et al.* The effect of elemental diet on intestinal permeability and inflammation in Crohn's disease. Gastroenterology 1991;101:84–9.
72. Ferguson A, Glen M, Ghoshi S. Crohn's disease: nutrition and nutritional therapy: Baillière's Clin Gastroenterol 1998;12:93–114.
73. Teahon K, Bjarnason I, Pearson M, Levi AJ. Ten years' experience with an elemental diet in the management of Crohn's disease. Gut 1990;31:1133–7.
74. Matsui U, Ueki M, Yamada M *et al.* Indications and options of nutritional treatment for Crohn's disease: a comparison of elemental and polymeric diets. J Gastroenterol 1995;30 (Suppl 8):95–7.
75. Seidman E. Nutritional therapy for Crohn's disease: lessons from the Ste.-Justine Hospital experience. Inflam Bowel Dis 1997;3:49–53.
76. Royall D, Jeejeebhoy KN, Baker JP *et al.* Comparison of aminoacid vs peptide based enteral diets in active Crohn's disease: clinical and nutritional outcome. Gut 1994;35:783–7.
77. Giaffer MH, North G, Holdsworth CD. Controlled trial of polymeric versus elemental diet in the treatment of active Crohn's disease. Lancet 1990;335:816–19.
78. Mansfield JC, Giaffer MH, Holdsworth CD. Controlled trial of oligopeptide versus aminoacid diet in the treatment of active Crohn's disease. Gut 1995;36:60–6.
79. Gorard DA, Hunt JR, Payne-James JJ *et al.* Initial response and subsequent course of Crohn's disease treated with elemental diet and prednisolone. Gut 1993;14:1198–202.
80. Raouf AH, Hildrey V, Daniel J *et al.* Enteral feeding as sole treatment for Crohn's disease: controlled trial of whole protein *v* amino acid based feed and a case study of dietary challenge. Gut 1991;32:702–7.
81. Rigaud D, Cosnes J, Le Quintrec Y, René E, Gendre JP, Mignon M. Controlled trial comparing two types of enteral nutrition in treatment of active Crohn's disease: elemental vs polymeric diet. Gut 1991;32:1492–7.
82. Okada M, Yao T, Takenaka K, Imamura K, Maeda K, Fujita K. Controlled trial comparing elemental diet with prednisolone in the treatment of active Crohn's disease. Hepatogastroenterology 1990;31:72–80.
83. Alun Jones V. Comparison of total parenteral nutrition and elemental diet in induction of remission of Crohn's disease: long-term maintenance of remission by personalized food exclusion diets. Dig Dis Sci 1987;32:100–7S.
84. Hiwatashi N. Enteral nutrition for Crohn's disease in Japan. Dis Colon Rectum 1997;40 (Suppl.):S48–53.
85. Middleton SJ, Rucker JT, Kirby GA, Riordan AM, Hunter JO. Long-chain triglycerides reduce the efficacy of enteral feeds in patients with active Crohn's disease. Clin Nutr 1995;14:229–36.
86. Verma S, Brown MH, Giaffer MH. Elemental versus polymeric diet in treatment of active Crohn's disease: a double blind randomised trial. Gut 1997; 41(Suppl. 3):P832.
87. Ueki M, Matsui Y, Yamada M *et al.* Jpn J Gastroenterol 1994;91:1415–25.
88. Fakuda Y, Kosaka T, Okui M, Hirakawa H, Shimoyama T. Efficacy of nutritional therapy for active Crohn's disease. J Gastroenterol 1995;30 (Suppl. 8):83–7.
89. Ruuska T, Savilahti E, Maki M, Örmälä T, Visakorpi JK. Exclusive whole protein diet versus prednisolone in the treatment of acute Crohn's disease in children. J Pediatr Gastroenterol Nutr 1994;19:175–80.
90. Greenberg GR, Fleming CR, Jeejeebhoy KN *et al.* Controlled trial of bowel rest and nutritional support in the management of Crohn's disease. Gut 1988;29:1309–15.
91. Bodemar G, Nilsson L, Smedh K, Larson J. Nasogastric feeding with polymeric, whole protein low fat diet in Crohn's disease. J Clin Nutr Gastroenterol 1991;6:75–83.
92. Coyle BL, Sladen GE. Whole protein diet in the treatment of acute uncomplicated Crohn's disease. J Hum Nutr Dietet 1989;2:25–30.

93. Gonzalez-Huix, F, de Leon R, Fernandez-Banares F *et al.* Polymeric enteral diets as primary treatment of active Crohn's disease; a prospective steroid controlled trial. Gut 1993;34:778–82.
94. Fernandez-Bañares F, Cabré E, Esteve-Comas M, Gassull MA. How effective is enteral nutrition in inducing remission in active Crohn's disease? A meta-analysis of the randomized clinical trials. J Parent Ent Nutr 1995;19:356–64.
95. Fernandez-Bañares F, Cabré E, Gonzalez-Huix F, Gassull MA. Enteral nutrition as primary therapy in Crohn's disease. Gut 1994(Suppl. 1):S55–9.
96. Wilchanski M, Sherman P, Pencharz P, Davis L, Corey M, Griffiths A. Supplementary enteral nutrition maintains remission in paediatric Crohn's disease. Gut 1996;38:543–8.
97. Koga H, Iida M, Aoyagi K, Matsui T, Fujishima M. Long-term efficacy of low residue diet for the maintenance of remission in patients with Crohn's disease. Nippon Shokakibyo Gakkai Zasshi 1993;90:1882–8.
98. Walker-Smith JA. Mucosal healing in Crohn's disease. Gastroenterology. 1998;114:419–20.

Section VII
New therapeutic approaches

Moderator: **C. N. Williams,** Halifax

22
Antibodies to proinflammatory cytokines

L. C. KARP AND S. R. TARGAN

ABSTRACT

Tumour necrosis factor-alpha (TNF-α) is a key molecule in T-helper-1 (Th1) type mucosal inflammation. Results of studies demonstrate variable increases in TNF-α production in the mucosa of patients with active Crohn's disease (CD) but not ulcerative colitis (UC). Recently published trials have demonstrated the efficacy of treatment with monoclonal antibodies to TNF-α in patients with steroid-dependent, chronically active CD. Sixty-five per cent of patients exhibit improved symptoms with anti-TNF-α treatment. Approximately 50% of responding patients achieve clinical remission. The utility of anti-TNF-α for treatment of fistulas was studied in another trial, in which 50% of patients experienced complete closure of their fistulas. Clinical improvement with anti-TNF-α can be prolonged by additional infusions of this monoclonal antibody. Nevertheless, some patients are not responsive to anti-TNF-α. Short-term toxicity to these chimaeric antibodies appears to be relatively minor; however, hypersensitivity/serum sickness reactions can arise with long-term interval treatments. Since anti-TNF-α became available for general use, open-label studies have corroborated efficacy results from the controlled trials, with approximately 60% of patients responding to treatment. The fact that not all patients respond to this therapy suggests the existence of more than one form of inflammation among subsets of CD patients. The hypothesis that mucosal Th1 cytokines are critical in a subpopulation of CD patients will be further tested in upcoming trials of antibodies to interleukin (IL)-12 (important for Th1 responses) and thalidomide (a down-regulator of TNF).

INTRODUCTION

Elevated levels of a large variety of inflammatory mediators, including lipid mediators, neuropeptides, oxygen metabolites and cytokines, have been measured in mucosal tissue samples from patients with ulcerative colitis (UC) and Crohn's diease (CD)[1]. Recent therapeutic developments have centred on selective inhibition of expression and/or activity of these mediators of inflammation. Over recent years numerous studies and extended clinical experience with anti-TNF-α highlight the utility of cytokine therapy and support the hypothesis that Th1 (proinflammatory) cytokines are critical to the inflammatory process of at least a subpopulation of patients with CD. This chapter summarizes the clinical experience to date with anti-TNF-α and discusses the future of this and other proinflammatory molecule manipulation in the treatment of mucosal inflammation.

CYTOKINES AND MUCOSAL INFLAMMATION

Normal mucosa is in a state of perpetually orchestrated inflammation, characterized by an intricate balance of immune mediators in response to various antigenic stimuli in a genetically regulated environment[2]. Failure of normal regulatory mechanisms, and perhaps persistent antigen presence, may result in a lack of down-regulation of inflammation. Inflammatory bowel disease pathogenesis may be the result of an abnormal immune response to a common antigen or may represent a failure to suppress the 'normal' immune response.

Th1 cells and macrophages produce proinflammatory cytokines, including IL-1, IL-6, IL-8, IL-12, TNF-α, and gamma-interferon (IFN-γ) – all of which incite inflammation[3,4]. Production of Th1-type cytokines is stimulated by TNF-α, particularly in the mucosa[5-8].

It is feasible that the therapeutic effect of cytokines in the regulation of inflammation may be to re-set the immune response to a 'normal' level of balanced Th1 and Th1 cytokine secretion. The regulatory properties of cytokines may persist beyond the point that the therapeutic cytokine can be measured in the case of cytokine therapy, or the absence thereof detected, as with the use of anti-cytokines. Therefore, alteration of the basic mechanism of inflammation can result in long-term regulation.

CLINICAL UTILITY OF ANTIBODIES TO PROINFLAMMATORY CYTOKINES: ANTI-TNF-α

Recent clinical trials[9-12], in which patients were treated successfully with intravenous infusions of anti-TNF-α, highlights the importance of TNF-α in the inflammatory process of the majority of patients with CD. Approximately two-thirds of patients responded to treatment, as measured by changes in the Crohn's Disease Activity Index (CDAI) and/or closure of fistulas. Differences among types of mucosal inflammation may account for the disparity in response among the studied populations. Parallel laboratory investigations show that enhanced levels of Th1-type cytokines were found in mucosal samples from the group of responsive patients.

Because TNF plays a central role in the inflammation present in inflammatory bowel disease, other anti-TNF therapies have been developed and are in the early stages of development[13]. These include recombinant TNF receptors (designed to bind TNF and prevent its subsequent effects) and the humanized IgG$_4$ antibody CDP571. CDP571 demonstrated promising results in a short-term (2-week) efficacy trial conducted in 31 patients with CD[14]; however, long-term efficacy and safety have not yet been established.

An initial open-label study of 10 patients with steroid-resistant, active CD assessed clinical benefit of a single infusion of anti-TNF-α. Eight of 10 patients showed improvement, as measured by CDAI and endoscopy, at 2 weeks, and achieved clinical remission by week 4[9].

In a multicentre, double-blind, placebo-controlled 12-week trial of anti-TNF-α in medically resistant, moderate to severe CD[10], 81% of patients treated with a single infusion of 5 mg/kg of anti-TNF-α were significantly improved compared to placebo at the end of 4 weeks. In the same trial, 64% of patients treated with 20 mg/kg of anti-TNF-α also demonstrated significant clinical improvement at week 4. Thirty-three per cent of trial participants achieved remission.

In another study, Rutgeerts et al.[15] performed a study of 30 patients to assess endoscopic and histological effects of treatment with anti-TNF-α. At 4 weeks after treatment patients underwent ileocolonoscopy with biopsies. Using the Crohn's Disease Endoscopic Index of Severity (CDEIS), investigators noted a significant decrease in patients treated with anti-TNF-α. No endoscopic improvement was seen in patients receiving placebo. Histologically, samples from patients receiving anti-TNF-α showed a disappearance of the inflammatory infiltrate, but the same response was not seen in placebo treated patients.

Multiple infusions of anti-TNF-α were studied in 73 patients who initially responded to a single anti-TNF-α infusion[16]. These patients received four infusions of anti-TNF-α at a dose of 10 mg/kg or placebo, at 8-week intervals starting at 12 weeks following the initial anti-TNF-α infusion. At the end of 44 weeks 66% of patients were able to maintain a clinical response to anti-TNF-α, and 51% were able to be maintained in remission, compared to 35% and 21%, respectively, of patients treated with placebo. There was also an additional increase in the number of patients who achieved remission over the 12–44-week treatment period. These encouraging results support the use of multiple infusions of anti-TNF-α to maintain disease response and remission following initial treatment with anti-TNF-α.

Anti-TNF-α has also been studied for the treatment of fistulas[17] in a 14-week trial of 94 patients with active, fistulizing CD. Patients were administered three infusions of anti-TNF-α at 5 mg/kg or 10 mg/kg, or placebo. Sixty-eight per cent and 56% of fistulas were 50% closed, respectively, versus only 26% of those treated with placebo. A statistically significant 55% and 38% of fistulas treated with 5 mg/kg per day or 10 mg/kg per day, respectively, of anti-TNF-α completely resolved by the end of the study. Improvement in fistulas was often observed within 2 weeks of treatment, and lasted a median of at least 3 months. These results show that anti-TNF-α may be a rapid and effective treatment for fistulizing CD, and a promising alternative for those who do not respond to standard therapy.

As mentioned above, an interesting feature of treatment with anti-TNF-α is the potential for a long duration of response even after cessation of therapy.

In one trial, responses were shown as long as 1 year after a single initial dose[10]. In a study of the extended response to infliximab, Hanauer *et al.* found that relapse occurred later in patients receiving higher doses of the medication and in those treated concomitantly with azathioprine[18]. Furthermore, patients treated with multiple infusions had longer remissions than those treated with a single infusion, particularly in the presence of 6-mercaptopurine or azathioprine[18].

More recently, data have come to the fore regarding the potential for delayed hypersensitivity reactions among patients treated with anti-TNF-α. In contrast to the simpler infusion reaction, which can be managed in most patients without discontinuation of treatment, the delayed hypersensitivity reaction requires immediate cessation of anti-TNF-α. In one study as many as 25% of patients experienced serum sickness characterized by myalgia, polyarthralgia, fever, pruritus, urticaria, facial oedema, and dysphagia. Since anti-TNF-α has become more widely available, the incidence of such delayed hypersensitivity reactions is much lower, less than 19%. Nevertheless, patients experiencing delayed hypersensitivity reaction may require hospitalization and high-dose steroids.

THE ROLE OF TNF-α IN MUCOSAL INFLAMMATION AND INFLAMMATORY BOWEL DISEASE PATHOGENESIS

Several studies have detected increased TNF-α protein and mRNA levels in mucosal biopsies from patients with Crohn's disease[19,20], while other studies have generated confounding conclusions[21,22]. Several recent trials of intravenously administered anti-TNF-α monoclonal antibody therapy have shown dramatic responses in CD[10,11]. These results demonstrate a primary role for TNF-α in the mediation of altered mucosal immune function and inflammation in this disease. The extended duration of clinical responses (up to 1 year) in patients treated with a single infusion of anti-TNF-α implicates the elimination of soluble TNF-α and/or blockage of transmembrane TNF-α function, or the elimination of a cell(s) expressing transmembrane TNF-α, in induction of prolonged periods of remission. Thus, the removal of TNF-α for a relatively short period of time by anti-TNF-α antibodies results in a prolonged and sustained down-regulation of the hyperactive inflammatory state. Anti-TNF-α therapy in human CD has been shown to retain its effect long after elimination of the antibodies. This finding suggests that the most important effect of blocking TNF-α is a protracted adjustment of the level of immune response(s) within the mucosa.

The mechanism by which TNF-α regulates inflammation in the gut of CD patients is likely to be complex and multifactorial. A series of *in-vitro* experiments was performed using specimens from patients participating in clinical trials of anti-TNF-α to determine the role of TNF-α in induction of the hyperactive T-cell state known to be present in Crohn's mucosa[23,24]. In one small study nine of 10 patients were evaluated at baseline and 4 weeks after administration of a single infusion of anti-TNF-α monoclonal antibody. Nine attained clinical and endoscopic remission, and six of the nine patients maintained remission for 8 weeks. The leucocyte chemoattractant, RANTES, derived from activated T cells, was detectable in biopsy specimens taken at baseline, but not in samples taken 4 weeks after the infusion[23]. These results demonstrate that anti-TNF-α down-regulates the number, or activation state, of mucosal T cells, and suggest that TNF-α is critical for maintenance of the hyperactive T cell state in CD. The lengthy duration of response to one infusion of anti-TNF-α monoclonal antibody was examined in another series of *in-vitro* studies performed in conjunction with an open-label trial. Among patients responsive to treatment with anti-TNF-α, there was sequential down-regulation of TNF-α and IFN-γ production in the mucosa. Th1 T cells were not eliminated; rather their function was reduced in inflamed mucosa to a level comparable with what is seen in uninflamed mucosa. This reduction in Th1 cytokines suggests that TNF-α-*augmented* Th1 function, not simply Th1 function, was critical for disease pathogenesis. This decrease in Th1 cell function persisted through the entire duration of the clinical response[24]. The studies demonstrate that anti-TNF-α therapy has a profound effect on the level and function of activated T cells within the mucosa, and confirms that the hyperactive T cell state and Th1 cytokine enhancement is central to CD pathogenesis. The presence of soluble or transmembrane TNF-α in the mucosa plays a critical role in the maintenance of this heightened and shifted T cell response. Finally, the data suggest that the prolonged clinical benefit seen with anti-TNF-α therapy may indeed be effected through partial reversal of these altered processes.

Monocytes[25], macrophages and T cells[25] are the major producers of TNF-α. Increased TNF-α levels are associated with sequential increases of IL-1, IL-6, and IL-8[26], and vice-versa. This correlative response suggests that TNF-α functions early in the inflammatory cascade. TNF-α appears to have an important role in regulation of the inflammation that characterizes CD[24,27-32]. Patients with inflammatory bowel disease have greater numbers of mucosal TNF-α-producing cells[32-35] and higher levels of mucosal TNF-α[28-32] than healthy individuals.

THE FUTURE OF THERAPEUTIC ANTIBODIES TO PROINFLAMMATORY CYTOKINES IN THE TREATMENT OF INFLAMMATORY BOWEL DISEASES

As described in the sections above, cytokine and anti-cytokines show great promise for the treatment of inflammatory bowel disease. Anti-TNF-α has been demonstrated to be beneficial, albeit for varying percentages of the affected populations, as has been IL-10. More recently on the horizon is thalidomide, which appears to have beneficial anti-inflammatory and immunomodulatory effects for a wide variety of severe conditions, including erythema nodosum leprosum (for which thalidomide is FDA-approved)[36-38], rheumatoid arthritis[39] and Behçet's syndrome[40,41]. Thalidomide down-regulates TNF-α production and inhibits production of IL-12, an important immunoregulatory cytokine critical to the development of cellular immune responses[42]. Blockage of IL-12 by anti-IL-12 antibody therapy has been shown to ameliorate mucosal inflammation in an animal model of colitis[43]. This inhibition of TNF-α production resulting in reduction of the elevated levels of TNF-α makes thalidomide of

Table 1 Potential sequences and combinations for future cytokine and anti-cytokine therapy of inflammatory bowel diseases

Modality	Sequential/combination	Modality
Anti-TNF-α	→	6-MP
Anti-TNF-α	→	anti-IL-12, anti-IL-18
Anti-TNF-α	→	Antigen manipulation
Anti-TNF-α	+	IL-10
Anti-TNF-α	+	Down-regulatory cells/TR3 (IL-10)

Anti-sense-cytokine specific
Induction of antigen-specific regulatory cells

potential therapeutic importance in any disease state in which high TNF-α levels cause primary problems or secondary complications. In an early study of 12 patients, Vasiliauskas *et al.*[44] found that disease activity improved consistently in all patients during weeks 1–4: 58% response, 17% remission. Clinical improvement was generally maintained despite steroid taper during weeks 5–12. All patients were able to reduce steroids by ≥50%. Forty-four per cent discontinued steroids entirely. In weeks 5–12, 70% of patients responded and 20% achieved remission. Side-effects were mild and mostly transient, with the most common being drowsiness, peripheral neuropathy, oedema, and dermatitis[44].

Data from laboratory science investigations performed in parallel with the clinical trials indicate that it may be possible to determine which patients will respond to a particular modality. Furthermore, the magnitude and duration of the response may also be predictable. At present a panel of tests to detect the presence of specific serum immune markers associated with ulcerative colitides and CD is being evaluated for their usefulness in this regard.

While the evidence for the use of cytokines and anti-cytokines individually is encouraging, perhaps their greatest potential will be realized in combination or sequential administration. Additional laboratory and clinical investigation will help to define the appropriate combinations and the patients most likely to respond to the therapy. Table 1 presents potential cytokine/anti-cytokine combinations which, based on their effects on the immune system, may prove to be highly beneficial.

The use of antibodies to proinflammatory cytokines may be to re-set the immunoregulatory functions of the gut, while another, less potent immunomodulator can then be used to maintain it. Alternatively, based on a cytokine profile of an individual patient, a combination of cytokines/anti-cytokines may be indicated. Once antigen culprits have been further identified, disease may be brought under control by cytokines/anti-cytokines and then maintained by antigen manipulation. Alternatively, an agent such as anti-TNF-α can be used to down-regulate Th1 function and then another agent employed for its potent anti-inflammatory effects.

Serological markers, in combination with genetic and immunological profiles, will allow specific characterization of patients and implicate certain therapeutics.

For example, a patient who is shown to produce limited IFN-γ will be most likely to respond to anti-TNF-α. As more characteristics are defined, the available therapeutic armamentarium will increase.

References

1. McAlindon ME, Mahida YR. Pro-inflammatory cytokines in inflammatory bowel disease. Aliment Pharmacol Ther 1996;10(Suppl. 2):72–4.
2. Stenson WF. Inflammatory bowel disease. In: Yamada T, editor. Textbook of Gastroenterology, 2nd edn. Philadelphia, PA: JB Lippincott; 1995:1748–806.
3. Mosmann TR, Coffman RL. Th1 and Th2 cells: different patterns of lymphokine secretion lead to different functional properties. Annu Rev Immunol 1989;7:145–73.
4. Powrie F, Coffman RL. Cytokine regulation of T-cell function: potential for therapeutic intervention. Immunol Today 1993;14:270–4.
5. Flesch IEA, Hess JH, Huang S et al. Early interleukin 12 production by macrophages in response to mycobacterial infection depends on interferon γ and tumor necrosis factor α. J Exp Med 1995;181:1615.
6. Hernandez-Pando R, Rook GAW. The role of TNF-α in T-cell mediated inflammation depends on the Th1/Th2 cytokine balance. Immunology 1994;82:591–5.
7. Halpern MD, Kurlander RJ, Pisetsky DS. Bacterial DNA induces murine interferon-γ production by stimulation of interleukin-12 and tumor necrosis factor-α. J Immunol 1996;167:72–8.
8. Prehn J, Landers CJ, Targan SR. A soluble factor produced by lamina propria mononuclear cells is required for TNF-alpha enhancement of IFN-gamma production by T-cells. J Immunol 1999 (In press).
9. van Dulleman HM, van Deventer SIH, Hommes DW et al. Treatment of Crohn's disease with anti-tumor necrosis factor chimeric monoclonal antibody (cA2). Gastroenterology 1995;109:129–35.
10. Targan SR, Hanauer SB, van Deventer SJ et al. A short-term study of chimeric monoclonal antibody cA2 to tumor necrosis factor-alpha for Crohn's disease. Crohn's Disease cA2 Study Group. N Engl J Med 1997;337:1029–35.
11. van Deventer SJ, Elson CO, Fedorak RN. Multiple doses of intravenous interleukin 10 in steroid-refractory Crohn's disease. Crohn's Disease Study Group. Gastroenterology 1997;113:383–9.
12. Schreiber S, Fedorak RN, Nielsen OH et al. Safety and efficacy study of recombinant human interleukin-10 (rHuIL-10) treatment in 329 patients with chronic active Crohn's disease. Gastroenterology 1998;114:4423.
13. Sands BE. Biologic therapy for inflammatory bowel disease. Inflam Bowel Dis 1997;3:95–113.
14. Stack WA, Mann SD, Roy AJ et al. Randomised controlled trial of CDP571 antibody to tumour necrosis factor-α in Crohn's disease. Lancet 1997;349:521–4.
15. D'Haens G, van Deventer S, van Hogezand R et al. Endoscopic and histological healing with infliximab anti-tumor necrosis factor antibodies in Crohn's disease. Gastroenterology 1999;116:1029–34.
16. Rutgeerts P et al. Retreatment with anti-TNF-α chimeric antibody (cA2) effectively maintains cA2-induced remission in Crohn's disease. Gastroenterology 1997;92:A1078.
17. Present D et al. Anti-TNF-alpha chimeric antibody (cA2) is effective in the treatment of the fistulae of Crohn's disease: a multicenter, randomized, double-blind, placebo-controlled study. Am J Gastroenterol 1997;112:A648.
18. D'Haens GR, Aerden I, van Hogezand R et al. Duration of response following cessation of infliximab therapy for active or fistulizing Crohn's disease. Gastroenterology 1999;116:A696.
19. MacDonald TT, Hutchings P, Choy M-Y, Murch S, Cooke A. Tumor necrosis factor-alpha and interferon gamma production measured at the single cell level in normal and inflamed human intestine. Clin Exp Immunol 1990;81:301–5.
20. Murch SH, Braegger CP, Walker-Smith JA, MacDonald TT. Location of tumour necrosis factor α by immunohistochemistry in chronic inflammatory bowel disease. Gut 1993;34:1705–9.
21. Isaacs KL, Sartor RB, Haskill S. Cytokine messenger RNA profiles in inflammatory bowel disease mucosa detected by polymerase chain reaction amplification. Gastroenterology 1992;103:1587–95.

22. Stevens C, Walz G, Singaram C *et al*. Tumor necrosis factor-α, interleukin-1β, and interleukin-6 expression in inflammatory bowel disease. Dig Dis Sci 1992;37:818–26.
23. Radema SA, van Dullemen HM, Mevissen M, Tytgat GNJ, van Deventer SJH. Anti-tumor necrosis factor therapy decreases production of the chemokines rantes, MCP, and MIP-2 in patients with Crohn's disease. Gastroenterology 1995;108:A898.
24. Plevy SE, Landers CJ, Prehn J *et al*. A role for TNF-α and mucosal T helper-1 cytokines in the pathogenesis of Crohn's disease. J Immunol 1997;159:6276–82.
25. Vassalli P. The pathophysiology of tumor necrosis factors. Annu Rev Immunol 1992;10:411–52.
26. Feldmann M, Elliott MJ, Woody JN, Maini RN. Anti-tumor necrosis factor-α therapy of rheumatoid arthritis. Adv Immunol 1997;64:283–350.
27. van Deventer SJH. Tumour necrosis factor and Crohn's disease. Gut 1997;40:443–8.
28. Murch SH, Braegger CP, Walker-Smith JA, MacDonald TT. Distribution and density of TNF immunoreactivity in chronic inflammatory bowel disease. Adv Exp Med Biol 1995;371B:1327–30.
29. MacDonald TT, Hutchings P, Choy M-Y, Murch S, Cooke A. Tumour necrosis factor-alpha and interferon-gamma production measured at the single cell level in normal and inflamed human intestine. Clin Exp Immunol 1990;81:301–5.
30. Reimund J-M, Wittersheim C, Dumont S *et al*. Mucosal inflammatory cytokine production by intestinal biopsies in patients with ulcerative colitis and Crohn's disease. J Clin Immunol 1996;16:144–50.
31. Reimund J-M, Dumont S, Muller CD *et al*. Increased production of tumour necrosis factor-α, interleukin-1β, and interleukin-6 by morphologically normal intestinal biopsies from patients with Crohn's disease. Gut 1996;39:684–9.
32. Reinecker H-C, Steffen M, Witthoeft T *et al*. Enhanced secretion of tumour necrosis factor-alpha, IL-6, and IL-1β by isolated lamina propria mononuclear cells from patients with ulcerative colitis and Crohn's disease. Clin Exp Immunol 1993;94:174–81.
33. Breese EJ, Michie CA, Nicholls SW *et al*. Tumor necrosis factor α-producing cells in the intestinal mucosa of children with inflammatory bowel disease. Gastroenterology 1994;106:1455–66.
34. Braegger CP, Nicholls S, Murch SH, Stephens S, MacDonald TT. Tumour necrosis factor alpha in stool as a marker of intestinal inflammation. Lancet 1992;339:89–91.
35. Narula SK, Cutler D, Grint P. Immunomodulation of Crohn's disease by interleukin-10. Agents Actions Suppl 1998;49:57–65.
36. Iyer CG, Languillon J, Ramanujam K *et al*. WHO co-ordinated short-term double-blind trial with thalidomide in the treatment of acute lepra reactions in male lepromatous patients. Bull World Health Org 1971;45:719–32.
37. Waters MF. An internally-controlled double blind trial of thalidomide in severe erythema nodosum leprosum. Lepr Rev 1971;42:26–42.
38. WHO Expert Committee on Leprosy: Sixth Report. Technical Report Series 768. Geneva: World Health Organization; 1988.
39. Gutiérrez-Rodriguez O, Starusta-Bacal P, Gutiérrez-Montes O. Treatment of refractory rheumatoid arthritis – the thalidomide experience. J Rheumatol 1989;16:158–63.
40. Larsson H. Treatment of severe colitis in Behçet's syndrome with thalidomide (CG-217). J Intern Med 1990;228:405–7.
41. Hamuryudan V, Mat C, Saip S *et al*. Thalidomide in the treatment of the mucocutaneous lesions of the Behçet syndrome. A randomized, double-blind, placebo-controlled trial. Ann Intern Med 1998;128:443–50.
42. Moller DR, Wysocka M, Greenlee BM *et al*. Inhibition of IL-12 production by thalidomide. J Immunol 1997;159:5157–61.
43. Neurath MF, Fuss I, Kelsall BL, Presky DH, Waegell W, Strober W. Experimental granulomatous colitis in mice is abrogated by induction of TGF-β-mediated oral tolerance. J Exp Med 1996;183:2605–16.
44. Vasiliauskas EA, Kam LY, Abreu MT *et al*. An open-label, stepwise dose-escalating pilot study of *low-dose* thalidomide in chronically-active, steroid-dependent Crohn's disease. Gastroenterology 1999;117:1271–7.

23
Immunomodulation of Crohn's disease

C. VAN MONTFRANS, T. TEN HOVE AND S. J. H. VAN DEVENTER

ABSTRACT

Crohn's disease is characterized by a relapsing inflammation of the gastrointestinal tract. Current standard treatment consists mainly of application of anti-inflammatory drugs, in particular corticosteroids. Although still the mainstay of therapy, the mode of action of corticosteroids is incompletely understood, side-effects are a common problem, and the therapy does not modify the natural course of disease. Knowledge of the immunopathogenesis of Crohn's disease has increased in recent years, and substantial evidence indicates an important role for uncontrolled T lymphocyte activation. Subsequently, new targets for therapy have been identified, including antibodies against the proinflammatory cytokine tumour necrosis factor-alpha (TNF-α) and the anti-inflammatory cytokine interleukin-10 (IL-10), either delivered as a recombinant cytokine or as the gene encoding for IL-10, and are now intensively studied.

INTRODUCTION

For several decades corticosteroids were the only potent anti-inflammatory agents effective and available for treatment of active Crohn's disease[1]. Corticosteroids act rapidly and have a wide range of anti-inflammatory activities, but do not alter the natural course of the disease, do not consistently heal intestinal ulcers, and are associated with many side-effects. Azathioprine has therapeutic activity in patients with active Crohn's disease, and maintains remissions, and methotrexate has steroid-sparing effects. Despite treatment with these drugs, may patients still have active disease. Recent data suggest that uncontrolled mucosal T lymphocyte activation has a central role in the pathogenesis of Crohn's disease. As a result, production of several proinflammatory cytokines is increased within the intestinal compartment[2-5] and several immunomodulating therapies specifically target these cytokines. Such therapeutic strategies include blockade of proinflammatory cytokines (TNF-α, IL-12, interferon-gamma (IFN-γ)) and administration of anti-inflammatory cytokines (IL-10, IL-11). Most published data concern treatment with anti-TNF-α, antibodies or administration of recombinant human IL-10, which will be discussed here. We will also briefly address the possibility of administration of cytokines to the mucosal compartment by means of gene therapy.

MONOCLONAL ANTI-TNF-α ANTIBODIES

TNF-α is a pleiotropic cytokine that is produced mainly by monocytes and T lymphocytes and seems to have a pivotal role in Crohn's disease[6]. Its relevant biological activities include recruitment of inflammatory cells to the tissue, induction of oedema, activation of the coagulation system and granuloma formation[7]. The number of TNF-α-secreting cells is increased in the lamina propria of Crohn's disease patients and TNF-α protein concentrations were also found to be increased in the stool of children with IBD[8,9].

Several antibodies have been generated that bind and neutralize human TNF-α. In addition, several designer molecules (constructed by grafting two TNF receptor-binding domains on an immunoglobulin G tail) have been clinically investigated. In Crohn's disease the best-studied antibody is a mouse–human chimaeric IgG1 antibody (infliximab) that is able to bind soluble as well as membrane-bound TNF-α. In a placebo-controlled trial of 108 patients with moderate to severe Crohn's disease, treatment with a single dose resulted in a clinical response at 4 weeks in 65% and a complete remission in 33% of the patients. In contrast, in the placebo-treated group the figures were respectively 17% and 4%[10]. Importantly, infliximab effectively induced clinical responses in patients that were refractory to other treatment. This study also showed that retreatment (infusion of the antibody at a dose of 10 mg/kg every 8 weeks) maintained the initial treatment benefit and had low incidence of immunogenicity. A recent study reported that in patients with enterocutaneous fistulas treatment with infliximab resulted in closure of fistulas in 55% of the subjects, whereas this occurred in only 13% of the standard-treated patients[11]. The median duration of fistula closure was 3 months.

A striking feature of anti-TNF antibody therapy is that within a few days several inflammatory processes are down-regulated. A reduction in C-reactive protein level and normalization of intravascular thrombin formation occurs in responders[12]. In addition, a rapid suppression of mucosal inflammation can be observed, as indicated by a decrease in the number of TNF-α-producing lamina propria cells, a reduction of RANTES and MIP-1α-positive cells and the disappearance of the mucosal inflammatory infiltrate[13–15]. However, the sustained improvements cannot be explained by these observations, implying a disease-modifying effect that outlives the persistence of the antibody.

Two recent studies have reported that Crohn's disease is characterized by resistance to apoptosis induction of T lymphocytes, which is a major mechanism of peripheral T lymphocyte tolerance[16,17]. We have recently demonstrated that infliximab greatly accelerates apoptosis induction of activated T lymphocytes;

in a study of 10 patients treated with infliximab apoptosis of mucosal T lymphocytes was apparent within 24 h after the infusion[18]. Such effects have the potential to modify the natural course of disease and may explain the long duration of the effect of infliximab treatment.

The long-term effects of regular or intermittent use are currently under investigation. Side-effects of infliximab treatment include the induction of human anti-chimaeric antibodies (HACA) and anti-double-stranded DNA antibodies, but treated patients do not seem to be more susceptible to infections.

INTERLEUKIN-10

Another candidate for therapeutic suppression of mucosal inflammation in Crohn's disease is the anti-inflammatory cytokine IL-10. This cytokine, which was identified in 1989 as cytokine synthesis inhibitory factor (CSIF), is mainly produced by monocytes and T lymphocytes[19,20]. The ability of IL-10 to down-regulate the antigen-presenting and accessory cell function of monocytes, together with its direct inhibitory effect on T lymphocyte activation and proinflammatory cytokine production, renders this cytokine a potent suppressor of the immune response[21-25]. Exposure of T lymphocytes to high-dose IL-10 during antigen-dependent stimulation results in the formation of a regulatory T lymphocyte (named Tr-1) that itself mainly produces IL-10[26,27] In experimental models of inflammatory bowel disease IL-10 has anti-inflammatory effects, and a lack of IL-10 is sufficient to induce colitis in susceptible mouse strains[26-31].

In the clinical setting, recombinant human IL-10 (rIL-10) has proved safe, well tolerated and showed an anti-inflammatory effect[32-36]. The therapeutic efficacy of rIL-10 in patients with Crohn's disease has been studied in various controlled randomized trials. A phase II dose-escalating study in 46 steroid-refractory patients with active Crohn's disease indicated the safety of a 1-week daily intravenous infusion of 0.5–25 µg/kg rIL-10. The therapy was well tolerated and, although the study was not designed to assess efficacy, 50% of the rIL-10-treated patients versus 23% of the placebo-patients had a complete clinical remission during the 3-week follow-up period[37]. Two subsequent trials investigated the efficacy of subcutaneous administration of rIL-10 in mild to moderate and chronic active Crohn's disease patients. Patients treated with a low dose of rIL-10 (5 µg/kg) had a better outcome than placebo-treated subjects, but effect was lost at higher doses, resulting in a 'bell-shaped' dose–response curve[38,39]. Recent data indicate that high doses of IL-10 (e.g. 20 µg/kg) can stimulate IFN-γ as well as TNF-α production, thereby limiting its anti-inflammatory activities[40,41] Side-effects of systemic cytokine-based therapies include the possible induction of allergic reactions, antibody formation to the 'foreign' peptides and increased susceptibility to opportunistic infections. Finally, the short half lives of recombinant cytokines may necessitate a frequent dosing regimen.

FUTURE STRATEGIES

An alternative approach, to specifically deliver immunomodulatory signals to the region of interest, is to use gene transfer. Initially gene therapy was developed to treat inherited diseases with a single gene defect but at present most of the approved clinical protocols involve cancer patients. However, gene therapy has also been explored in inflammatory and autoimmune disease[42]. Hence, although Crohn's disease does not result from a single genetic mutation, the enhanced local expression of anti-inflammatory cytokine genes within the intestinal mucosa provides an exciting outlook.

Gene transfer to target cells is hampered by a number of technical issues, including low gene transfer efficiencies into target cells, short duration or low expression, and immune responses to novel protein products of the introduced genes. The characteristics of the vector used for gene transfer determine the duration and distribution of the transferred gene expression[43].

Murine retroviral vectors are commonly used for *ex-vivo* delivery as their capacity for genomic integration results in persistence of the transferred gene, but they have a low transduction efficiency[44,45]. A promising strategy to overcome the low transduction efficiency of retroviral vectors is the selection of transduced cells. The enhanced green fluorescent protein (EGFP) is a feasible marker to select the genetically modified cells[46–50].

At present the engineering of peripheral blood $CD4^+$ T lymphocytes in order to yield a 'Tr-1-like' cell, is studied to improve IL-10-based immune therapy. Culturing of Tr-1 cells is cumbersome and has low yields. Recently, a replication-defective murine retroviral vector was generated containing both human IL-10 gene and the gene encoding for EGFP[51,52]. Selected $CD4^+$ T cells, transduced with this vector, produced high levels of IL-10 after a CD3/CD28 double stimulation compared to control $CD4^+$ T cells[53]. Hence, human T lymphocytes can be efficiently transduced to express IL-10, and experiments are in progress to examine the possibility of autologous grafting of these engineered cells in order to down-regulate mucosal inflammation in Crohn's disease. In other Th1-mediated models retroviral gene delivery has already proved effective. Local delivery of IL-4 by retroviral-transduced T lymphocytes ameliorated experimental autoimmune encephalomyelitis (EAE), that is caused by $CD4^+$ basic myelin protein-specific T lymphocytes[54]. Retrovirus-mediated transfer of viral IL-10 gene prolonged murine cardiac allograft survival[55].

A second approach is to use an adenoviral vector that does not insert into the genome and is therefore transiently expressed. Intraperitoneal administration of adenoviral IL-10 prevented the occurrence but did not reverse experimental colitis in rats[56]. Injection of adenoviral IL-4 significantly inhibited tissue damage in experimental colitis[57]. In other models of Th1-mediated disease adenoviral gene transfer also proved effective[58,59]. The use of adeno-associated vectors forms another option for in-vivo gene therapy of Crohn's disease, as these vectors may cause less side-effects than adenoviral vectors.

CONCLUSIONS

The therapeutic management of patients with Crohn's disease remains a clinical and scientific challenge. Experimental and clinical studies indicate that inhibition of specific inflammatory pathways may reduce severity of inflammatory bowel disease. Controlled clinical trials showed the potential benefit of anti-TNF-α antibodies in treatment-resistant Crohn's disease patients and in patients with enterocutaneous fistulas. Administration of IL-10 was less efficient in active disease. The rapid onset and the long-term effects of infliximab may be explained by the ability of anti-TNF-α antibodies to induce apoptosis of activated T lymphocytes. A more targeted delivery of IL-10 by means of viral vector-based gene transfer holds much promise for future clinical application. Preliminary data suggest that engineered regulatory T lymphocytes are a potential source for autologous grafting to maintain a non-inflammatory state of the gut in Crohn's disease. Direct intrarectal administration of adenoviral or adeno-associated IL-10 might also be a feasible approach.

In conclusion, several potent new players have appeared on the therapeutic stage, that have the potential to change therapeutic management of Crohn's disease.

References

1. Summers RW, Switz DM, Sessions JTJ et al. National Cooperative Crohn's Disease Study: results of drug treatment. Gastroenterology 1979;77:847–69.
2. Sartor RB. Cytokines in intestinal inflammation: pathophysiological and clinical considerations. Gastroenterology 1994;106:533–9.
3. Sartor RB. Current concepts of the etiology and pathogenesis of ulcerative colitis and Crohn's disease. Gastroenterol Clin N Am 1995;24:475–507.
4. Monteleone G, Biancone L, Marasco R et al. Interleukin 12 is expressed and actively released by Crohn's disease intestinal lamina propria mononuclear cells. Gastroenterology 1997;112:1169–78.
5. Parronchi P, Romagnani P, Annunziato F et al. Type 1 T-helper cell predominance and interleukin-12 expression in the gut of patients with Crohn's disease. Am J Pathol 1997;150:823–32.
6. Van Deventer SJ. Tumour necrosis factor and Crohn's disease [see comments]. Gut 1997;40:443–8.
7. Lukacs NW, Chensue SW, Strieter RM, Warmington K, Kunkel SL. Inflammatory granuloma formation is mediated by TNF-alpha-inducible intercellular adhesion molecule-1. J Immunol 1994;152.
8. Breese EJ, Michie CA, Nicholls SW et al. Tumor necrosis factor alpha-producing cells in the intestinal mucosa of children with inflammatory bowel disease. Gastroenterology 1994;106:1455–66.
9. Braegger CP, Nicholls S, Murch SH, Stephens S, MacDonald TT. Tumour necrosis factor alpha in stool as a marker of intestinal inflammation [see comments]. Lancet 1992;339:89–91.
10. Targan SR, Hanauer SB, Van Deventer SIH et al. A short-term study of chimeric monoclonal antibody Ca2 to tumor necrosis factor alpha for Crohn's disease. N Engl J Med 1997;337:1029–35.
11. Present DH, Rutgeerts P, Targan S et al. Infliximab for the treatment of fistulas in patients with Crohn's disease. N Engl J Med 1999;340:1398–405.
12. Hommes DW, van Dullemen HM, Levi M et al. Beneficial effect of treatment with a monoclonal anti-tumor necrosis factor-a antibody on markers of coagulation and fibrinolysis in patiens with active Crohn's disease. Haemostasis 1997;27:269–77.
13. Radema SA, van Dullemen H, Mevissen M, Jansen J, Tytgat GNJ, van Deventer SJH.

Anti-TNF therapy decreases production of chemokines in patients with Crohn's disease. Immune activation and neutropihl migration in inflammatory bowel disease. Thesis, 1996.

14. D'Haens G, van Deventer S, van Hogezand R *et al*. Endoscopic and histological healing with infliximab anti-tumor necrosis factor antibodies in Crohn's disease: a European multicenter trial. Gastroenterology 1999;116:1029–34.

15. Baert FJ, D'Haens GR, Peeters M *et al*. Tumor necrosis factor alpha antibody (infliximab) therapy profoundly down-regulates the inflammation in Crohn's ileocolitis. Gastroenterology 1999;116:22–8.

16. Boirivant M, Marini M, Di Felice G *et al*. Lamina propria T cells in Crohn's disease and other gastrointestinal inflammation show defective CD2 pathway-induced apoptosis. Gastroenterology 1999;116:557–65.

17. Ina K, Itoh J, Fukushima K *et al*. Resistance of Crohn's disease T cells to multiple apoptotic signals is associated with a Bcl-2/Bax mucosal imbalance. J Immunol 1999;163.

18. ten Hove T *et al*. Infliximab treatment induces apoptosis of activated lamina propria T-lymphocytes in Crohn's disease. (Submitted).

19. Fiorentino DF, Bond MW, Mosmann TR. Two types of mouse T helper cell. IV. Th2 clones secrete a factor that inhibits cytokine production by Th1 clones. J Exp Med 1989;170:2081–95.

20. Moore KW, O'Garra A, de Waal Malefyt R, Vieira P, Mosmann TR, Interleukin-10. Annu Rev Immunol 1993;11:165–90.

21. de Waal Malefyt R, Abrams J, Bennett B, Figdor CG, de Vries JE. Interleukin 10(IL-10) inhibits cytokine synthesis by human monocytes: an autoregulatory role of IL-10 produced by monocytes. J Exp Med 1991;174:1209–20.

22. de Waal Malefyt R, Haanen J, Spits H *et al*. Interleukin 10 (IL-10) and viral IL-10 strongly reduce antigen-specific human T cell proliferation by diminishing the antigen-presenting capacity of monocytes via downregulation of class II major histocompatibility complex expression. J Exp Med 1991;174:915–24.

23. de Waal Malefyt R, Yssel H, de Vries JE. Direct effects of IL-10 on subsets of human CD4+ T cell clones and resting T cells. Specific inhibition of IL-2 production and proliferation. J Immunol 1993;150:4754–65.

24. Koppelman B, Neefjes JJ, de Vries JE, de Waal Malefyt R. Interleukin-10 down-regulates MHC class II alphabeta peptide complexes at the plasma membrane of monocytes by affecting arrival and recycling. Immunity 1997;7:861–71.

25. Goldman M, Marchant A, Schandené L. Endogenous interleukin-10 in inflammatory disorders: regulatory roles and pharmacological modulation. Ann NY Acad Sci 1996; 796:282–93.

26. Groux H, Ogarra A, Bigler M *et al*. A CD4(+) T-cell subset inhibits antigen-specific T-cell responses and prevents colitis. Nature 1997;389:737–42.

27. Asseman C, Powrie F. Interleukin 10 is a growth factor for a population of regulatory T cells. Gut 1998;42:157–8.

28. Kuhn R, Lohler J, Rennick D, Rajewsky K, Muller W. Interleukin-10-deficient mice develop chronic enterocolitis. Cell 1993;75:263–74.

29. Rennick DM, Fort MM, Davidson NJ. Studies with IL-10–/– mice: an overview. J Leuk Biol 1997;61:389–96.

30. Powrie F, Correa-Oliveira R, Mauze S, Coffman RL. Regulatory interactions between CD45RBhigh and CD45RBlow CD4+ T cells are important for the balance between protective and pathogenic cell-mediated immunity. J Exp Med 1994;179:589–600.

31. Hagenbaugh A, Sharma S, Dubinett SM *et al*. Altered immune responses in interleukin 10 transgenic mice. J Exp Med 1997;185:2101–10.

32. Huhn RD, Radwanski E, O'Connell SM *et al*. Pharmacokinetics and immunomodulatory properties of intravenously administered recombinant human interleukin-10 in healthy volunteers. Blood 1996;87:699–705.

33. Schreiber S, Heinig T, Thiele HG, Raedler A. Immunoregulatory role of interleukin 10 in patients with inflammatory bowel disease. Gastroenterology 1995;108:1434–44.

34. Keystone E, Wherry J, Grint P. IL-10 as a therapeutic strategy in the treatment of rheumatoid arthritis. Rheum Dis Clin N Am 1998;24:629–39.

35. Chernoff AE, Granowitz EV, Shapiro L *et al*. A randomized, controlled trial of IL-10 in humans. Inhibition of inflammatory cytokine production and immune responses. J Immunol 1995;154:5492–9.

36. Pajkrt D, Camoglio L, Tiel-van Buul MC *et al*. Attenuation of proinflammatory response by

recombinant human IL-10 in human endotoxemia: effect of timing of recombinant human IL-10 administration. J Immunol 1997;158:3971–7.

37. van Deventer SH, Elson CO, Fedorak RN. Multiple doses of intravenous interleukin 10 in steroid-refractory Crohn's disease. Crohn's Disease Study Group. Gastroenterology 1997;113:383–9.

38. Fedorak RN, Gangl A, Elson CO *et al.* Safety, tolerance and efficacy of multiple doses of subcutaneous interleukin-10 in mild to moderate active Crohn's disease. Gastroenterology 1998;114:A9074 (abstract).

39. Schreiber S, Fedorak RN, Nielsen OH *et al.* A safety and efficacy study of recombinant interleukin-10 (rHuIL-10) in 329 patients with chronic active Crohn's disease (CACD). Gastroenterology 1998;114:A1080 (abstract).

40. van Montfrans C, van den Ende A, Fedorak RN *et al.* Anti-and proinflammatory effects of IL-10 in mild to moderate Crohn's disease. Gastroenterology (abstracts) 1999.

41. Tilg H *et al.* Induction of neopterin and interferon gamma sythesis during recombinant interleukin-10 treatment of Crohn's disease. (Submitted)

42. Anderson WF. Human gene therapy. Nature 1998;392:25–30.

43. Sokol DL, Gewirtz AM. Gene therapy: basic concepts and recent advances. Crit Rev Eukaryot Gene Expr 1996;6:29–57.

44. Havenga M, Hoogerbrugge P, Valerio D, van Es HH. Retroviral stem cell gene therapy. Stem Cells 1997;15:162–79.

45. Miller AD. Human gene therapy comes of age. Nature 1992;357:455–60.

46. Chalfie M, Tu Y, Euskirchen G, Ward WW, Prasher DC. Green fluorescent protein as a marker for gene expression. Science 1994;263:802–5.

47. Bierhuizen MF, Westerman Y, Visser TP, Dimjati W, Wognum AW, Wagemaker G. Enhanced green fluorescent protein as selectable marker of retroviral-mediated gene transfer in immature hematopoietic bone marrow cells. Blood 1997;90:3304–15.

48. Limón A, Briones J, Puig T *et al.* High-titer retroviral vectors containing the enhanced green fluorescent protein gene for efficient expression in hematopoietic cells. Blood 1997;90:3316–21.

49. Persons DA, Allay JA, Allay ER *et al.* Retroviral-mediated transfer of the green fluorescent protein gene into murine hematopoietic cells facilitates scoring and selection of transduced progenitors *in vitro* and identification of genetically modified cells *in vivo*. Blood 1997;90:1777–86.

50. Dardalhon V, Noraz N, Pollok K *et al.* Green fluorescent protein as a selectable marker of fibronectin-facilitated retroviral gene transfer in primary human T lymphocytes. Human Gene Ther 1999;10:5–14.

51. Kinsella TM, Nolan GP. Episomal vectors rapidly and stably produce high-titer recombinant retrovirus. Human Gene Ther 1996,7.1405–13.

52. Heemskerk MHM, Hooijberg E, Ruizendaal JJ *et al.* Enrichment of antigen-specific T cell response by retrovirally transduced human dendritic cells. Cell Immunol 1999;195:10–17.

53. van Montfrans C, Hooijberg E, Vanwetswinkel S, Spits H, te Velde AA, van Deventer SJH. Towards T-lymphocyte directed IL-10 gene therapy of Crohn's disease. Immunol Lett 1999;69:159 (abstract).

54. Shaw MK, Lorens JB, Dhawan A *et al.* Local delivery of interleukin 4 by retrovirus-transduced T lymphocytes ameliorates experimental autoimmune encephalomyelitis. J Exp Med 1997;185:1711–14.

55. Qin L, Chavin KD, Ding Y *et al.* Retrovirus-mediated transfer of viral IL-10 gene prolongs murine cardiac allograft survival. J Immunol 1996;156:2316–23.

56. Barbara G, Gauldie J, Collins SM. Amelioration of experimental colitis by interleukin-10 gene transfer. 6th United European Gastroenterology Week, 1997 (abstract).

57. Hogaboam CM, Vallance BA, Kumar A *et al.* Therapeutic effects of interleukin-4 gene transfer in experimental inflammatory bowel disease. J Clin Invest 1997;100:2766–76.

58. Parks E, Strieter RM, Lukacs NW *et al.* Transient gene transfer of IL-12 regulates chemokine expression and disease severity in experimental arthritis. J Immunol 1998;160:4615–19.

59. Qin L, Ding Y, Pahud DR, Robson ND, Shaked A, Bromberg JS. Adenovirus-mediated gene transfer of viral interleukin-10 inhibits the immune response to both alloantigen and adenoviral antigen. Human Gene Ther 1997;8:1365–74.

24
Application of recombinant DNA technology to the identification of novel therapeutic targets in inflammatory bowel disease

G. E. WILD, J. HASAN, M. J. ROPELESKI, K. A. WASCHKE,
C. COSSETTE, L. DUFRESNE, B. Q. H. LE AND
A. B. R. THOMSON

ABSTRACT

Our knowledge base pertaining to the pathogenesis of inflammatory bowel disease (IBD) has greatly expanded over the past decade, owing to dramatically improved animal models of enterocolitis and major advances in mucosal immunology and recombinant DNA technology. The current model pertaining to the pathogenesis of IBD emphasizes the important interactions among genetic, immune and environmental factors and underscores the observation that each mucosal cell type functions as effector and target cells.

The identification of differentially expressed genes in the intestine has added to our understanding of the cellular mechanisms associated with the regulation of gene expression in this biological system. Abnormal intestinal cell gene products and responses play a central role in the pathogenesis of IBD. However, the identification and differential expression of potentially aberrant genes remains to be defined.

Of the estimated 100 000 genes encoded by the genome of higher eukaryotic cells, approximately 10–20% are expressed by the average cell, and this subset is the major determinant of the phenotype of a particular cell under physiological conditions and in a diverse array of pathological processes. Two revolutionary approaches to high-throughput analysis and profiling of gene expression have been recently described: differential display PCR and cDNA expression analysis.

The technique of differential display polymerase chain reaction (DDPCR) is a powerful and widely used method for studying differential gene expression. DDPCR merges the technologies of reverse transcriptase PCR and random polymorphic DNA mapping strategies to sequentially select mRNA subpopulations which are subsequently amplified and displayed by polyacrylamide gel electrophoresis. Individual cDNAs that visually indicate differentially regulated mRNAs are used as probes to confirm differential gene expression by conventional Northern analysis. The resultant cDNAs are sequenced directly and compared with DNA databases. The determination of the complete gene sequence coupled with data regarding regulation of the gene allows for an analysis of the function of genes isolated by DDPCR.

Nucleic acid arrays and their applications have been recently described. The cDNAs are grouped into functional classes (e.g. cell proliferation, transcription factors, growth factors, cytokines, etc.). Thus, a single hybridization experiment generates an expression profile allowing the simultaneous comparison of the levels of expression of cDNAs prepared from two different RNA populations (e.g. normal and diseased tissue), representative of the spectrum of differential gene expression characteristic of a particular tissue or experimental condition.

These novel and complementary molecular strategies constitute a powerful framework for the analysis of differential gene expression in the intestinal mucosa in IBD. Data pertaining to the differential expression of novel and known genes may be examined in the context of clinical parameters and disease activity in an attempt to define phenotypic markers associated with relapse, or uncover markers associated with response to therapy or maintenance of clinical remission. The discovery of phenotypic markers may define markers which serve as signposts for novel therapeutic approaches.

INTRODUCTION

The past decade has witnessed a growing understanding of the mechanisms underlying the pathogenesis of Crohn's disease (CD) and ulcerative colitis (UC). The techniques of recombinant DNA technology have played a pivotal role in defining these mechanisms. The tools of molecular biology have been used along with sophisticated immunological techniques to define a number of genetically engineered models of intestinal inflammation. The critical analysis of these and other models of intestinal inflammation has generated important insights into the pathogenesis of IBD and has led to the identification of a variety of novel therapeutic targets. The latter part of this decade has witnessed the translation of the insights derived from these studies into a framework for the rational design of specific biological therapies for IBD, and this growing molecular tool set has been applied in areas of drug discovery and production. This chapter will focus on selected and recent developments in the analysis of differential gene expression. The objective of this review is to examine the potential impact of this technology to further define the pathophysiology of IBD and unveil novel therapeutic targets.

GENETIC ANALYSIS OF DISEASE HETEROGENEITY IN IBD

There is a growing body of evidence obtained from clinical, epidemiological, and molecular biological typing studies which underscores the importance of genetic factors as pivotal determinants of the susceptibility to both CD and UC[1]. The current model which has emerged from these data supports the working hypothesis that HLA and cytokine gene polymorphisms, important in the regulation of inflammation, contribute to determining the severity of the disease. Environmental factors trigger the inflammatory response, and evidence is accumulating that this response is abnormal in IBD[2].

The presence of subgroups of IBD patients with varied disease presentations, defined solely by clinical parameters, has long been recognized. The recent findings of particular HLA associations, variations in expression of antienutrophil cytoplasmic antibody (ANCA) and the presence of cytokine gene polymorphisms have provided a novel set of genetic and mucosal markers[1,2]. It is anticipated that the subgrouping of patients, incorporating genetic and molecular markers, which reflect the emerging concepts pertaining to the molecular pathophysiology of the inflammatory process, will be of great importance in identifying patients who would benefit from treatment with the appropriate therapeutic modality and in a timely manner. It follows that the expression of these markers may also serve to identify those patient subgroups resistant to a particular therapy.

IBD AS A PARADIGM OF ABERRANT DIFFERENTIAL GENE EXPRESSION

The traditional view of the pathophysiology of IBD assigned was focused largely on the destruction of non-immune mucosal cells by soluble mediators (i.e. cytokines, reactive oxygen metabolites) released from activated immune effector cells which were thought to play the dominant role in orchestrating the inflammatory response[3]. It has become increasingly apparent that this traditional paradigm has substantial limitations. The growing body of evidence describing overlapping functions between immune and non-immune cells (i.e. epithelial, endothelial, nerve and muscle cells, and fibroblasts) is congruent with a paradigm in which reciprocal cellular signalling among cells residing in distinct compartments shapes the inflammatory response in IBD[2].

In physiological states the generation and maintenance of the diverse cell phenotypes (i.e. absorptive, goblet, endocrine cells) which comprise the intestinal mucosa constitutes a paradigm of differential gene expression along temporal and spatial (i.e. aboral and crypt-villus) gradients[4,5]. The identification and characterization of differentially expressed genes (e.g. sucrase isomaltase, Na^+/glucose cotransporter) has added to our understanding of the cellular mechanisms associated with the regulation and adaptation of gene expression in this biological system[4–7]. While gene expression may be regulated at diverse control points (i.e. transcription, translation and post-translational modification), the control of transcription through the interaction of transcription factors with intestine-specific gene-regulatory elements represents a particularly critical control point in differential gene expression[4–7].

A variety of cytokines have been shown to be overexpressed in the inflamed intestinal mucosa in CD and UC specimens[2,8]. Cytokines interact with other mediators derived from the cellular and cellular components of the intestinal mucosa and the patterns of cellular responses lead to mucosal inflammation. It is tempting to speculate that the pathogenesis of IBD is a sequential process wherein the mucosal inflammatory response is determined by differential gene expression between cells in diseased and normal areas of the intestinal mucosa. However, the identification and characterization of profiles of differentially expressed genes await definition. Several techniques have recently been described which provide a novel framework to facilitate the identification of genes whose expression has changed during physiological and pathological processes.

METHODOLOGICAL APPROACHES TO THE ANALYSIS OF DIFFERENTIAL GENE EXPRESSION

Approximately 10–20% of the estimated 100 000 genes encoded by the genome of higher eukaryotic cells are expressed by the average cell[9,10]. This subset is the major determinant of the phenotype of a particular cell under physiological conditions and changes in expression of this subset (e.g. induction or repression) occur in pathological processes. The Human Genome Project has generated partial sequence data (i.e. ESTs) for thousands of genes[11–13]. However, the roles that these genes play in mediating cellular processes remain to be elucidated. A key step towards defining these roles is focused on determining profiles of gene expression (i.e. comparing the patterns of gene expression) in different tissues and developmental stages, in normal and in pathological states, or in different *in-vitro* conditions. The analysis of differential gene expression is a major theme that is shared across a variety of disciplines, including developmental biology, oncology and immunology. Moreover, the identification of differentially expressed genes is a primary objective shared by large-scale genomic projects.

While the conventional gel-based techniques (e.g. Northern blotting, reverse transcriptase-based PCR reactions, immunoblotting) are widely used in comparative analyses of gene expression, only limited numbers of samples can be analysed at a time. Alternatively, the differential screening of cDNA libraries as a means to identify genes that differ between control and experimental conditions represents a 'brute-force' approach that involves the screening of thousands of isolated colonies on duplicate colony lifts to identify cDNAs more strongly expressed in one of the two cDNA pools[14]. This technique is limited by problems with signal sensitivity and specificity. To overcome these problems subtractive hybridization protocols have been developed and successfully applied to the analysis of differential gene expression in a variety of biological systems including the gastrointestinal tract[15,16]. The technique involves the synthesis of double-stranded cDNA–cRNA hybrids which are physically separated on hydroxyapatite columns to remove mRNAs shared between control ('driver') and experimental ('target') cells. The cDNAs that are unique to the experiment are ligated into a vector to make a subtracted cDNA library. As with the technique of differential screening, subtractive hybridization methods require large quantities of mRNA and yield few clones of interest.

The 1990s witnessed the development of two novel, high-throughput approaches to the analysis and profiling of gene expression – differential display

PCR and hybridization array technologies. Both approaches have revolutionized the analysis of differential gene expression, and their applications and refinements continue to grow at an incredible pace.

Differential display PCR

In 1992 differential display polymerase chain reaction (DDPCR) was described as an alternative to differential screening and subtractive hybridization methodology[17]. In the ensuing years DDPCR has been extensively cited in the literature, and there have been several hundred reports of its successful application in a broad spectrum of experimental systems[18–20]. Several refinements have been incorporated into the original concept of DDPCR which make this technique a robust and powerful approach to study differential gene expression[18–20].

DDPCR merges the technologies of reverse transcriptase PCR (i.e. anchored 3' oligo-dT primers) and random polymorphic DNA mapping strategies (i.e. arbitrary 5' oligomers) to sequentially select mRNA subpopulations which are subsequently amplified. The resulting 50–100 cDNA bands (ESTs of 100–500 bp), which represent the 3' end of the cDNA, are displayed by polyacrylamide gel electrophoresis (PAGE). This facilitates the side-by-side comparisons of cDNAs obtained from different experimental conditions. The various steps in the DDPCR process are depicted in Figure 1.

Individual cDNAs that visually indicate differentially regulated mRNAs are recovered from the gel, subcloned and used as probes to confirm differential gene expression by conventional Northern analysis or by 'reverse' Northern analysis[22] (Figure 2). The resultant ESTs are sequenced directly and compared with DNA databases, and a match at the 3' untranslated region can often lead to coding information at the 5' end. The cataloguing of DDPCR derived ESTs is a unique approach, as the ESTs represent the 3' end of the mRNA which is the most unique region and establishes the orientation of poly-A tail. Importantly, data obtained from DDPCR provide regulatory information (i.e. up-or down-regulation) pertaining to a particular cDNA.

The subsequent determination of the complete gene sequence, coupled with data regarding regulation of the gene, allows for an analysis of the function of the genes isolated by DDPCR. A comparison of the features of DDPCR and subtractive hybridization is summarized in Table 1. While DDPCR was initially used to detect differences in gene expression between transformed and non-transformed cells, later studies focused on the identification of developmentally or hormonally regulated genes in a variety of model systems of cell growth and differentiation[17–21].

Differentiation is a complex cellular process wherein the acquisition of the mature phenotype is determined by the regulated expression of specific genes. The elucidation of many of the cellular processes leading to normal enterocyte differentiation has relied on clues obtained from several human colon cancer cell lines[23,24]. For example, Caco-2 cells spontaneously differentiate to an enterocyte phenotype as indicated by the presence of brush-border microvilli, dome formation and the expression of a variety of intestinal hydrolases at the apical cell brush-border membrane after the cells form a confluent monolayer[23,24]. DDPCR has recently been used in the Caco-2 *in-vitro* model

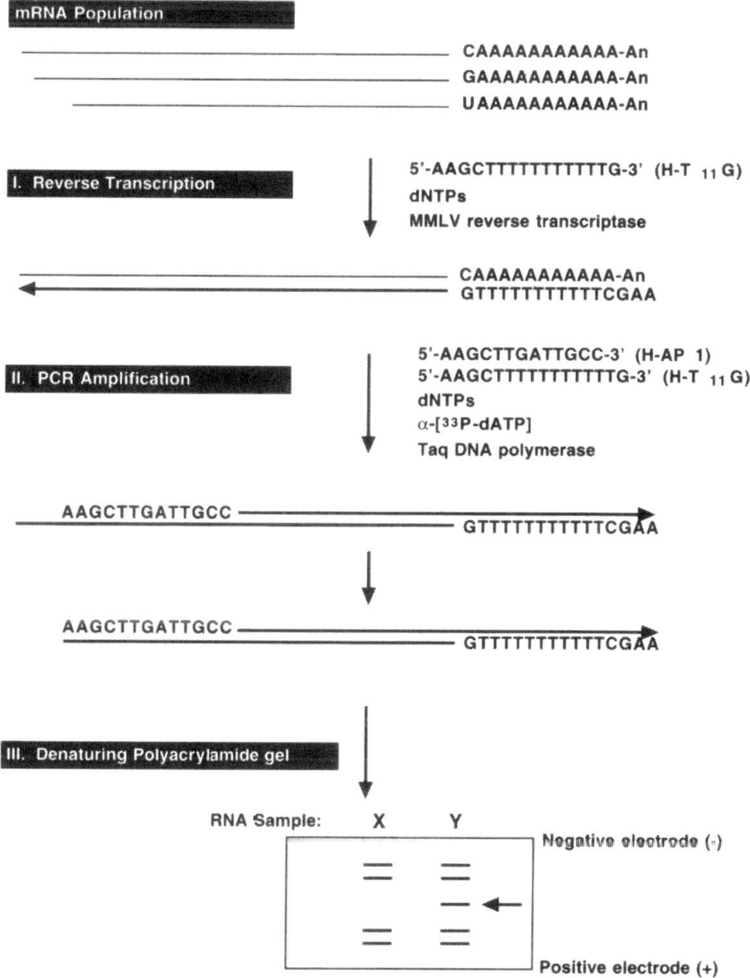

Figure 1 Schematic representation of mRNA differential display technique. Three one-base anchored oligo-dT primers are used in combination with a series of arbitrary 13 mers to reverse transcribe and amplify cellular mRNA. The resulting cDNA populations are resolving on conventional polyacrylamide gels

of enterocyte differentiation to identify new molecular markers for differentiation. The novel differentiation related cDNA *Drg1* (Genbank accession number X92845) encodes a 43 kDa protein expressed in the cytoplasm of enterocytes. The expression of *Drg1* is up-regulated during enterocyte differentiation[25]. A novel 1.2 kb cDNA, termed enterocyte differentiation associated factor (*EDAF*, Genbank accession number U62136), encodes a 16.4 kDa nuclear protein which appears to be a marker of cellular differentiation in this *in-vitro* model of the crypt–villus axis[26].

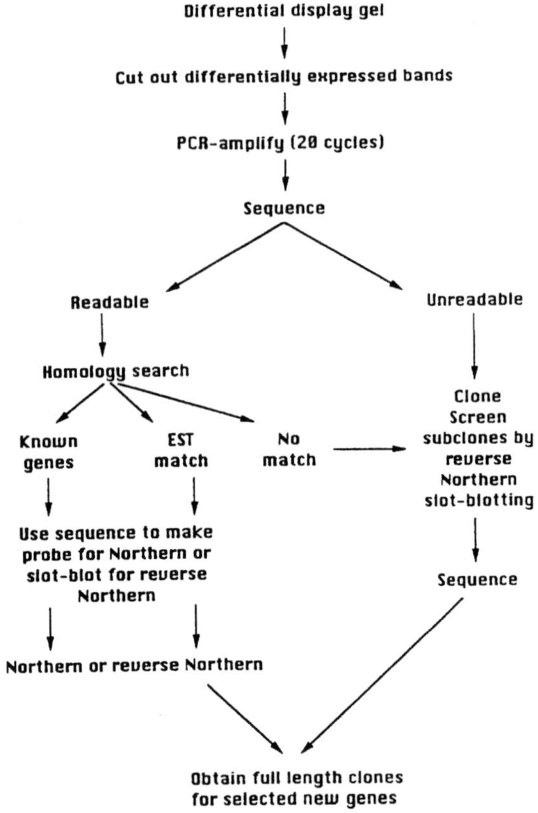

Figure 2   Flowchart illustrating the steps to further characterize differentially expressed cDNAs

Recently, DDPCR methodology has been extended to include an analysis of differences in gene expression in the intact intestinal mucosa. A variety of genes whose expression is modulated in the small intestinal mucosa in a rodent model of zinc deficiency have been identified by DDPCR[27,28]. One of these cDNAs encodes the rat uroguanylin precursor. Increased levels of uroguanylin precursor mRNA abundance were detected in the small intestinal mucosa in zinc-deficient rats and these data constitute the first report of gene regulation of this hormone[27,28].

Intestinal secretory phospholipase A2 was successfully cloned by DDPCR using intact intestinal epithelial cells as a source of RNA and subsequent *in-situ* hybridization experiments revealed a preferential expression of this transcript in Paneth cells[29]. These data underscore the use of complementary approaches to determine the cell-specific origin of cDNAs isolated from complex tissues.

The application of DDPCR to the identification and characterization of genes differentially expressed in the intestinal mucosa has provided a unique framework to initiate an examination of the role of differential gene expression

Table 1 Comparison of differential display and subtractive hybridization

	Differential display	*Subtractive hybridization*
RNA required	5 µg total RNA	1–5 µg poly-A RNA
Prevalence of mRNA surveyed	Abundant and rare	Abundant and rare
Type of differences	≥2-fold	All or none
Type of redundancy found	Primer sequence dependent	mRNA abundance dependent
Optimal application	Seeking rapid output and/or simultaneous evaluation of several experimental conditions	Targeting mRNAs with large (>10×) changes in concentration
Considerations	Usually clone short 3' untranslated region	One-way comparisons; technically difficult

in the intestinal mucosa during the pathogenesis of IBD. The isolation and partial characterization of cDNAs from involved and uninvolved mucosa in colectomy from a patient with UC and from patients with CD have recently been reported[30,31]. The levels of differentially expressed ESTs representing known and unknown sequences cDNAs isolated from the UC colectomy specimen have not been further characterized[30]. By contrast, a 1065 bp PCR product isolated from CD resection specimens hybridized to a unique 3.1 kb RNA species that was specific to CD[31]. The role of this transcript in the pathogenesis of inflammation awaits definition.

It is noteworthy that the differential expression of cDNAs in the intestinal mucosa in patients refractory to medical therapy may not be representative of the spectrum of differential gene expression characteristic of the pathogenesis of IBD (i.e. Berkson's bias). To this end we have recently initiated an analysis of differential gene expression, using DDPCR, in colonic mucosal biopsies from inflamed and normal-appearing mucosa obtained endoscopically from patients with quiescent UC and at relapse and from patients with CD[32]. An example of a differentially expressed cDNA isolated an area of active inflammation in UC with 3' anchored primer–13 mer combination G-A2 is illustrated in Figure 3.

The 161 bp EST identified in the inflamed colonic mucosa in UC (Figure 3), was subsequently sequenced and a Genebank search disclosed extensive homology with the fibronectin gene (Figure 4).

Slot–blot analysis confirmed the increased levels of expression in the inflamed mucosa in UC (Figure 5) and *in-situ* hybridization studies with a riboprobe prepared from the GA17 PCR-TRAP plasmid construct revealed increased gene expression in colonic mucosal epithelial cells in inflamed versus non-inflamed UC mucosal biopsies (Figure 6). Signal was absent in colonic mucosal biopsies from CD.

Fibronectin is a key extracellular matrix (ECM) protein. The differential expression of this cDNA in UC is consistent with previous reports that T cell adherence and mucosal injury in colitis, mediated by the recruitment of leucocytes, involves an integrin–fibronectin interaction[33,34]. Our preliminary

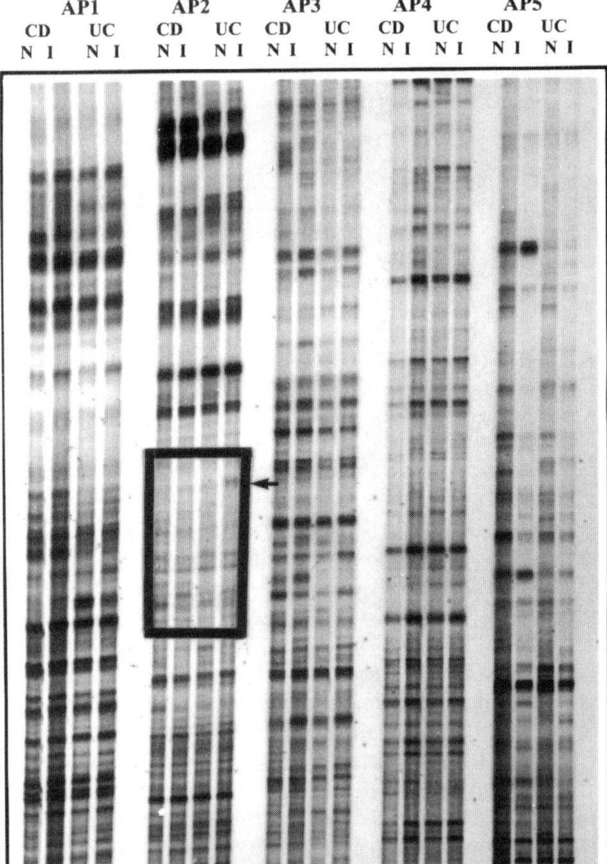

Figure 3 Representative section of a DDPCR map prepared from RNA isolated from biopsies taken from endoscopically normal (N) and inflamed (I) areas of the colon. An example of a differentially expressed cDNA, termed G2a17, isolated with 3 anchored primer–13 mer combination G-A2 is depicted in the inset

findings have defined transcriptional regulation as an important cellular mechanism associated with the up-regulation of fibronectin gene expression in active UC.

Hybridization array technologies

As the Human Genome Project reaches its target of sequencing the 3×10^9 base pairs that comprise the human genome, an array of new techniques and

A.

1   <u>GACCGCTTGT</u> GGAGGTATGT AATCAATGCT CAAGATCTGG

41   CAGCTTTGCC TCAGCTAAGA CACCGGGAGC TTTTATTCTT

81   TTCACAGATT TTATCATTTT ACACTATCAT ACACTATCAT

121   TTTCAAAAAA TCCTTTAACC TTTCTCAGTA TAATCTGGTG

161   TC<u>CCAAAAAA AAAAAAA</u>

B.

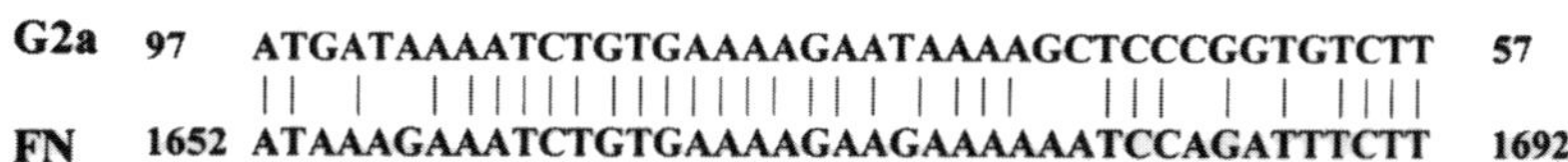

Figure 4 Nucleotide sequence of the G2a17 EST. The sequences of the flanking primers ($T_{12}MG$ and AP_2) are underlined (**A**). Nucleotide sequence homology of the G2a17 EST with the human fibronectin (FN) (**B**)

tools have been invented to screen genes rapidly. The overall goal is to obtain functional biological information concerning gene expression[35]. The advent of DNA chip array (also known as biochips, oligonucleotide arrays and hybridization arrays) assays has revolutionized the manner in which large amounts of genetic information are analysed[36–40]. The Affymetrix Corporation (http:www.affymetrix.com) created the GeneChip® technology which is based on high-density DNA probe arrays that contain DNA sequences as a platform to analyse genetic information in the human genome.

DNA chip arrays are constructed using one of two available methods. One method begins with the synthesis of oligonucleotide arrays onto glass slides with an array density of 106 probes per square centimetre. Fluorescent-labelled DNA probes are hybridized to the oligonucleotide array and the complementary sequences are detected by fluorescent scanning and analysed by pattern recognition software. The alternative format involves the hybridization of fluorescent-labelled probes to cDNA 'printed' onto the glass slide. The currently available GeneChip® contains probes interrogating 40 000 human genes and ESTs. While these applications have attempted to include as many cDNAs as possible in a single array, the sophisticated fluorescence detection equipment and costly dedicated unit required for automated oligonucleotide array analysis are not readily accessible to the average research group.

Nucleic acid cDNA arrays and their applications have been previously described in the literature[41–44]. These methods of gene profiling were restricted in the range of applications, and the signal detection and data analysis requirements limited their widespread use.

The CLONTECH™ (http:www.clontech.com) cDNA expression arrays

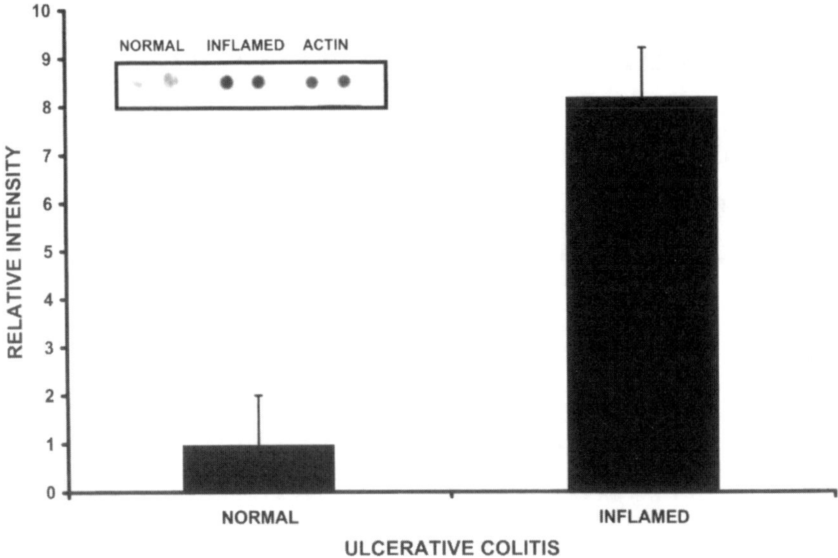

Figure 5   Relative levels of fibronectin mRNA abundance in colonic mucosal biopsies taken from endoscopically normal and inflamed areas of the colon. The relative abundance of this transcript was estimated by slot–blot analysis using digoxigenin, the labelled G2a17 EST, as a cDNA probe and compared with β-actin mRNA levels used as a reference

are the first commercially available nucleic acid arrays[45]. These arrays are constructed to obtain a visual expression profile of 588 human cDNAs (10 ng, 200–500 bp each) immobilized in six quadrants of a hybridization membrane along with housekeeping genes (e.g. GAPDH) for normalizing mRNA abundance. A broad set of genes including oncogenes, transcription factors, cell cycle regulators, intracellular signalling genes, growth factors and cytokines, along with their receptors, cell adhesion molecules, apoptosis-related genes and cell–cell communication genes, are represented in these arrays. Thus, a single hybridization experiment generates an expression profile allowing the simultaneous comparison of the expression levels of cDNAs prepared from two different RNA populations (e.g. normal and diseased tissue) (Figure 7).

Broad-scale expression profiling allows the exploration of interrelationships among genes, thereby providing an insight into how gene expression results in a complex phenotype. Expression levels can be compared between different tissues, at different stages of cell growth and development, or from different experimental time points. From a diagnostic standpoint cDNA expression arrays can be used to identify and characterize disease-related genes. Finally, expression arrays are powerful tools to probe phenotypic differences between normal and transgenic or knockout mice. The recent availability of these cDNA expression arrays has been met with enthusiasm from the research community, as witnessed by the growing numbers of reports that have been published in the oncology literature during the short interval since the availability of this method of profiling gene expression[45–51].

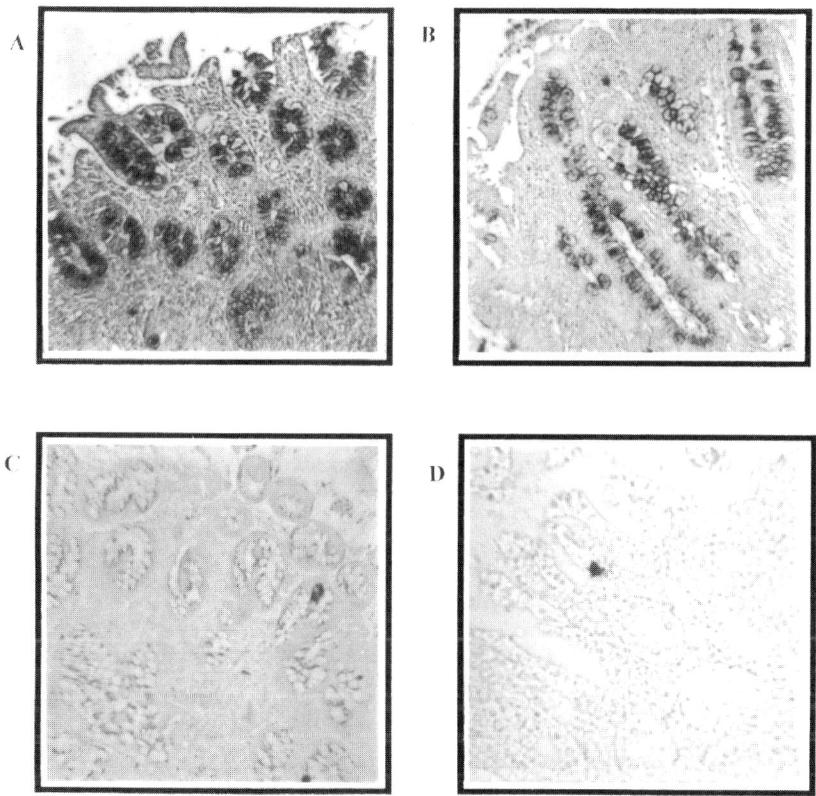

Figure 6 Localization of fibronectin expression by *in-situ* hybridization using a G2a17 antisense riboprobe. Regions of inflamed colonic mucosa in ulcerative colitis (**A** and **B**) revealing fibronectin transcripts in epithelial cells. The transcripts were not detected in endoscopically normal-appearing colonic mucosa (**C**). Tissue section from inflamed mucosa incubated with G2A17 sense riboprobe as a control (**D**)

The comparison of gene expression profiles of phenotypically immature cells and their differentiated counterparts is a powerful strategy in the identification and characterization of genes that determine or are expressed at specific stages during cellular differentiation. The Caco-2 cell line is a well-characterized *in-vitro* model of enterocyte differentiation[23,24]. A representative cDNA expression array in the Caco-2 model of enterocyte differentiation is illustrated in Figure 8.

NUCLEAR FACTOR κ B PLEIOTROPIC TRANSCRIPTION FACTOR AND THERAPEUTIC TARGET IN IBD

Nuclear factor κ B (NF-κB) is a ubiquitous transcription factor which has been the focus of intense investigation since it was first discovered by Sen and

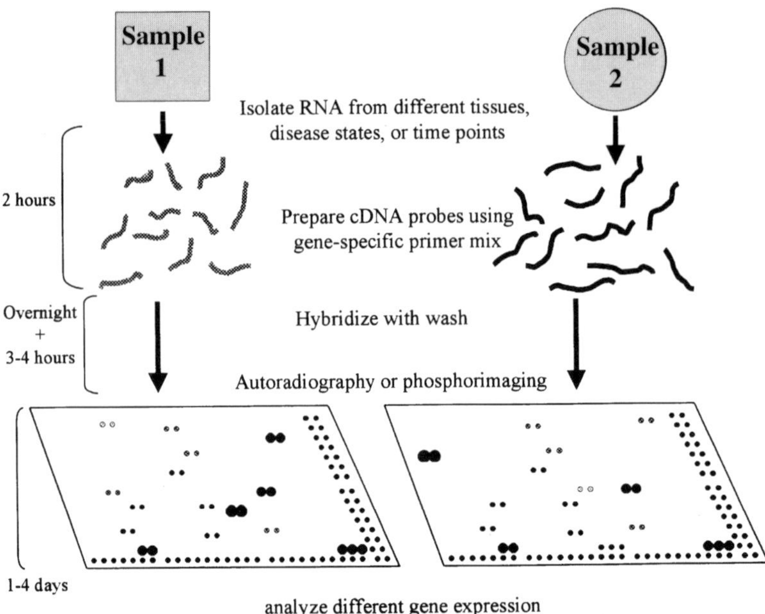

Figure 7 Broad-scale gene expression profiling with cDNA expression arrays. Sid-by-side hybridizations with complex cDNA probes prepared from two different RNA populations allow the simultaneous comparison of the levels of expression of all the cDNAs contained on the array

Baltimore in 1986[52]. A large body of evidence assigns a central role to NF-κB in enhancing the function of a diverse array of genes involved in apoptosis, growth control and most importantly immunological and inflammatory processes[53]. NF-κB is required for the maximal transcription of many cytokine genes including tumour necrosis factor-alpha (TNF-α), IL-1, IL-6 and IL-8, all of which are important in the generation of acute inflammatory disease. NF-κB is also rapidly activated in response to many signals including bacterial and viral products, inflammatory cytokines, parasites, and oxidative stress. This transcription factor orchestrates the pathogenesis of many chronic inflammatory diseases by increasing the expression of the cytokines and adhesion molecules, molecules that recruit inflammatory cells from circulation to the site of inflammation that are critical in the pathogenesis of these types of diseases.

NF-κB resides in the cytoplasm as an inactive complex with unprocessed precursor or I-κB proteins. Activation of cells by a host of signals initiates a signalling cascade leading to disruption of the inactive complex and release of NF-κB. Upon activation, NF-κB is translocated to the nucleus where it binds with high affinity to consensus DNA sequences (p65/p50) which leads to the activation of transcription of a variety of cytokine genes (e.g. IL-1, interferon-gamma (IFN-γ), IL-2, IL-6, IL-12) in lymphocytes, monocytes and epithelial cells. Recent evidence suggests that NF-κB is important in regulating the

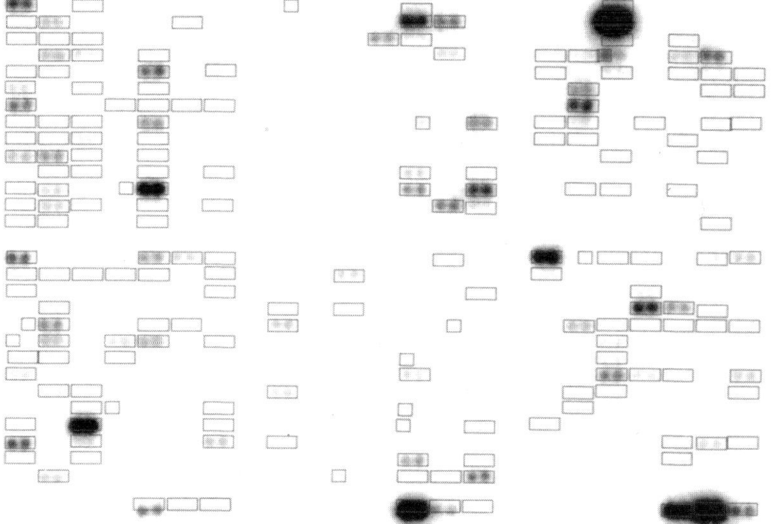

Figure 8   Representative Caco-2 cDNA expression array (Clontech™) hybridized with cDNA probes prepared from RNA isolated from proliferating and differentiated Caco-2 cells.

expression of intracellular adhesion molecule expression in the intestine[54]. The cellular events associated with NF-κB activation are illustrated in Figure 9.

Recent studies have shown that, in both CD and UC, increased activation of NF-κB may be involved in the regulation of the inflammatory response in IBD[55–57]. These observations suggest that NF-κB is an attractive target for therapeutic interventions. In this regard it has recently been shown that the blockade of NF-κB activation by steroids is one of the mechanisms by which steroids inhibit the inflammatory cascade in IBD[55]. These findings are consistent with observations pertaining to the action of steroids in other biological systems[59]. Both sulphasalazine and 5-aminosalicylic acid have recently been shown to block NF-κB activation in intestinal epithelial cells, suggesting that part of the function of these agents includes the disruption of critical cell signalling events required for the perpetuation of chronic inflammation[58,60].

In summary the down-regulation of NF-κB activity emerges as a potential key target in IBD, and strategies that target NF-κB more specifically have been examined in intestinal epithelial cells and in animal models of colitis[57,61]. Such strategies include antisense DNA targeting of the p65 NF-κB subunit and the inhibition of NF-κB by adenoviral I-κB expression vectors. The applicability of these findings to the therapeutic arena in IBD awaits definition[57,61].

CONCLUSIONS

The application of the insights and tools from the disciplines of cell and molecular biology has led to a tremendous expansion of the knowledge base

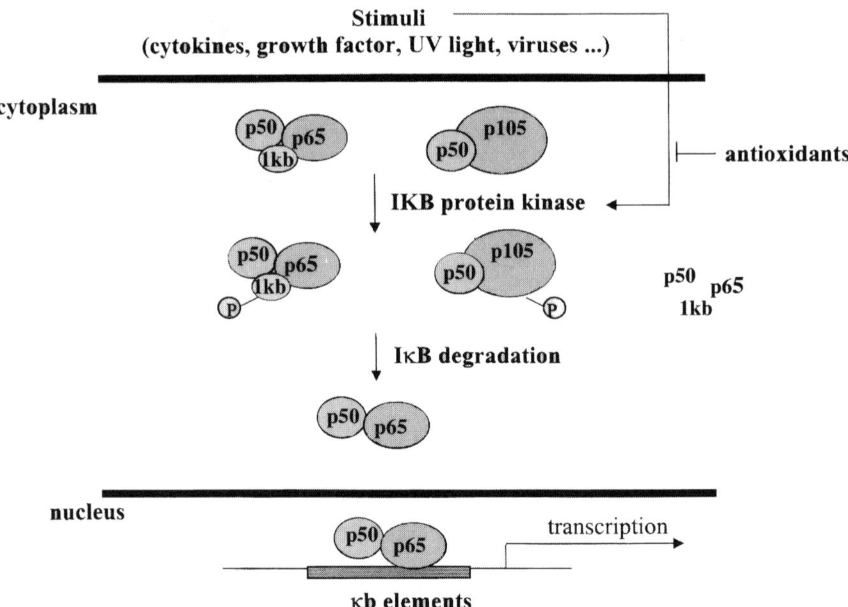

Figure 9 Schematic representation of NF-κB activation and translocation to the nucleus. Activating stimuli promote degradation of I-κB and the subsequent release of NF-κB which translocates to the nucleus. The functionally active NF-κB binds to specific sites in inflammation gene promoters and stimulates transcription

pertaining to the pathogenesis of IBD. The specificity of the therapeutic agents derived from the application of this new knowledge is unprecedented and has provided proof of concept regarding the relative importance of each therapeutic target in the pathogenesis of CD and UC. It is clear that drug discovery has undergone a major paradigm shift from a technology-driven process to an indication-driven process.

The growing use of the technology of gene expression profiling affords the opportunity to identify changes in the patterns of expression of functional classes of genes (e.g. signalling genes, oncogenes, cytokines, etc.) in the clinical context of inflammation. As more data regarding the profiles of gene expression in IBD emerge, it is imperative that these data be examined in the context of clinical parameters and disease activity, in an attempt to relevant surrogate markers associated with response to therapy or maintenance of clinical remission.

Acknowledgements

This work was funded by an operating grant from the Crohn's and Colitis Foundation of Canada. Dr Mark J. Ropeleski is the recipient of a Canadian Association of Gastroenterology–Medical Research Council of Canada Fellowship and Dr Gary Wild is a senior clinician scientist of Les Fonds de la Recherche en Santé du Québec.

References

1. Pena AS. Genetics of inflammatory bowel disease. The candidate gene approach: susceptibility versus disease heterogeneity. Dig Dis 1998;16:356–63.
2. Fiocchi C. Inflammatory bowel disease: etiology and pathogenesis. Gastroenterology 1998;115:182–205.
3. Fiocchi C. Intestinal inflammation: a complex interplay of immune and nonimmune cell interactions. Am J Physiol 1997;273:G769–75.
4. Podolsky DK. Regulation of intestinal epithelial proliferation: a few answers, many questions. Am J Physiol 1993;264:G179–86.
5. Simon TC, Gordon JI. Intestinal epithelial cell differentiation: new insights from mice, flies and nematodes. Curr Opin Genet Dev 1995;5:577–86.
6. Thomson ABR, Wild GE. Adaptation of intestinal nutrient transport in health and disease. Dig Dis Sci 1997;42:453–88.
7. Traber PG, Silberg DG. Intestine-specific gene transcription. Annu Rev Physiol 1996;58:275–97.
8. Fiocchi C, Podolsky DK. Cytokines and growth factors in inflammatory bowel disease. In: Kirsner JB, Shorter RG, editors. Inflammatory Bowel Disease. Baltimore MD: Williams Wilkins; 1995:252–80.
9. Axel R, Feigelson P, Schutz G. Analysis of the complexity and diversity of mRNA from chicken liver and oviduct. Cell 1976;7:247–54.
10. Bishiop JO, Morton JG, Rosbash M, Richardson M. Three abundance classes in HeLa cell messenger RNA. Nature 1974;250:199–204.
11. Aaronson JS, Eckman B, Blevins RA *et al.* Toward the development of a gene index to the human genome: an assessment of the nature of high-throughput EST sequence data. Genome Res 1996;6:829–45.
12. Hillier LD *et al.* Generation and analysis of 280,000 human expressed sequence tags. Genome Res 1996;6:807–28.
13. Marra MA, Hillier L, Waterston RH. Expressed sequence tags–ESTablishing bridges between genomes. Trends Genet 1998;14:4–7.
14. Cochran BH, Reffel AC, Stiles CD. Molecular cloning of gene sequences regulated by platelet-derived growth factor. Cell 1983;33:939–47.
15. Barila DC, Murgia C, Nobili F, Gaetani, S, Perozzi G. Subtractive hybridization cloning of novel genes differentially expressed during intestinal development. Eur J Biochem 1994;223:701–9.
16. Sykes DE, Weiser MM. The identification of genes specifically expressed in epithelial cells of the rat intestinal crypts. Differentiation 1992;50:41–6.
17. Liang P, Pardee AB. Differential display of eukaryotic messenger RNA by means of the polymerase chain reaction. Science 1992;257:967–71.
18. Sunday ME. Differential display RT-PCR for identifying novel gene expression in the lung. Am J Physiol 1995;269:L273–84.
19. Liang P, Pardee AB. Recent advances in differential display. Curr Opinion Immunol 1995;7:274–80.
20. Matz MV, Lukyanov SA. Different strategies of differential display: areas of application. Nucleic Acids Res 1998;26:5537–43.
21. Hu E, Spiegeiman BM. Identification of novel genes involved in adipose differentiation by differential display. Methods Mol Biol 1997; 85:195–204.
22. Zhang H, Zhang R, Liang P. Differential screening of differential display cDNA products by reverse northern. Methods Mol Biol 1997;85:87–94.
23. Zweibaum A, Laburthe M, Grasset E, Louvard D. Use of cultured cell lines in studies of intestinal cell differentiation and function. In: Schultz SG, editor. Handbook of Physiology, Section 6: The Gastrointestinal System. Volume IV. Bethesda MD: American Physiological Society; 1991:223–55.
24. Thomson ABR, Wild GE. Cell culture systems in the elucidation of cellular and molecular mechanisms associated with intestinal adaptation. J Nutr Biochem 1995;6:240–5.
25. van Belzen N, Dinjens VNM, Diesveld MPG *et al.* A novel gene which is up-regulated during colon epithelial cell differentiation and down-regulated in colorectal neoplasms. Lab Invest 1997;77:85–92.

26. Faria J, Wild GE. Isolation and characterization of a marker of intestinal absorptive cell differentiation using an *in-vitro* model of the crypt–villus axis. Surg Forum 1996;47:200–2.

27. Blanchard RK, Cousins RJ. Differential display of intestinal mRNAs regulated by dietary zinc. Proc Natl Acad Sci USA 1996;93:6863–8.

28. Blanchard RK, Cousins RJ. Upregulation of rat intestinal uroguanylin mRNA by dietary zinc restriction. Am J Physiol 1997;272:G972–8.

29. Keshav S, McKnight AJ, Arora R, Gordon S. Cloning of intestinal phospholipase A2 from intestinal epithelial RNA by differential display PCR. Cell Prolif 1997;30:369–83.

30. Zuo L, Ogle CK, Fischer JE, Nussbaum MS. mRNA differential display of colonic mucosa cells in ulcerative colitis. J Surg Res 1997;69:119–27.

31. Lafontaine DA, Mercure S, Perreault JP. Identification of a Crohn's specific transcript with potential as a diagnostic marker. Gut 1998;42:878–82.

32. Hasan J, Faria J, Ropeleski M, Wild G. Analysis of gene expression in inflammatory bowel disease by differential display PCR of colonocyte mRNA. Can J Gastroenterol 1998;12:96A.

33. Ito M, Hirata S, Arai S, Takahashi T. T cell adherence and mucosal injury in ulcerative colitis: involvement of integrin–fibronectin interaction *in situ*. J Gastroenterol 1995;30:70–2.

34. Hirata K, Nagata N, Hiranuma K *et al.* The healing process of chronic colitis in rats, induced by 2,4,6-trinitrobenzene sulfonic acid, with special reference to the role of fibronectin. Scand J Gastroenterol 1994;29:624–9.

35. Okubo K, Hori N, Matoba R *et al.* Large scale cDNA sequencing for analysis of quantitative and qualitative aspects of gene expression. Nature Genet 1992;2:173–9.

36. Marshall A, Hodgson J. DNA chips: an array of possibility. Nature Biotechnol 1998;16:27–31.

37. Ramsay G. DNA chips: state-of-the art. Nature Biotechnol 1998;16:40–4.

38. Lipsshultz R, Morris D, Chee M *et al.* Using oligonucleotide probe arrays to probe genetic diversity. Bio Techniques 1996;19:442–7.

39. Schena M, Shalon D, Davis R, Brown P. Quantitative monitoring of gene expression patterns with a complementary DNA microarray. Science 1995;270:467–70.

40. Alon U, Barkai N, Notterman DA *et al.* Broad patterns of gene expression revealed by clustering analysis of tumour and normal colon tissues probed by oligonucleotide arrays. Proc Natl Acad Sci USA 1999;96:6745–50.

41. Chalifour LE, Fahmy R, Holder EL *et al.* A method for the analysis of gene expression patterns. Anal Biochem 1994;216:299–304.

42. DeRisi J, Penland L, Brown PO *et al.* Use of a cDNA microarray to analyse gene expression patterns in human cancer. Nature Genet 1996;14:457–60.

43. Heller RA, Schena M, Chai A *et al.* Discovery and analysis of inflammatory disease related genes using cDNA microarrays. Proc Natl Acad Sci USA 1997;94:2150–5.

44. Pietu G, Alibert O, Guichard V *et al.* Novel gene transcripts preferentially expressed in human muscles revealed by quantitative hybridization of a high density cDNA array. Genome Res 1996;6:492–503.

45. Zhang W, Chenick A, Chen S, Siebert P, Rhee CH. Molecular profiling of human gliomas by cDNA expression array. J Genet Med 1997;1:57–9.

46. Shim C, Zhang W, Rhee CH, Lee JH. Profilling of differentially expressed genes in human primary cervical cancer by complementary DNA expression array. Clin Cancer Res 1998;4:3045–50.

47. Rhee CH, Hess K, Jabbur J *et al.* cDNA expression array reveals heterogeneous gene expression profiles in three glioblastoma cell lines. Oncogene 1999;18:2711–17.

48. Rhee CH, Ruan S, Chen S *et al.* Characterization of cellular pathways involved in glioblastoma response to the chemotherapeutic agent 1,3-bis (2-chloroethyl)-1-nitrosourea (BCNU) by gene expression profiling. Oncol Rep 1999;6:393–401.

49. Hilsenbeck SG, Friedrichs WE, Schiff R *et al.* Statistical analysis of array expression data as applied to the problem of tamoxifen resistance. J Natl Cancer Inst 1999;91:453–9.

50. Komarova EA, Diatchenko L, Rokhlin OW *et al.* Stress-induced secretion of growth inhibitors. Oncogene 1998;17:1089–96.

51. Hoch RV, Thompson DA, Baker RJ, Weigel RJ. GATA-3 is expressed in association with estrogen receptor in breast cancer. Int J Cancer 1999;84:122–8.

52. Sen R, Baltimore D. Inducibility of κ immunoglobulin enhancer-binding protein NFκB. Cell 1986;47:921–8.

53. Barnes PJ, Karin M. Nuclear factor κB: a pivotal transcription factor in chronic inflammatory diseases. N Engl J Med 1997;336:1066–71.
54. Jobin C, Hellerbrand C, Licato LL, Brenner DA, Sartor RB. Mediation by NF-κB of cytokine induced expression of intracellular adhesion molecule 1 in an intestinal epithelial cell line, a process blocked by proteasome inhibitors. Gut 1998;42:779–87.
55. Ardite E, Panes J, Miranda M *et al*. Effects of steroid treatment on activation of nuclear factor kappaB in patients with inflammatory bowel disease. Br J Pharmacol 1998;124:431–3.
56. Schreiber S, Nikolaus S, Hampe J. Activation of nuclear factor κB in inflammatory bowel disease. Gut 1998;42:477–84.
57. Neurath MF, Pettersson S, Meyer zum Büschenfelde KH, Strober W. Local administration of antisense phosphorothioate oligonucleotides to the p65 subunit of NFκB abrogates established experimental colitis in mice. Nature Med 1996;2:998–1004.
58. Kaiser GC, Yan F, Polk DB. Mesalamine blocks tumour necrosis factor growth inhibition and nuclear factor κB activation in mouse colonocytes. Gastroenterology 1999;116:602–9.
59. Auphan N, DiDonato JA, Rosette C, Helmberg A, Karin M. Immunosuppression by glucocorticosteroids: inhibition of NF-κB activity through induction of IκB synthesis. Science 1995;270:286–90.
60. Wahl C, Liptay S, Adler G, Schmid RM. Sulphasalazine: a potent and specific inhibitor of nuclear factor kappa B. J Clin Invest 1998;101:1163–74.
61. Jobin C, Panja A, Hellerbrand C *et al*. Inhibition of proinflammatory molecule production by adenovirus-mediated expression of a nuclear factor κB superrepressor in human intestinal epithelial cells. J Immunol 1998;160:410–18.

25

The use of probiotics in inflammatory bowel disease

M. CAMPIERI, P. GIONCHETTI, F. RIZZELLO AND A. VENTURI

ABSTRACT

A body of evidence from clinical and experimental observations indicates a role for intestinal microflora in the pathogenesis of inflammatory bowel disease (IBD). Probiotics are defined as 'living organisms, which upon ingestion in certain numbers, exert health benefits beyond inherent basic nutrition'. Recent evidence supports the potential role of probiotics in IBD therapy.

Our own experience was recently focused on the use of a new probiotic preparation (VSL#3) containing 300 billion/g of viable lyophilized bacteria of four strains of lactobacilli, three strains of bifidobacteria, and one strain of *Streptococcus salivarius* subsp. *thermophilus*.

First a pilot study using VSL#3 as maintenance treatment in patients allergic or intolerant to SASP or 5-aminosalicylic acid (5-ASA) was carried out. Twenty patients received 6 g a day of VSL#3 for 12 months and were periodically assessed. Microbiological determination showed a significant increase in concentration of lactobacilli, bifidobacteria and *Streptococcus salivarius* subsp. *thermophilus*, faecal pH was significantly reduced, and the great majority of patients (75%) remained in remission. Subsequently efficacy of this new oral probiotic preparation was tested versus placebo in the maintenance treatment of chronic relapsing pouchitis. Forty patients who obtained clinical and endoscopic remission after 1 month antibiotic treatment were randomized to receive VSL#3 6 g daily or an identical-appearing placebo for 9 months. Of the 20 patients who received the placebo, all relapsed, whereas 17 of the 20 patients treated with VSL#3 were still in remission after 9 months. All these 17 patients, after suspension of the treatment, had a relapse within 4 months. Faecal concentration of lactobacilli, bifidobacteria and *Streptococcus salivarius* supsp. *thermophilus* significantly increased. A controlled study evaluating the efficacy of treatment with antibiotics and probiotics vs mesalazine in the prevention of postoperative recurrence in patients with Crohn's disease is now in progress.

These findings suggest that probiotics may be of therapeutic benefit in maintenance treatment of IBD.

INTRODUCTION

The presence of the indigenous flora is crucial for maturation of the immune system and development of normal intestinal morphology, and to maintain a chronic and immunologically balanced intestinal inflammatory response ('physiological inflammation').

Earlier in the century the Russian Nobel Prize Laureate, Elie Metchnikoff, first hypothesized that large numbers of lactobacilli were important in the intestinal flora for health and longevity in humans[1]. In the same period it was speculated that infant diarrhoea could be treated by giving large doses of bifidobacteria orally[2].

The term 'probiotic' dates from 1965 when Lilly and and Stilwell[3] used it to describe any substance or organism that contributes to intestinal microbial balance, primarily of farm animals. Fuller[4] subsequently stressed the need for a live microbial feed supplement. Even more recently, probiotics have been defined as 'living organisms, which upon ingestion in certain numbers, exert health benefits beyond inherent basic nutrition'[5]. This definition emphasizes the need for a sufficient population of live microorganisms, and further implies that benefits such as improvement of microbial balance may be associated with other health effects, such as immunomodulation.

Most probiotics belong to a large group of bacteria, empirically designated as lactic acid bacteria (lactobacilli, streptococci and bifidobacteria), that are important components of the human gastrointestinal microflora, where they exist as harmless commensals. New probiotics also include other microbes, such as yeast (e.g. *Saccharomyces boulardii*) and other types of bacteria (*Clostridium, Bacillus subtilis*). Probiotic strains must be of human origin, because some health-promoting effects may be species-specific. They also must be acid- and bile-resistant, and have the ability to be metabolically active within the intestinal lumen where, ideally, they should survive, but not persist for the long term. These strains are presumed to be antagonistic against pathogenic bacteria through the production of antimicrobial substances and promoting a reduction of luminal colonic pH. Obviously they must be safe and tested for human use, and should maintain their viability and beneficial properties after processing, culture and storage[6]. The 'probiotic concept', however, remains controversial, mainly because the mechanisms by which probiotic bacterial strains antagonize pathogenic gastrointestinal microorganisms, or exert other beneficial effects in the host *in vivo*, have not yet been fully defined. It is possible that they promote non-specific stimulation of the host immune system, including immune cell proliferation, enhanced phagocytic activity and increased production of secretory immunoglobulin A. Wagner *et al*. have reported that oral administration of either of four probiotic strains (*Lactobacillus acidophilus, Lactobacillus GG, Lactobacillus reuteri* and *Bifidobacterium animalis*) to immunodeficient euthymic or athymic beige mice decreases *Candida albicans* systemic dissemination with concomitant reduction of mortality, emphasizing the complexity of mechanisms involved in host defence against pathogens[7].

Unfortunately, to date the beneficial effects of probiotics have been shown, almost exclusively, under defined experimental conditions, and the number of well-designed, double-blind clinical controlled trials, supporting the many health-promoting claims, is small.

PROBIOTICS IN IBD

A body of evidence from clinical and experimental observations indicates a role for intestinal microflora in the pathogenesis of IBD. The distal ileum and the colon are the areas with highest luminal bacterial concentration, and represent the sites of inflammation in IBD. Similarly, pouchitis, a non-specific inflammation of the ileal reservoir, appears to be associated with a bacterial overgrowth and dysbiosis. Enteric bacteria and their products have been detected within the inflamed mucosa of patients with Crohn's disease (CD). Recent studies have shown convincing evidence of a breakdown of tolerance to the normal commensal flora in active IBD, supporting the theory that hyper-reactivity to ubiquitous antigens from the intestinal microflora is implicated at least in perpetuation of IBD[8,9]. Suppression of the microflora with antibiotics, faecal stream diversion and bowel rest decrease activity of CD, but have less effect in patients with ulcerative colitis (UC)[10,11]. Patients with pouchitis may also be effectively treated with antibiotics. Purified bacterial products are able to determine and perpetuate experimental inflammation; lipopolysaccharide and FMLP can induce an acute enterocolitis, while peptidoglycan–polysaccharide injected into the gut wall of rats produces a transmural inflammation which resembles CD. Additionally, it has recently been shown that luminal contents have the ability to trigger postoperative recurrence of CD in the neoterminal ileum within a few days[12]. The importance of normal luminal bacterial flora is further emphasized by the absence of spontaneous intestinal inflammation in many transgenic and knockout mutant murine models of colitis in the germ-free environment.

Very few data are available on the role of probiotics in IBD. Fabia *et al.* have shown a significant decrease in lactobacilli concentration in colonic biopsies from patients with active ulcerative colitis[13]. In patients with CD a decrease of bifidobacteria fecal concentration has been reported[14] and oral administration of *Lactobacillus GG* determined an increase in gut IgA immune response[15]. Recently a reduced faecal concentration of lactobacilli and bifidobacteria has also been shown in patients with active pouchitis[16]. Exogenous administration of *Lactobacillus reuteri*, either as pure bacterial suspension or as fermented oatmeal soup, was shown to prevent the development of acetic acid-induced colitis[17] or methotrexate-induced colitis[18] in rats. This latter could be even more effectively attenuated by *Lactobacillus plantarum*. More recently, treatment with *Lactobacillus* sp. was able to prevent the development of spontaneous colitis in interleukin-10 (IL-10)-deficient mice[19], and *Lactobacillus plantarum* was able to attenuate an established colitis in the same knockout model[20].

In two recent controlled studies, patients with UC were given oral mesalazine or capsules containing a non-pathogenic strain of *Escherichia coli* as maintenance treatment. No significant difference in relapse rate was observed between the two treatments[21,22].

OUR CLINICAL EXPERIENCE

We have recently evaluated the use of a new probiotic preparation (VSL#3, Yovis, Sigma-Tau, Pomezia, Italy) containing 300 billion/g of viable lyophilized bacteria of four strains of lactobacilli (*L. casei, L. plantarum, L. acidophilus,* and *L. delbruekii* subsp. bulgaricus), three strains of bifidobacteria (*B. longum, B. breve* and *B. infantis*), and one strain of *Streptococcus salivarius* subsp. *thermophilus*. This preparation possesses two main innovative characteristics: a very high bacterial concentration, and the presence of a mixture of different bacterial species with potential synergistic relations to enhance suppression of potential pathogens[23]. Different strains of probiotics possess very different and specialized metabolic activities[24], such that claims made for one strain of an organism cannot necessarily be applied to another. Theoretically, a composite mixture of a large number of probiotic strains may be the ideal.

A pilot study using VSL#3 as maintenance treatment in patients allergic or intolerant to sulphasalazine or mesalazine was carried out. Twenty patients received 6 g a day of VSL#3 for 12 months and were periodically assessed; stool culture and determination of faecal pH were also performed at various intervals. Microbiological determination showed a significant increase in concentration of lactobacilli, bifidobacteria and *Streptococcus salivarius* subsp. *thermophilus*, which was evident after 10 days and persisted throughout the treatment period; no significant modifications were seen in the concentrations of the other bacterial species (Figure 1). Faecal pH was significantly reduced by the treatment (Figure 2), and most patients (75%) remained in remission[25].

Subsequently, the efficacy of this new oral probiotic preparation was compared with placebo in the maintenance treatment of chronic relapsing pouchitis. Forty patients who obtained clinical and endoscopic remission after 1 month antibiotic treatment (rifaximin 1 g twice daily plus ciprofloxacin 500 mg twice daily), were randomized to receive VSL#3 6 g daily or an identical-appearing placebo for 9 months. Of the 20 patients who received the placebo,

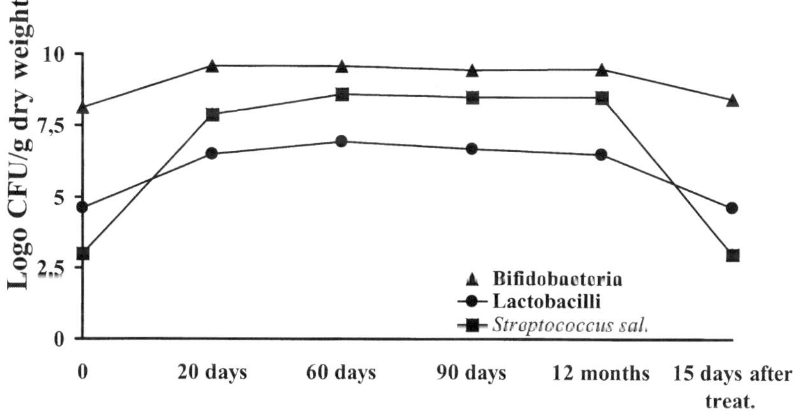

Figure 1 Faecal concentration of lactobacilli (●), bifidobacteria (▲) and *Streptococcus salivarius* subsp. *thermophilus* (■) in patients with ulcerative colitis during treatment with VSL#3

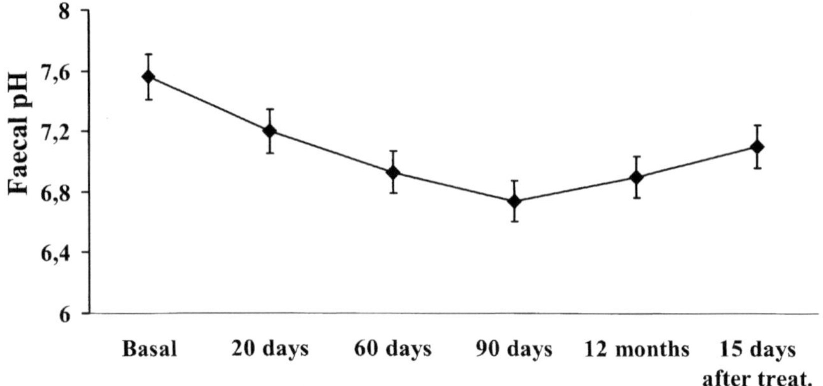

Figure 2 Variation of faecal pH during maintenance treatment with VSL#3 in patients with ulcerative colitis

all had a relapse, eight within 2 months, seven within 3 months and the remaining five within 4 months. In contrast, 17 of the 20 patients treated with VSL#3 were still in remission after 9 months. All these 17 patients had a relapse within 4 months after suspension of the treatment. Faecal concentration of lactobacilli, bifidobacteria and *Streptococcus salivarius* subsp. *thermophilus* significantly increased within 1 month after starting VSL#3 treatment and remained stable throughout the study (Figure 3)[26]. As regards the mechanisms of action of VSL#3, we have recently found that continuous treatment of patients with chronic pouchitis with this probiotic preparation determines a significant increase of tissue levels of IL-10 while concentration of tumour necrosis factor-alpha (TNF-α) and interlukein-1β (IL-1β) remained unchanged (Figure 4)[27].

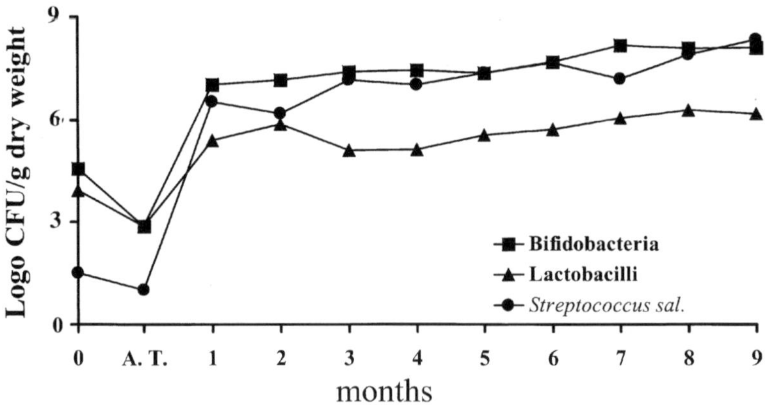

Figure 3 Faecal concentration of lactobacilli (●), bifidobacteria (▲) and *Streptococcus salivarius* subsp. *thermophilus* (■) in patients with chronic pouchitis. A.T. = Data after antibiotic therapy

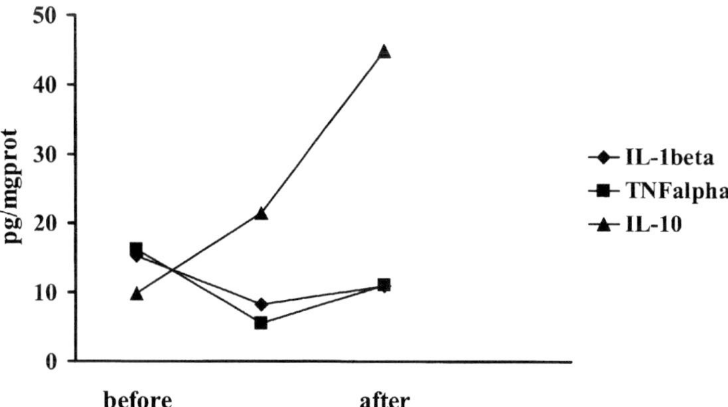

Figure 4 Modification of IL-10, TNF-α and IL-1 tissue levels in patients with pouchitis during VSL#3 treatment

We have carried out a pilot study to evaluate the efficacy of 3 months treatment with rifaximin (1.8 g/day) a non-absorbable rifamicyn derivative with a wide antibacterial spectrum, followed by 9 months treatment with VSL#3 6 g/day, in prophylaxis of postoperative recurrence of CD. Patients were assessed endoscopically and histologically after 3 and 12 months, and clinically every 3 months for 1 year. Only one patient had a severe endoscopic recurrence at 3 months. At 12 months one of 10 had a clinical relapse, together with a severe endoscopic recurrence. These preliminary results suggest that the combination of antibiotics and probiotics may be of benefit in prevention of postoperative recurrence of CD; a controlled trial vs mesalazine is now in progress.

CONCLUSIONS

These findings suggest that probiotics could represent a form of treatment valuable, for instance, in patients with pouchitis.

Whether bacteriotherapy would also be effective where the inflammation is well established for a long-term period, such as in UC or CD, needs to be further assessed.

Future research needs to be centred on obtaining more precise information on the mechanisms by which probiotics exert their beneficial effects *in vivo*. This will provide a scientific rationale for the selection of the best probiotic strains to carry out large, double-blind, controlled clinical trials.

References

1. Metchnikoff E. In: Mitchell C, editor. The Prolongation of Life: Optimistic Studies. London; William Heinemann; 1907:161–83.
2. Tissier H. Traitement des infections intestinales par la méthode de la flore bactérienne de l'intestin. C R Soc Biol 1906;60:359–61.
3. Lilly DM, Stillwell RH. Probiotics: growth promoting factors produced by microorganisms. Science 1965;47:747–8

4. Fuller R. Probiotics in human medicine. Gut 1991;32:439–42.
5. Schaafsma G. State of the art concerning probiotic strains in milk products. IDF Nutr Newsl 1996;5:23–4.
6. Lee YK, Salminen S. The coming age of probiotics. Trends Food Sci Technol 1995;6:241–5.
7. Wagner ED, Warner T, Roberts L, Farmer J, Balish E. Colonization of congenitally immunodeficient mice with probiotic bacteria. Infect Immun 1997;65:3345–51.
8. Duchmann R, Kaiser I, Hermann E, Mayet W, Ewe K, Meyer zum Büschenfelde K-H. Tolerance exists towards resident intestinal flora but is broken in active inflammatory bowel disease (IBD). Clin Exp Immunol 1995;102:448–55.
9. Macpherson A, Khoo UY, Forgacs I, Philpott-Howard J, Bjarnason I. Mucosal antibodies in inflammatory bowel disease are directed against intestinal bacteria. Gut 1996;38:365–75.
10. Rutgeerts P, Hiele M, Geboes K et al. Controlled trial of metronidazole treatment for prevention of Crohn's recurrence after ileal resection. Gastroenterology 1995;108:1617–21.
11. Rutgeerts P, Geboes K, Peeters M et al. Effect of faecal stream diversion on recurrence of Crohn's disease in the neoterminal ileum. Lancet 1991;338:771–4.
12. D'Haens GR, Geboes K, Peeters M, Penninckx F, Rutgeerts P. Early lesions of recurrent Crohn's disease caused by infusion of intestinal contents in excluded ileum. Gastroenterology 1998;114:771–4.
13. Fabia R, Ar'Rajab A, Johansson ML et al. Impairment of bacterial flora in human ulcerative colitis and experimental colitis in the rat. Digestion 1993;54:248–55.
14. Favier C, Neut C, Mizon C, Cortot A, Colombel JF, Mizon J. Fecal β-D-galactosidase production and bifidobacteria are decreased in Crohn's disease. Dig Dis Sci 1997;42:817–22.
15. Malin M, Suomalainen H, Saxelin M, Isolauri E. Promotion of IgA immune response in patients with Crohn's disease by oral bacteriotherapy with *Lactobacillus GG*. Ann Nutr Metab 1996;40:137–45.
16. Ruseler-van-Embden JGH, Schouten WR, van Lieshout LMC. Pouchitis: result of microbial imbalance? Gut 1994;35:658–64.
17. Fabia R, Ar'Rajab A, Johansson M-L et al. The effect of exogenous administration of *Lactobacillus reuteri* R2LC and oat fiber on acetic acid-induced colitis in the rat. Scand J Gastroenterol 1993;28:155–62.
18. Mao Y, Nobaek S, Kasravi B, et al. The effects of *Lactobacillus* strains and oat fibre on methotrexate-induced enterocolitis in rats. Gastroenterology 1996; 111:334–44.
19. Madsen KL, Tavernini MM, Doyle JSG, Fedora RN. *Lactobacillus* sp. prevents development of enterocolitis in interleukin-10 gene-deficient mice. Gastroenterology 1999;116: 1107–14.
20. Schultz M, Veltkamp C, Dieleman LA, Wyrick, PB, Tonkonogy SL, Sartor RB. Continuous feeding of *Lactobacillus plantarum* attenuates established colitis in interleukin-10 deficient mice. Gastroenterology 1998;114:A1081.
21. Rembacken BJ, Snelling AM, Hawkey PM, Axon ATR. A double blind trial of non pathogenic *E. coli* vs mesalazine for the treatment of ulcerative colits Gut 1997;41(Suppl. 3):3911.
22. Kruis W, Schuts E, Fric P, Fixa B, Judmaier G, Stolte M. Double-blind comparison of an oral *Escherichia coli* preparation and Mesalazina in maintaining remission of ulcerative colitis. Aliment Pharmacol Ther 1997;11:853–8.
23. Mackowiak PA. The normal microbial flora. N Engl J Med 1982;307:83–93.
24. Bengmark S. Econutrition and health maintenance. A new concept to prevent GI inflammation, ulceration and sepsis. Clin Nutr 1996;15:1–10.
25. Venturi A, Gionchetti P, Rizzello F et al. Impact on the faecal flora composition of a new probiotic preparation. Preliminary data on maintenance treatment of patients with ulcerative colitis (UC) intolerant or allergic to 5-aminosalicylic acid (5-ASA). Aliment Pharmacol Ther 1999 (In press).
26. Gionchetti P, Rizzello F, Venturi A et al. Maintenance treatment of chronic pouchitis: a randomized, placebo-controlled, double-blind trial with a new probiotic preparation. Gastroenterology 1998;114:G4037.
27. Gionchetti P, Rizzello F, Cifone G et al. *In vivo* effect of a highly concentrated probiotic on IL-10 pelvic ileal pouch tissue levels. Abstract book Digestive Diseases Week, Orlando, Florida, 16–19 May 1999;a743:4093.

Index

Aeromonas hydrophilus 82
aetiology 4, 25–6
alendronate 169
alkaline phosphatase 149, 167
aminosalicylates 109, 111
5-aminosalicylic acid (5-ASA) 109, 125,
    129–31, 137, 138, 142–3
ANCA *see* antineutrophil cytoplasmic
    antibodies
ANDA 236
animal models 29, 42, 49, 50, 61, 64–6
ankylosing spondylitis 17
anorexia 90
anti-inflammatory treatment 142–3
anti-tumour necrosis factor
    (infliximab) 128, 134, 138, 220–2,
    228–9
antibiotics 81, 101, 122, 133, 142
antibodies
    autoimmunity 49
    proinflammatory cytokines 219–26
antibody to *Saccharomyces cerevisiae*
    (ASCA) 73, 76–7, 87, 89
antineutrophil cytoplasmic antibodies
    (ANCA) 73, 77, 81–2
    perinuclear 50, 87, 89, 187–9
aphthous ulcer 140
apoptosis 48, 228
5-ASA *see* 5-aminosalicylic acid
ASCA *see* antibody to *Saccharomyces
    cerevisiae*
aspirin 57, 59, 80
attachment insecurity 187–9
autoimmunity 46 51, 65
avascular necrosis *see* osteonecrosis
AZA *see* azathioprine
azathioprine (AZA) 19, 88, 92, 123, 132–3,
    137, 151

B cells 42, 44, 48
bacterial factors 39–45, 67
biological agents 133 4

biopsies 75, 79, 82
bisphosphonates 163, 164, 166, 169
BMD *see* bone mineral density
body weight 152
bone disease 93–4, 147
    see also osteoporosis
    drug therapy 168–70
    management 163–72
    prevalence 154–6
    risk factors 148–54, 166–8
bone growth 164–5
bone mineral density (BMD) 94, 147,
    148–9, 154–5, 163
bone resorption 167
bowel rest 111
budesonide 130, 137, 143
butyrate 209

caecal patch 83
calcitonin 163, 166
calcium 151, 153, 167, 168
CAM *see* complementary and alternative
    medicine
Campylobacter jejuni 82
Canadian lawsuits 173–84
Candida albicans 77
candidate genes 8–9, 62
carboxy terminal telopeptide of type 1
    collagen (ICTP) 150
cat's claw 198–9, 201, 204
CCR5 gene 18
CD4$^+$ lymphocytes 64
CD14 expression 39, 41, 44
CD *see* Crohn's disease
CDAI *see* Crohn's Disease Activity Index
CDEIS *see* Crohn's Disease Endoscopic
    Index of Severity
cDNA expression analysis 234
chemoattractants 56
chemokines 41, 56, 66, 69
children, Crohn's disease 87–94
cigarette smoking 81, 108, 153

ciprofloxacin 82, 101, 122, 133
Clostridium difficile 82, 96, 98
coeliac disease 32
colectomy 80
colonoscopy 83, 89
colorectal cancer 100
complementary and alternative medicine (CAM) 109, 194–200, 201–6
conditioning factors 23
consent 174–5
constipation 108
corticosteroids 98, 101, 107, 109, 131–2
  bone disease 150–1, 169
Crohn's disease (CD)
  autoimmunity 46, 50, 65
  bone disease 152, 156
  children 87–94
  curative surgery 139
  diagnosis 73, 74–7, 82
  elderly 96–7, 100–2
  genetics 5, 9, 15, 18, 63
  HLA 17
  immunomodulation 227–33
  induction therapy 128–36
  neoterminal ileum 140–3
  nutrition 208
  postoperative 143
  recurrence 139
  relapse 139
  remission maintenance 137–46
  T cells 61
  TNF-α 222–3
Crohn's Disease Activity Index (CDAI) 76, 129
Crohn's Disease Endoscopic Index of Severity (CDEIS) 221
crypt abscesses 54, 55
curative resections 139–40
cyclosporin 107, 112, 113, 124, 132
cytokines 9, 56, 66, 69, 78, 219–26, 236–7

DDPCR *see* differential display polymerase chain reaction
deoxypyridoline (DPD) 150
DEXA *see* dual-energy X-ray absorptiometry
diagnosis 73–86, 88–91
diet 153, 208, 209, 210–11
dietary factors 108
differential display polymerase chain reaction (DDPCR) 234–5, 238–42
distal colitis 118
DNA chip arrays 243
Doppler sonography 87, 90–2
DPD *see* deoxypyridoline
drug therapy
  see also antibiotics
  anti-tumour necrosis factor

(infliximab) 128, 134, 138, 220–2, 228–9
  azathioprine 88, 92, 123, 132–3
  bone disease 168–70
  complications 99
  corticosteroids 98, 101, 107, 131–2
  cyclosporin 107, 112, 113, 124, 132
  inductive 107
  LXS$_4$ analogues 54
  6-mercaptopurine 88, 92, 123, 132–3
  mesalamine 114, 129–31
  sulphasalazine 109, 117, 129–31
dual-energy X-ray absorptiometry (DEXA) 94

elderly 96–104
elemental diets 208, 210–11
endoscopy 75, 79, 82, 141
environmental factors 18, 24, 28, 65
Escherichia coli O157:H7 96, 98
etidronate 169
exclusion diets 209
exercise 152
expression profiling 244
extensive colitis, treatment 119–22

FACS *see* fluorescence-activated cell sorting
familial incidence 13–16
ω-3 fatty acids 138
fibre 208, 209
fibronectin 241
fluorescence-activated cell sorting (FACS) 41
fluoride 166
fractures 147
fulminant colitis 112–13

GCS *see* glucocorticosteroids
gene therapy 230
genetics 18–20, 24, 26, 33, 67
  candidate genes 8–9, 62
  genomic screening 62–3
  linkage analysis 5–7, 13–14, 29, 63, 67
  multiplicity 28
  osteoporosis 154
  spontaneous mutations 27
  susceptibility genes 3, 9, 13, 29–30, 44
genistein 201, 203
gliadin 33
glucocorticosteroids (GCS) 118, 137, 152
gluten-sensitive enteropathy 32
growth failure 88, 90

haematochezia 89
herbal medicine *see* complementary and alternative medicine (CAM)
heterogeneity 24–5, 28
HLA antigens 8, 16–17, 31, 32–3, 82, 236

hormone replacement therapy (HRT)   163
HRT *see* hormone replacement therapy
hybridization array technologies   242–5

ICAM-1   9
ICTP *see* carboxy terminal telopeptide of
        type 1 collagen
IL *see* interleukin
ileum   75–6
immune function   24, 31–3, 64
immunomodulation   138, 139, 227–33
immunosuppressive agents   132–3, 144
infections   81
infliximab *see* anti-tumour necrosis factor
inheritance patterns   14–15
innate immune response   39, 42–4
interleukin-1 (IL-1)   17
interleukin-8 (IL-8)   56, 58
interleukin-10 (IL-10)   229
interleukin-12 (IL-12)–interferon gamma
        pathway   39, 44, 65
intestinal flora   39–40
intestinal inflammation
    animal models   42
    CD14 expression   41
    down-regulation   57–9
    induction   55–6
intravenous steroids   111
ischaemic colitis   98

joint complications   17

'knockout mice'   42

lactobacilli   253, 255
lactose   108
lesions   75, 140–1
linkage analysis   5–7, 13–14, 29, 63, 67
lipid A binding protein (LBP)   40
lipoproteins   40
lipopolysaccharides (LPS)   39–41
lipoteichoic acids (LTA)   39–40
lipoxin A$_4$ (LXA$_4$)   54, 57–8
LPB *see* lipid A binding protein
LPS *see* lipopolysaccharides
LTA *see* lipoteichoic acids
luminal factors   141
lupus erythematosus   46
LXS$_4$ *see* lipoxin A$_4$

macrophage chemotactic protein-1
        (MCP-1)   58
malignancy   100
MCP-1 *see* macrophage chemotactic
        protein-1
measles   16
medical negligence, Canada   173–84
mental status   99

6-mercaptopurine (6-MP)   88, 92, 123,
        132–3, 137, 144
mesalamine   114, 142–3
methotrexate   132, 151
metronidazole   82, 101, 133, 141–2
microsatellite markers   13, 62
mortality   80, 98
mouth ulceration   17
6-MP *see* 6-mercaptopurine
mucosal barrier   61, 64, 68
mucosal inflammation   219, 222–3
mucosal repair   69
mucosal–cell interactions   68
mutaflor   122
myasthenia gravis   46

neoterminal ileum   140–3
neutrophils, transmigration   54–5
NF-κB   54, 201, 245–7
nicotine   122
non-steroidal anti-inflammatory drugs
        (NSAID)   80–1, 109
nucleic acid arrays   235
nutrition   207–16

oestrogen   151–2, 154, 163
ON *see* osteonecrosis
oral contraceptives   81
osteocalcin   149, 167
osteomalacia   168
osteonecrosis (ON), steroid
            induced   173–84
osteopenia   149, 154, 165–6
osteoporosis   93–4, 108, 147–9, 165–6, 168

paediatric IBD   87–95, 150
pain   78
pamidronate   169
pANCA *see* perinuclear antineutrophil
        cytoplasmic antibodies
pancolitis   119–22
parathyroid hormone (PTH)   149, 166, 168
parenteral nutrition   107
pathogen-elicited epithelial chemoattractant
        (PEEC)   56
pathogenesis   19
peak bone mass (PBM)   164
PEEC *see* pathogen-elicited epithelial
        chemoattractant
peptidoglycans (PGN)   40
perinuclear antineutrophil cytoplasmic
        antibodies (pANCA)   50, 87, 89,
        187–9
PET *see* positron emission tomography
PGN *see* peptidoglycans
pharmacogenetics   19
PICP *see* pro-collagen-carboxy terminal
        propeptide

polyarteritis nodosa   49
polyclonal activation   47
polygenicity   27
polymorphonuclear neutrophil leucocyte
    (PMN) *see* neutrophils
n-3 polyunsaturated fatty acids
    (PUFA)   210
positional cloning   5–7
positron emission tomography (PET)   76
pouchitis   82, 108, 209, 254
pregnancy   124
primary sclerosing cholangitis (PSC)   16
pro-collagen-carboxy terminal propeptide
    (PICP)   149
probiotics   252–8
proinflammatory cytokines,
    antibodies   219–26
psychoanalysis   186
psychosocial disease risk   187–9
psychotherapy   185–93
PTH *see* parathyroid hormone
PUFA *see* n-3 polyunsaturated fatty acids
purine analogues   132, 151

raloxifene   166
recombinant DNA technology   234–51
remission   108
retroviral vectors   230
risk factors   15–16

Salmonella typhimurium   54, 56
sangre de grado   201, 205
SASP *see* sulphasalazine
scintigraphy   76
sclerosing cholangitis   108
screening tests   90
SE *see* supportive-expressive group
    psychotherapy
secretory diarrhoea   54, 55
selective oestrogen receptor modulators
    (SERMs)   163, 166
self-tolerance   47
SERMs *see* selective oestrogen receptor
    modulators
serological assays   89
sigmoidoscopy   79
single-nucleotide polymorphisms (SNP)   18
SNP *see* single-nucleotide polymorphisms
soluble mediators   69

spontaneous mutations   27
standard of care   175
steroids   209
stress   81, 186
subgroups   29
subtractive hybridization protocols   237
sulphasalazine (SASP)   109, 117, 129–31,
    142–3
supportive-expressive (SE) group
    psychotherapy   185, 189–91
surgery   99, 101
susceptibility genes   3, 9, 13, 29–30, 44, 62

T cells   42, 44, 50, 61, 67–8, 228–9
TDT *see* transmission by descent test
thalidomide   219, 223–4
thiopurine methyltransferase (TPMT)   88,
    92
TNF *see* tumour necrosis factor
Toll receptors   41
topical treatments   109, 114
toxic megacolon   112–13
TPMT *see* thiopurine methyltransferase
transmission by descent test (TDT)   6, 18
trauma   152
traveller's diarrhoea   108
tumour necrosis factor (TNF)   9, 20, 138,
    219, 228
    antibody   128, 134, 138, 220–2, 228–9

UC *see* ulcerative colitis
ulcerative colitis (UC)
    attachment insecurity   187–9
    autoantibodies   46, 50, 65
    diagnosis   73, 74, 78–82
    distal   109–10, 119
    elderly   96–100
    extensive   110–12, 119–22
    genetics   5, 9, 15, 18, 63
    HLA   16
    nutrition   209
    psychoanalysis   186
    refractory   113–14
    remission induction   107–16
    remission maintenance   117–27
ulcerative proctitis   80, 119

vancomycin   82
vitamin D   149, 153–5, 167, 168